# Behavioral Sport Psychology

James K. Luiselli · Derek D. Reed
Editors

# Behavioral Sport Psychology

Evidence-Based Approaches
to Performance Enhancement

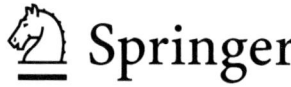

*Editors*
James K. Luiselli
May Institute
Pacella Park Drive 41
Randolph, MA 02368, USA
jluiselli@mayinstitute.org

Derek D. Reed
Department of Applied Behavioral Science
University of Kansas
Sunnyside Avenue 1000
Lawrence, KS 66045, USA
dreed@ku.edu

ISBN 978-1-4614-0069-1     e-ISBN 978-1-4614-0070-7
DOI 10.1007/978-1-4614-0070-7
Springer New York Dordrecht Heidelberg London

Library of Congress Control Number: 2011933552

© Springer Science+Business Media, LLC 2011
All rights reserved. This work may not be translated or copied in whole or in part without the written permission of the publisher (Springer Science+Business Media, LLC, 233 Spring Street, New York, NY 10013, USA), except for brief excerpts in connection with reviews or scholarly analysis. Use in connection with any form of information storage and retrieval, electronic adaptation, computer software, or by similar or dissimilar methodology now known or hereafter developed is forbidden.
The use in this publication of trade names, trademarks, service marks, and similar terms, even if they are not identified as such, is not to be taken as an expression of opinion as to whether or not they are subject to proprietary rights.

Printed on acid-free paper

Springer is part of Springer Science+Business Media (www.springer.com)

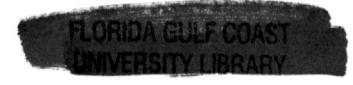

# Preface

Sport psychology is a topic of growing interest. Many professionals read journals such as *The International Journal of Sports, Journal of Sport Behavior, Journal of Applied Sport Psychology, Research Quarterly for Exercise and Sport*, and *The Sport Psychologist*. Division 47 of the American Psychological Association is devoted to "the scientific, educational, and clinical foundations of exercise and sport psychology." The North American Society for the Psychology of Sport and Physical Activity (NASPSPA) and the Association for the Advancement of Applied Sport Psychology (AAASP) convene conferences each year to present scientific findings and new developments in a rapidly expanding field. The AAASP and other organizations also qualify professionals as certified sport and exercise psychology consultants. Finally, a visit to any bookstore will reveal the lay public's fascination with sports, as revealed in numerous self-help books and guides to perfecting athletic performance.

Behavioral psychologists have studied sport psychology for more than three decades (Martin, Thompson, & Regehr, 2004). *Applied behavior analysis* (ABA), in particular, has been an instrumental approach to behavioral coaching in many sports, including *baseball* (Osborne, Rudrud, & Zezoney, 1990), *basketball* (Kladopoulos & McComas, 2001), *figure skating* (Ming & Martin, 1996), *football* (Stokes, Luiselli, & Reed, 2010; Stokes, Luiselli, Reed, & Fleming, 2010; Ward & Carnes, 2002), *ice hockey* (Rogerson & Hrycaiko, 2002), *soccer* (Brobst & Ward, 2002), *swimming* (Hume & Crossman, 1992), and *tennis* (Allison & Ayllon, 1980). ABA stresses the application of learning theory principles, objective measurement of athletic skills, controlled outcome evaluation, and socially significant behavior change. *Cognitive behavior therapy*, or CBT, also has been a dominant approach to psychological intervention in sports (Meyers, Whelan, & Murphy, 1996; Weinberg & Comar, 1994). CBT addresses athletic performance through cognitive-change methods combined with behavioral practice and environmental modifications. Additionally, there have been many advances in sports-related behavioral, cognitive, and neuropsychological assessment methods (Donahue, Silver, Dickens, Covassin, & Lancer, 2007; Webbe & Salinas, 2010).

*Behavioral Sport Psychology: Evidence-Based Approaches to Performance Enhancement* was written for academic professionals, practicing psychologists and consultants, and general readers interested in athletics. We focused on several criteria when selecting chapters for the book. First, our objective was to assemble chapters authored by recognized experts in sport psychology and performance management. We also wanted chapters to reflect the most contemporary clinical and experimental findings. Most important, the chapters contain many recommendations for improving behavioral sport psychology applications, advancing research, and refining the performance of youth, amateur, and elite athletes. A book of this type cannot cover every relevant topic, but hopefully, we have addressed many of the dominant areas that make up the sport psychology landscape.

We are, first and foremost, clinical psychologists, but also avid sport enthusiasts. Dr. Luiselli acknowledges the many coaches who shaped his athletic pursuits in middle school, high school, and college: James C. Murphy, Michael Donato, Richard Sterndale, Jerry Splaine, Louis Gnerre, Rocky Carzo, and Herb Erikson. My father, the late James "Jack the Barber" Luiselli, was my finest coach, always there in the stands, consistently positive, and helping me in ways he probably never realized – I am forever indebted to him. I thank my wife, Dr. Tracy Evans Luiselli, for enduring my tales of athletic conquests long gone and commiserating with me during Patriots, Celtics, Bruins, and Red Sox games. Our daughter, Gabrielle Luiselli, has given us so much pleasure watching her perform on the ice and landing those combination jumps. And to our son, Thomas Luiselli, your exploits on the hockey rink and the lacrosse field fill us with pride – you and your sister are true champions!

Dr. Reed acknowledges his father, David Reed, for being a patient trainer, an understanding coach, and most importantly, an unconditional fan and supporter. I thank my mentors, Dr. Thomas Critchfield, Dr. Brian Martens, and my co-editor, Dr. James Luiselli, for supporting my efforts to study the behavioral processes underlying athletic performance. Finally, I thank my wife, Dr. Florence DiGennaro Reed, for humoring me when I claim that my playing of football video games is for the sake of science.

## References

Allison, M. G., & Ayllon, T. (1980). Behavioral coaching in the development of skills in football, gymnastics, and tennis. *Journal of Applied Behavior Analysis, 13*, 297–314.

Brobst, B., & Ward, P. (2002). Effects of public posting, goal setting, and oral feedback on the skills of female soccer players. *Journal of Applied Behavior Analysis, 35*, 247–257.

Donahue, B., Silver, N. C., Dickens, Y., Covassin, T., & Lancer, K. (2007). Development and initial psychometric evaluation of the sport interference checklist. *Behavior Modification, 31*, 937–957.

Hume, K. M., & Crossman, J. (1992). Musical reinforcement of practice behaviors among competitive swimmers. *Journal of Applied Behavior Analysis, 25*, 665–670.

Kladopoulos, C. N., & McComas, J. J. (2001). The effects of form training on foul-shooting performance in members of a women's college basketball team. *Journal of Applied Behavior Analysis, 34*, 329–332.

Martin, G. L., Thompson, K., & Regehr, K. (2004). Studies using single-subject designs in sport psychology: 30 years of research. *The Behavior Analyst, 27*, 123–140.

Meyers, A., Whelan, J., & Murphy, S. (1996). Cognitive behavioral strategies in athletic performance enhancement. *Progress in Behavior Modification, 30*, 137–164.

Ming, S., & Martin, G. L. (1996). Single-subject evaluation of a self-talk package for improving figure skating performance. *The Sport Psychologist, 10*, 227–238.

Osborne, K., Rudrud, E., & Zezoney, F. (1990). Improved curveball hitting through the enhancement of visual cues. *Journal of Applied Behavior Analysis, 23*, 371–377.

Rogerson, L. J., & Hrycaiko, D. W. (2002). Enhancing competitive performance of ice hockey goal tenders using centering and self-talk. *Journal of Applied Sport Psychology, 14*, 14–26.

Stokes, J. V., Luiselli, J. K., & Reed, D. D. (2010). A behavioral intervention for teaching tackling skills to high school football athletes. *Journal of Applied Behavior Analysis, 43*, 509–512.

Stokes, J. V., Luiselli, J. K., Reed, D. D., & Fleming, R. K. (2010). Behavioral coaching to improve offensive line blocking skills of high school football athletes. *Journal of Applied Behavior Analysis, 43*, 463–472.

Ward, P., & Carnes, M. (2002). Effects of posting self-set goals on collegiate football players' skill execution during practice and games. *Journal of Applied Behavior Analysis, 35*, 1–12.

Webbe, F. M., & Salinas, C. (2010). Pediatric sport neuropsychology. In A. S. Davis (Ed.), *Handbook of pediatric neuropsychology*. New York: Springer.

Weinberg, R., & Comar, W. (1994). The effectiveness of psychological interventions in competitive sport. *Sports Medicine, 18*, 406–418.

# Contents

**Part I    Introduction**

1   **Overview of Behavioral Sport Psychology** . . . . . . . . . . . . . . 3
Garry L. Martin and Kendra Thomson

**Part II    Assessment and Measurement**

2   **Actigraphy: The Ambulatory Measurement of Physical Activity** . . 25
Warren W. Tryon

3   **Quantitative Analysis of Sports** . . . . . . . . . . . . . . . . . . . . 43
Derek D. Reed

4   **Single-Case Evaluation of Behavioral Coaching Interventions** . . . 61
James K. Luiselli

5   **Cognitive Assessment in Behavioral Sport Psychology** . . . . . . . 79
Bradley Donohue, Yani L. Dickens, and Philip D. Del Vecchio III

**Part III    Performance Enhancement**

6   **Goal Setting and Performance Feedback** . . . . . . . . . . . . . . . 99
Phillip Ward

7   **Cognitive–Behavioral Strategies** . . . . . . . . . . . . . . . . . . . . 113
Jeffrey L. Brown

8   **Establishing and Maintaining Physical Exercise** . . . . . . . . . . . 127
Christopher C. Cushing and Ric G. Steele

9   **Behavioral Momentum in Sports** . . . . . . . . . . . . . . . . . . . 143
Henry S. Roane

**Part IV    Special Topics**

10  **Developing Fluent, Efficient, and Automatic Repertoires
of Athletic Performance** . . . . . . . . . . . . . . . . . . . . . . . . . 159
Brian K. Martens and Scott R. Collier

| 11 | Sport Neuropsychology and Cerebral Concussion | 177 |
|---|---|---|
| | Frank M. Webbe | |
| 12 | Aggression in Competitive Sports: Using Direct Observation to Evaluate Incidence and Prevention Focused Intervention | 199 |
| | Chris J. Gee | |
| 13 | Behavioral Effects of Sport Nutritional Supplements: Fact or Fiction? | 211 |
| | Stephen Ray Flora | |
| 14 | Cognitive–Behavioral Coach Training: A Translational Approach to Theory, Research, and Intervention | 227 |
| | Ronald E. Smith and Frank L. Smoll | |
| 15 | Conclusions and Recommendations: Toward a Comprehensive Framework of Evidenced-Based Practice with Performers | 249 |
| | Gershon Tenenbaum and Lael Gershgoren | |
| Index | | 263 |

# Contributors

**Jeffrey L. Brown**  Harvard Medical School, Boston, MA, USA, jeffrey_brown@hms.harvard.edu

**Scott R. Collier**  College of Health Sciences, Appalachian State University, Boone, NC, USA, colliersr@appstate.edu

**Christopher C. Cushing**  Clinical Child Psychology Program, University of Kansas, Lawrence, KS, USA, christophercushing@ku.edu

**Philip D. Del Vecchio III**  Claremont Graduate University, Claremont, CA, USA, philip.delvecchio@cgu.edu

**Yani L. Dickens**  University of Nevada, Reno, NV, USA, ydickens@unr.edu

**Bradley Donohue**  University of Nevada, Las Vegas, NV, USA, bradley.donohue@gmail.com

**Stephen Ray Flora**  Youngstown State University, Youngstown, OH, USA, srflora@ysu.edu

**Chris J. Gee**  Department of Exercise Sciences, University of Toronto, Toronto, ON, Canada, chris.gee@utoronto.ca

**Lael Gershgoren**  Florida State University, Tallahassee, FL, USA, lg07e@fsu.edu

**James K. Luiselli**  May Institute, Randolph, MA, USA, jluiselli@mayinstitute.org

**Brian K. Martens**  Department of Psychology, Syracuse University, Syracuse, NY, USA, bkmarten@syr.edu

**Garry L. Martin**  University of Manitoba, Winnipeg, MB, Canada, gmartin@cc.umanitoba.ca

**Derek D. Reed**  Department of Applied Behavioral Science, University of Kansas, Lawrence, KS, USA, dreed@ku.edu

**Henry S. Roane**  Department of Pediatrics and Psychiatry, SUNY Upstate Medical University, Syracuse, NY, USA, roaneh@upstate.edu

**Ronald E. Smith**  University of Washington, Seattle, WA, USA, resmith@uw.edu

**Frank L. Smoll** University of Washington, Seattle, WA, USA, smoll@uw.edu

**Ric G. Steele** Clinical Child Psychology Program, University of Kansas, Lawrence, KS, USA, rsteele@ku.edu

**Gershon Tenenbaum** Florida State University, Tallahassee, FL, USA, gtenenbaum@fsu.edu

**Kendra Thomson** University of Manitoba, Winnipeg, MB, Canada, thomsonk@cc.umanitoba.ca

**Warren W. Tryon** Fordham University, Bronx, NY, USA, wtryon@fordham.edu

**Phillip Ward** The Ohio State University, Columbus, OH, USA, Ward.116@osu.edu

**Frank M. Webbe** Florida Institute of Technology, Melbourne, FL, USA, webbe@fit.edu

# Part I
# Introduction

# Chapter 1
# Overview of Behavioral Sport Psychology

Garry L. Martin and Kendra Thomson

The term *behavior analysis* refers to the scientific study of laws that govern the behavior of human beings and other animals (Pear, 2001). *Behavioral sport psychology* involves the use of behavior analysis principles and techniques to enhance the performance and satisfaction of athletes and others associated with sports (Martin & Tkachuk, 2000). In this chapter, we trace the early development of the field, highlight five characteristics that tend to be evident in research and current practice in behavioral sport psychology, and summarize nine major areas of application in this field to date.

## The Early Development of Behavioral Sport Psychology

The field of sport psychology in general began to acquire status in the 1960s with the formation of the *International Society of Sport Psychology* in 1965, *The North American Society for the Psychology of Sport and Physical Activity* in 1967, and *The Canadian Society for Psychomotor Learning and Sport Psychology* in 1969. A prominent behaviorally oriented individual in this early history was Brent Rushall. In 1969, Rushall and Pettinger published a comparison of several different reinforcement contingencies on the amount of swimming performed by members of an age-group swimming team. In 1972, Rushall teamed up with physical educator Daryl Siedentop to publish *The Developmental and Control of Behavior in Sport and Physical Education*. This book was written within an operant conditioning framework, and it contained numerous practical strategies for teaching new sport skills, motivating sports persons to practice existing skills at a high level, and generalizing practice skills to competitive settings. In 1974, Thom McKenzie and Rushall published the first research in the *Journal of Applied Behavior Analysis* that took place in a sport setting, and it was the first study in behavioral sport psychology to use a single-subject design. Their research demonstrated the effectiveness of a self-monitoring package for improving practice performance of young competitive swimmers. Two other prominent individuals in behavioral sport psychology in the

G.L. Martin (✉)
University of Manitoba, Winnipeg, MB, Canada
e-mail: gmartin@cc.umanitoba.ca

1970s were Ron Smith and Frank Smoll at the University of Washington, where they conducted behavioral assessments and interventions in youth sports (for a review, see Smith, Smoll, & Christensen, 1996). Rushall, Siedentop, McKenzie, Smith, and Smoll were the early leaders for behaviorally oriented sport psychologists.

During the late 1970s and the early 1980s, publications in behavioral sport psychology included the following: (a) single-subject evaluations of strategies to improve performance of youth athletes in football, gymnastics, tennis, swimming, soccer, and figure skating, and college athletes in volleyball, baseball, basketball, and soccer (for a review of these studies, see Martin, Thompson, & Regehr, 2004); (b) an insightful book that offered a Skinnerian analysis of the contingencies that deter and promote participation in sports (Dickinson, 1977); (c) articles that described and examined behavioral strategies for coaches of young athletes (e.g., see Martin & Hrycaiko, 1983; Rushall & Smith, 1979; Smith, Smoll, & Curtis, 1979; Smoll, Smith, & Curtis, 1978); and (d) research on cognitive–behavioral strategies for improving athletic performance of adult athletes (e.g., Desiderato & Miller, 1979; Gravel, Lemieux, & Ladouceur, 1980; Kirchenbaum, Ordman, Tomarken, & Holtzbauer, 1982; and Weinberg, Seabourne, & Jackson, 1981). Many of the early studies were contained in a book of readings by Martin and Hrycaiko (1983). By the mid-1980s, behavioral sport psychology had a strong foundation and a promising future.

## Prominent Characteristics of Behavioral Sport Psychology

Preliminary to a discussion of the characteristics of behavioral sport psychology is a clarification of the meaning of the terms *behavior* and *stimulus*. In general, behavior is anything that a person says or does. Technically, behavior is any muscular, glandular, or electrical activity of an organism (Martin & Pear, 2011). Commonly used synonyms for behavior include "response," "action," "reaction," "performance," and "activity." *Overt behaviors* can be easily monitored by others, and examples are swimming, throwing a basketball, doing a spin in figure skating, yelling at a teammate, and arguing with a coach. *Covert behaviors* refer to activities that are internal and cannot be readily monitored by observers. Examples include a gymnast thinking, "I hope I don't fall"; a figure skater feeling nervous (e.g., increased heart rate, and rapid breathing) just before performing; and a diver mentally rehearsing a dive just before performing it. (Thinking and feeling are discussed later.) Stimuli (plural of stimulus) are the physical variables in one's immediate surroundings that impinge on one's sense receptors and that can affect one's behavior (Martin & Pear, 2011). Examples of external stimuli include the behavior and physical appearance of the coach and other athletes in the immediate vicinity, the characteristics of the playing field or facility, and the actions and sounds of spectators. One's private behavior, such as an athlete's feelings, self-talk, and imagery (discussed later in this chapter and in Chapter 8), can also serve as internal stimuli to influence subsequent behavior. When a stimulus precedes and influences a behavior, the stimulus is often called a "prompt," "signal," or "cue."

*The first characteristic* of behavioral sport psychology involves identifying target behaviors of athletes and/or coaches to be improved, defining those behaviors in a way so that they can be reliably measured, and using changes in the behavioral measure as the best indicator of the extent to which the recipient of an intervention is being helped (Martin, 2011). This characteristic is discussed further in Chapters 2, 3, and 5.

*A second characteristic* is that behavioral psychology treatment procedures and techniques are based on the principles and procedures of Pavlovian (or respondent) and operant conditioning and are ways of rearranging the stimuli that occur as antecedents and consequences of an athlete's behavior. Pavlovian conditioning is very important in influencing the physiological components of our emotions that we describe as our feelings.

Suppose, for example, that a young figure skater experiences several bad falls while attempting to learn the triple-toe jump, with each fall causing feelings of fear and considerable pain. The principle of Pavlovian conditioning states that if a neutral stimulus (practicing the triple-toe jump) is closely followed by an unconditioned stimulus (a bad fall), which elicits an unconditioned response (feelings of fear), then the previously neutral stimulus (practicing the triple-toe jump) will also tend to elicit that response (feelings of fear). The model for Pavlovian conditioning is shown in the top half of Fig. 1.1. Fortunately, a conditioned reflex (a CS–CR sequence), as illustrated in Fig. 1.1, can be eliminated through the process known as Pavlovian extinction. As illustrated in the bottom half of Fig. 1.1, the Pavlovian extinction procedure is the presentation of the CS without further pairings with the US, and the result is that the CS eventually loses the ability to elicit the CR. Pavlovian procedures for influencing desirable emotional reactions (e.g., calmness and relaxation) and for eliminating undesirable emotional reactions (e.g., fear and anxiety) are important intervention strategies in behavioral sport psychology (Martin, 2011).

Pavlovian conditioning is all about learned and unlearned reflexes – involuntary responses to prior stimuli. However, much of our behavior is referred to as voluntary. Examples of voluntary behavior among athletes include passing a basketball, performing a figure skating jump, swimming the backstroke, listening to a coach, and talking to a teammate. Skinner (1953) referred to such activities as operant behavior – behavior that operates on the environment to produce consequences, and, in turn, is influenced by those consequences. While Pavlovian conditioning causes individuals to involuntarily respond to stimuli due to pairings of antecedent stimuli before the response, operant conditioning teaches individuals to emit voluntary behavior to antecedent stimuli due to consequences for those behaviors. A simplified sport example is illustrated in Fig. 1.2. Suppose that a golfer is practicing putts of approximately 6–8 feet in length. At some places on the practice putting green, the surface around the hole is flat. At another place on the putting green, the surface around the hole is sloped. In the presence of the cues provided by a flat green, the golfer's behavior of aiming and hitting the ball directly at the hole will be positively reinforced by making the putt. In the presence of the cues when there is a slope on the green, however, the golfer's behavior of aiming and hitting the putt directly at

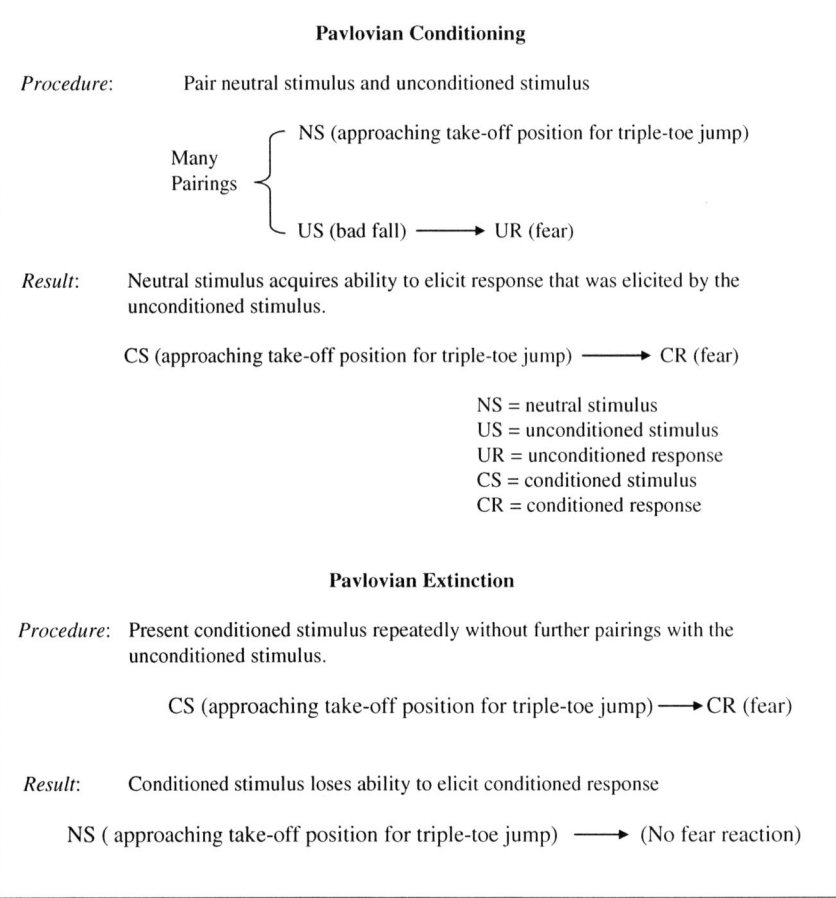

Fig. 1.1 An illustration of Pavlovian conditioning of fear while a figure skater is practicing a jump, and an illustration of Pavlovian extinction of that fear (adapted with permission from illustrations in Martin, 2011)

the hole will encounter operant extinction in that the behavior will not be reinforced by making the putt. As illustrated in Fig. 1.2, after several trials, the golfer learns to putt directly at the hole only when putting at a flat green.

Operant conditioning principles and procedures include methods for teaching new skills (e.g., shaping and chaining), strategies for maintaining existing skills and behaviors at desired levels (e.g., intermittent reinforcement), procedures for bringing new skills under the control of appropriate cues (e.g., stimulus discrimination training, modeling, and fading), and strategies for decreasing unwanted behaviors (e.g., operant extinction, response-cost punishment, and reinforcement of desirable alternative behavior).

Pavlovian and operant conditioning procedures are summarized with many sport examples in a single chapter in a book by Martin (2011) and are described in

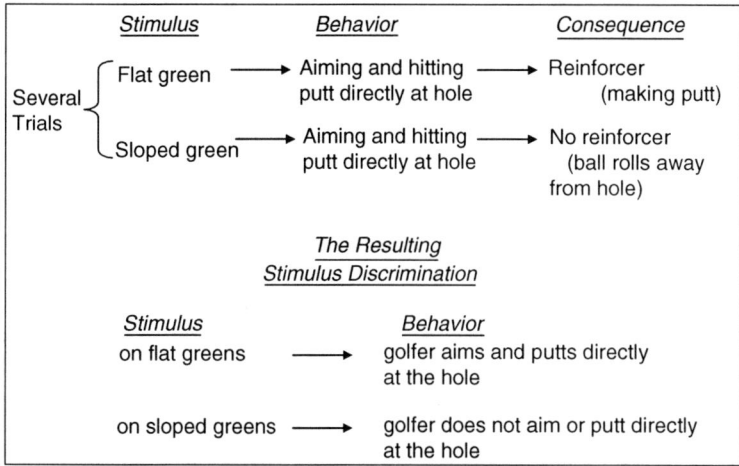

**Fig. 1.2** An illustration of stimulus discrimination training involving operant behavior of a golfer (adapted with permission from an illustration in Martin, 2011)

considerable detail in many chapters by Martin and Pear (2011). This second characteristic is discussed further in Chapters 3, 6, 7, 9, and 10.

*A third characteristic* of behavioral sport psychology is that many of the interventions with athletes have been developed by practitioners with a cognitive–behavioral orientation (e.g., see Smoll & Smith, 2010; Zinsser, Bunker, & Williams, 2006). Cognitive–behavior therapy typically focuses on cognitive processes frequently referred to as *believing, thinking, expecting, and perceiving.* Over the years, cognitively oriented sport psychologists have provided considerable evidence that inappropriate thinking by athletes can lead to poor performance and that appropriate or positive thinking can lead to good performance (Zinsser et al., 2006). From an applied behavior analysis (ABA) perspective, cognitive processes are referred to as covert verbalizations and/or imagery (both of which are discussed later in this chapter), and it is assumed that the behavioral principles and techniques that apply to overt behaviors are also applicable to covert behaviors (Martin & Pear, 2011). Cognitive–behavioral interventions in sports are discussed further in Chapters 5, 8, and 15.

*A fourth characteristic* of this approach is that researchers have relied heavily on the use of single-subject research designs. As expressed by Hrycaiko and Martin (1996) and Virués-Ortega and Martin (2010), single-subject designs have a number of features that render them "user-friendly" for practitioners to evaluate interventions in sport settings, including the following: (a) a focus on individual athletic performance across several practices and/or competitions; (b) acceptability by athletes and coaches because no control group is needed, few participants are needed, and sooner or later all participants receive the intervention; (c) easy adaptability to assess a variety of interventions in practices and/or competitions; and (d) effectiveness assessed through direct measures of sport-specific behaviors (e.g., jumps landed by figure skaters) or outcomes of behaviors (e.g., points scored by basketball players). For a review of research using single-subject designs in sport psychology, from the initial study by McKenzie and Rushall in 1974 through the next 30 years, see Martin et al. (2004). Single-subject designs are discussed further in Chapter 4.

*A final characteristic* of a behavioral approach, whether with athletes and coaches or with other populations, is that it places high value on accountability for everyone involved in the design, implementation, and evaluation of an intervention (Martin & Pear, 2011). In ABA, the term *social validation* refers to procedures to ensure that the techniques employed by a practitioner are selected and applied in the best interests of the clients. In behavioral sport psychology, social validation requires that the practitioner constantly seek answers to three questions: (a) What do the athletes (and perhaps the coach and parents) think about the goals of the intervention? (b) What do they think about the procedures recommended by the practitioner? (c) What do they think about the results produced by those procedures? Also, behavioral sport psychologists need to be aware of and behave consistently with the set of ethical principles to guide the actions of sport psychologists published in 1995 by the Association for the Advancement of Applied Sport Psychology, which, in 2006, became the Association for Applied Sport Psychology (AASP). (For the ethical principles of AASP, see the website http://appliedsportpsych.org.) Additional discussion of topics relevant to this characteristic can be found in Chapters 11, 12, 13, 14, and 15.

## Major Areas of Application of Behavioral Sport Psychology

### *Motivating Practice and Fitness Training*

Webster's unabridged dictionary defines motive as "some inner drive that causes a person to act in a certain way," and many people conceptualize motivation as some "thing" within us that affects behavior. A behavioral approach, on the other hand, encourages the use of the verb "to motivate" which has the advantage of providing coaches and athletes with a variety of strategies for motivating practice performance and endurance and fitness activities. Martin (2011) described the details of a behavioral approach to the topic of motivation and athletic performance, and summarized a variety of strategies for arranging antecedents and/or consequences to motivate athletic behavior in a variety of settings. For example, consider the problem of motivating speed skaters to work hard in practices. Members of the Manitoba Provincial Speed Skating Team, ranging in age from 12 to 17 years, were preparing for the Canada Winter Games. Three of the skaters, however, showed considerable off-task behavior and completed only 85% of the skating drills assigned by the coach. With the help of Connie Wanlin, a master's student at the University of Manitoba, the three skaters agreed to participate in a project to improve their motivation. The skaters agreed to set weekly written goals and daily goals for number of laps skated and practice drills completed, to record their daily performance in log books, and to meet with Connie once a week to discuss their progress and receive feedback. During the intervention, which lasted for several weeks, the three skaters showed an average of 73% increase in the number of laps skated per practice, and they completed an average of 98% of the drills assigned by the coach. Racing times obtained in practices and competitions improved for all three skaters (Wanlin, Hrycaiko, Martin, & Mahon, 1997). Additional examples in this area include motivating young competitive swimmers (Critchfield & Vargas, 1991), adult novice rowers (Scott, Scott, Bedic, & Dowd, 1999), and adult recreational athletes performing a gymnasium triathlon (Thelwell & Greenlees, 2003). Detailed discussion of motivational procedures is presented in Chapters 6, 7, 9, and 10.

## Teaching New Sport Skills

During the past 50 years, behavioral researchers have investigated a variety of behavioral principles and techniques for helping individuals in all walks of life to learn new skills, develop persistence, and eliminate bad habits. As described by Martin and Pear (2011), thousands of research reports have demonstrated the value of these principles and techniques for improving a wide variety of behaviors of thousands of individuals in diverse settings. It should not be surprising, then, that an important area of application of behavioral sport psychology is teaching new skills to athletes and/or coaches. In a review of 30 years of research using single-subject designs in sport psychology, 72% of the studies focused on improving athletic skills of athletes in a variety of sports (Martin et al., 2004). Examples include improving free throw shooting form in basketball (Kladopoulos & McComas, 2001), improving the correctness of compulsory figures in figure skating (Ming & Martin, 1996), improving offensive blocking in youth football (Allison & Ayllon, 1980), increasing arm extension in pole vaulting (Scott & Scott, 1997), teaching golf to beginners (Simek & O'Brien, 1981), improving positioning and tackling of linebackers in college football (Ward & Carnes, 2002), increasing correct tags of inline roller speed skaters (Anderson & Kirkpatrick, 2002), and improving freestyle and backstroke turns in youth swimming (Hazen, Johnstone, Martin, & Skrikameswaran, 1990).

For some details of an example, consider the problem of teaching novice tennis players to serve. In the Juniper High School tennis class, Linda Hill had devoted three classes in a row to instruction on how to serve. After each class, each player was given the chance to practice while Coach Hill observed and pointed out errors. With this strategy, the novice players showed little improvement and averaged only 13% correct across service attempts. With the help of Hillary Buzas, a doctoral candidate in clinical psychology at Georgia State University, Coach Hill agreed to try a different strategy. First, the specific components of the serve were listed and discussed with the players. Next, when the players practiced, Coach Hill watched for and praised components (from the checklist) that were performed correctly or near correctly. When an error occurred, the coach did not comment on it in any way. This approach, which involved the behavioral procedure of shaping, produced an improvement from 13% during baseline observations to almost 50% correct performance in only a few sessions. Moreover, the young players enjoyed it more and were eager to practice their skills (Buzas & Ayllon, 1981). For further discussion of behavioral procedures for teaching new skills, see Chapters 6, 7, and 11.

## *Decreasing Persistent Errors in Sport Skills*

Even after considerable practice, many young athletes will continue to make errors in the execution of athletic skills. As described by Martin (2011), there are numerous reasons why errors are repeated. Persistent errors in skills made by beginning athletes might be due to imitation of other young athletes who are making the same errors; lack of focus on the appropriate antecedent cues, as a strategy to obtain attention from the coach; lack of reinforcement for correct performance especially when the correct performance requires a lot of effort; and accidental positive reinforcement of an error when the young athlete is successful in spite of the error. Regarding the last point, when a skill results in early success for a young athlete, all of the components of that skill are strengthened, even if one of the components is flawed. For example, in a youth competitive swim team composed of 9- and 10-year-olds, if the swimmers swim 500 m of freestyle during a practice (a common occurrence), an error in their freestyle stroke will be repeated several hundred times per practice. Thus, it is not surprising that certain errors are difficult to decrease. Sandra Koop, a doctoral student in psychology at the University of Manitoba, was contacted by a coach of the Manitoba Marlins, a youth competitive swim club, to help decrease repetitive errors in some of the young swimmers. The errors had persisted for several weeks in spite of the usual coaching techniques. Sandra developed an intervention package that consisted of identification of errors and correct behaviors, awareness training regarding the errors and correct behaviors, instruction with key words, mastery criteria, and immediate feedback, and demonstrated the effectiveness of the package in a multiple-baseline design across participants and swimming strokes (Koop & Martin, 1983). Other examples of strategies for decreasing errors have been reported for play execution of the offensive backfield of a youth football team (Komaki & Barnett, 1977), performance of gymnastic skills with young gymnasts (Allison & Ayllon, 1980), execution of throw-ins and goal kicks in youth soccer (Rush & Ayllon, 1984), and performance of volleyball skills by college players (Landin & Hebert, 1999; McKenzie & Liskevych, 1983).

## *Decreasing Problem Behaviors of Athletes in Sport Environments*

Sport psychology consultants are sometimes asked for their advice to help coaches decrease problem behaviors exhibited by athletes. By problem behaviors we mean a variety of disruptive, non-athletic activities that are likely to interfere with athletic performance and/or create aversiveness for others, such as excessive socializing during athletic drills, temper tantrums, annoying and disruptive behaviors while the coach is talking to the team, and so forth. Examples of strategies to decrease problem behaviors include monitoring and the public posting of such behaviors (Galvan & Ward, 1998), using self-monitoring and charting to increase desirable alternative practice behaviors (Hume, Martin, Gonzalez, Cracklen, & Genthon, 1985), using group music reinforcement for desirable alternative behaviors (Hume & Crossman, 1992), and awareness training, competing response training, and arranging supporting contingencies (Allen, 1998).

## *Managing Emotions to Maximize Athletic Performance*

Martin and Pear (2011) suggested that emotions have three important characteristics: (a) the internal autonomic reaction that one feels during the experiencing of an emotion (such as the nervous sensations that an athlete feels just before the start of an important competition), which is influenced by respondent conditioning; (b) the way that one learns to express an emotion overtly (such as swearing and throwing things when angry), which is influenced by operant conditioning; and (c) the way that one becomes aware of and describes one's emotions (e.g., "I'm a little excited," as opposed to "I'm really nervous"), which is also influenced by operant conditioning. With this analysis in mind, two areas that have received attention from behavioral sport psychologists are as follows: (a) teaching athletes strategies to decrease excessive nervousness or fear that negatively affects athletic performance and (b) teaching athletes strategies to overcome excessive anger and aggression. A related area of research has examined the relationship between physiological arousal and athletic performance. We will briefly comment on all three of these areas.

Excessive nervousness or anxiety or fear is often identified by coaches and athletes to account for poor athletic performance. Goldberg (1998) suggested that "fear is probably the single biggest cause of choking in sports." Using the model of emotions summarized previously, Martin (2011) outlined four main reasons why excessive feelings of nervousness or fear can interfere with athletic performance. First, the physiological activity from excessive nervousness consumes energy, which can be problematic in endurance athletic activities. Second, because of our evolutionary history, experiencing nervousness can cause a narrowing of attention, so that fearful athletes may miss important external cues. Third, excessive nervousness causes the secretion of adrenaline, which can cause an athlete to rush a skilled routine and destroy the timing of it. Finally, if an athlete is relatively relaxed at practices and very nervous at a competition, the excessive nervousness adds additional stimuli that may interfere with stimulus generalization of a skill from practices to competitions. Strategies that have been applied by behavioral sport psychologists to help athletes cope with excessive nervousness or fear include teaching athletes to (a) recognize and change negative thinking that might cause the fear or nervousness, (b) restructure the environment to "tune out" and prompt relaxing thoughts, (c) practice a relaxing breathing technique called deep center breathing, (d) practice progressive muscle relaxation by alternatively tensing and relaxing various muscle groups and paying close attention to how the muscles feel when they are relaxed versus tense, (e) maintain a sense of humor, and (i) visualize relaxing scenes [these strategies are described in detail by Martin (2011) and Williams (2010)].

In the model of emotions described by Martin and Pear (2011), anger is caused by the withdrawal or the withholding of rewards such as a missed shot by a basketball player, a disallowed goal for a soccer player, or a penalty in football that wipes out a yardage gain. Several studies have described successful anger management procedures for athletes (Allen, 1998; Brunelle, Janelle, & Tennant, 1999; Connelly, 1988; Jones, 1993; Silva, 1982). Such studies commonly follow a four-step strategy including (a) helping the athlete to identify anger-causing situations, (b) teaching the athlete to perform substitute behaviors to compete with the anger, (c) prompting the athlete to practice the substitute behaviors using imagery and/or simulations and/or role-playing, and (d) encouraging the athlete to use the coping skills in competitive situations and to receive feedback. For further discussion of aggression in competitive sports, see Chapter 13.

Regarding the relationship between physiological arousal and athletic performance, many studies have suggested an inverted-U relationship between arousal and performance (Landers & Arent, 2010). To illustrate this relationship, consider the level of arousal as varying on a continuum from very low to medium to very high. When the level of physiological arousal is low, athletic performance is likely to be poor, and the athlete is likely to be described as being indifferent, disinterested, not being able to "get into the game," lacking intensity, etc. As the level of physiological arousal increases to some medium level, athletic performance is likely to increase to a peak, and the athlete is likely to be described as having lots of energy, having great anticipation, and being on top of his/her game. As the level of arousal continues to increase to a high level, athletic performance is likely to decrease, and the athlete is likely to be described as being excessively nervous, tense, or fearful and will show a high tendency to "choke." For discussion of strategies to help athletes achieve an optimal level of arousal, see Landers and Arent (2010) and Williams (2010).

## *Using Self-Talk and/or Imagery Training to Improve Athletic Performance*

As indicated previously, applied behavior analysts consider private behavior to include saying things to oneself (i.e., self-talk) and imagining (e.g., visualizing a clear blue sky), and assume that behavioral principles and procedures apply to private as well public behavior. Regarding self-talk, research has indicated that athletes can use self-talk to improve performance in a variety of areas, including controlling their emotions and/or mood, stopping negative thoughts, improving their focusing or concentration skills, problem solving or planning, and improving skill acquisition and performance (Zinsser et al., 2006). To take just one example, Ziegler (1987) reported that beginning tennis players practicing backhand shots showed little progress when simply told to "concentrate." However, they showed rapid improvement when they vocalized the word "ready" when the ball machine was about to present the next ball, the word "ball" when they saw the ball coming toward them from the machine, the word "bounce" as the ball contacted the surface of the court, and the word "hit" when they observed the ball contact their racquet while swinging their backhand.

From a behavioral perspective, Martin (2011) suggested that self-talk might serve four behavioral functions. First, self-talk can serve as a conditioned stimulus (due to prior respondent conditioning) to elicit various emotions, such as the gymnast who thinks "balance, graceful" just before stepping on the balance beam to elicit feelings of relaxation. Second, self-talk might function as a cue for attending or focusing on certain stimuli (such as a batter in baseball saying, "watch the ball," when the ball leaves the pitcher's hand). Third, in terms of operant conditioning, specific words commonly called *key words* in sports might serve as discriminative stimuli to prompt particular body positions for motor skills (such as a swimmer thinking "hips" during the backstroke as a prompt to keep his/her hips high in the water and as flat as possible). Fourth, self-talk can function as a conditioned reinforcer for desirable actions (such as a weight lifter thinking, "Good work, keep it up," after completing 10 repetitions of a particular weight exercise). For further discussion of self-talk to improve athletic performance, see Chapters 8 and 15.

Regarding imagery, cognitive–behavioral psychologists have made considerable use of imagery training to improve the performance of athletes (Vealey & Greenleaf, 2010). From a behavioral perspective, we learn to experience visual imagery through a process referred to by Skinner (1953) as "conditioned seeing," in other words, through respondent conditioning. For example, as we grew up, we experienced many trials in which the words "blue sky" were paired with actually looking at and seeing a blue sky. As a result, when we now close our eyes and imagine a blue sky, the activity elicited in our visual system enables us to experience the behavior of "seeing" a blue sky. Two behavioral psychologists, Malott and Whaley (1983), talked more generally about instances of conditioned sensing. Our long history of associating words with actual sights, sounds, and feelings enable us to experience inside activity when we imagine seeing, feeling, or hearing something. In sport psychology, the process of imagining and seeing oneself performing an activity is referred to as *mental rehearsal* or *mental practice*. In a survey of 235 Canadian Olympic athletes, 99% claimed to use mental rehearsal to enhance their performance (Orlick & Partington, 1988), and many studies have shown that various imagery training procedures can enhance athletic performance (Vealey & Greenleaf, 2010).

Strategies to use mental imagery to enhance practice performance include the following: (a) scheduling separate imagery sessions to imagine performing a skill (such as imagery practice to improve a basketball player's free throw shooting); (b) using imagery to energize before practices (for example, an athlete imagining that an important competition is about to start); (c) using imagery at practices before performing a previously learned skill in order to increase the likelihood of performing it correctly (such as a figure skater mentally rehearsing a jump at practices just before attempting it); (d) practicing instant mental replays following a correctly performed skill to help remember the feelings of performing it correctly; and (e) using visualization to simulate the competitive environment to promote stimulus generalization from practices to competitions [these strategies are discussed in detail by Martin (2011) and Zinsser et al. (2006)]. Strategies to use mental imagery to enhance competitive performance include the following: (a) use of imagery for emotional control just before and during competitions (such as an athlete who is excessively nervous athlete imagining that he/she is relaxing at the beach on a warm summer day); (b) mental rehearsal of a skill just before performing it such as reported by Jack Nicklaus before each of his shots when he was an active competitive golfer (Nicklaus, 1974); and (c) use of imagery to help tune out distracters [details of these strategies are described by Martin (2011) and Zinsser et al. (2006)]. For further discussion of imagery training to improve athletic performance, see Chapters 8 and 15.

## *Maximizing Confidence and Concentration for Peak Performance During Competitions*

Questionnaire studies with athletes have reported that the factor that most consistently distinguishes highly successful athletes from less successful ones is "confidence" (Weinberg & Gould, 2007; Zinsser et al., 2006). The ability to concentrate effectively has also been identified as a key ingredient of peak athletic performance (Nideffer & Sagal, 2006). The term *peak performance* is used to refer to an outstanding athletic performance, when an athlete "puts it all together" (Krane & Williams, 2010). How do behavioral psychologists talk about confidence and concentration? From a behavioral perspective, *confidence* is a term that is used to describe athletes who have performed well in recent practices and/or competitions and who show certain behavior patterns that would be described collectively as illustrating the belief that they will perform well in an upcoming competition (Martin, 2011). A behavioral interpretation of the term *concentration* suggests that two behavioral processes are involved (Martin, 2011). First, concentration includes behavior commonly referred to as observational, orienting, attending, or focusing – behavior that puts the individual in contact with important cues for further responding. For example, a batter in baseball who is "concentrating" is likely to focus on the pitcher, rather than attending to the first baseman. Second, following appropriate attending or focusing behavior, concentration refers to the extent to which particular cues exert effective stimulus control over skilled performance. For example, after a batter has focused on the pitcher, if the sight of the baseball approaching the strike zone exerts stimulus control over a solid swing and a hit by the batter, we would say that the batter has shown good concentration.

Strategies to improve confidence, concentration, and peak performance include teaching athletes to orient to proper cues (Nideffer & Sagal, 2006; Wilson, Peper, & Schmid, 2006), influencing athletes to perform well in simulations of competitive cues (Weinberg & Gould, 2007), using imagery to relive best performances (Orlick & Partington, 1988), encouraging athletes to focus on realistic goals for execution rather than worrying about outcome (Swain & Jones, 1995; Ward & Carnes,

2002), using facts and reasons to build a case against negative thinking (called countering; Bell, 1983), and encouraging athletes to prepare and follow specific competition plans (Rushall, 1979, 1992). For additional discussion on the topics of this subsection, see Chapters 5, 8, 11, and 15.

## Development of User-Friendly Behavioral Assessment Tools for Athletes

Behavioral assessment has been defined as the collection and analysis of information and data in order to identify and describe target behaviors, identify possible causes of the behavior, guide the selection of an appropriate behavioral treatment, and evaluate treatment outcome (Martin & Pear, 2011). Behavioral assessment began to emerge in clinical psychology in the 1970s in response to criticisms by behaviorally oriented practitioners against traditional diagnostic assumptions and approaches (Nelson & Hayes, 1979; Nelson, 1983). Behavioral assessment in sport psychology typically begins with a behavioral interview to help the athlete identify major problem areas, select one or two such areas for initial treatment, identify specific behavioral deficits or excesses within the targeted problem areas, attempt to identify controlling variables of the problem behavior, and identify some specific target behaviors for initial treatment (Orlick, 1989; Smith et al., 1996; Tkachuk, Leslie-Toogood, & Martin, 2003). User-friendly behavioral checklists for athletes have been developed to facilitate this process. One type of checklist is an *across-sport behavioral checklist*, which lists performance aspects of practices and/or competitions that apply to a number of different sports. For example, in the *Pre-competition and Competition Behavior Inventory* developed by Rushall (1979), an athlete is presented with such statements as, "I get nervous and tense before an important competition," "I mentally rehearse my competition plan before contests," and "When I am tired during a competition, I concentrate on my technique." The athlete is asked to respond to each statement by checking either Always, or Occasionally, or Never. Other examples of across-sport behavioral checklists include the *Post-competition Evaluation Form* (Orlick, 1996), the *Psychological Skills Inventory for Sport* (Mahoney, Gabriel, & Perkins, 1987), and the *Athletic Coping Skills Inventory-28* (Smith, Schutz, Smoll, & Ptacek, 1995).

A *within-sport behavioral checklist* lists performance aspects of practices and/or competitions for a particular sport. Such checklists contain behavioral descriptors and situational examples with terminology specific to a given sport. Martin, Toogood, and Tkachuk (1997) described within-sport behavioral checklists for 21 different sports. The within-sport checklists were positively reviewed (Smith & Little, 1998), and research on the checklists for basketball, swimming, running, volleyball, and figure skating has found them to have high face validity and high test–retest reliability (Leslie-Toogood & Martin, 2003; Lines, Schwartzman, Tkachuk, Leslie-Toogood, & Martin, 1999; Martin & Toogood, 1997). In one study, the within-sport checklists for assessing mental-skills strengths and weaknesses of athletes were completed by a sample of volleyball players, a sample of track athletes, and their respective coaches. Surprisingly, there was little agreement between volleyball coaches and the athletes that they coached, and between track coaches and the athletes that they coached, concerning the mental-skills strengths and weaknesses of those athletes. In spite of this evidence that the coaches in these samples did not know the mental skills of their athletes, the coaches showed a high degree of confidence in their ability to evaluate the mental-skills strengths and weaknesses of their athletes (Leslie-Toogood & Martin, 2003). Although more research is needed, results to date indicate that such checklists can facilitate behavioral sport psychology consulting.

Another type of behavioral assessment tool is the *Student–Athlete Relationship Instrument,* or SARI (Donohue, Miller, Crammer, Cross, & Covassin, 2007). The SARI was developed to assess sport-specific problems in the relationships of athletes with their coaches, teammates, families, and peers. The initial assessment of the SARI indicates that it has good reliability and validity and that it could be a very useful tool for assessing an important source of variability in the performance of athletes. Interestingly, in a study of the SARI with 198 high school and college athletes, the athletes on average reported strongest happiness with family relationships and least happiness in their relationships with their coaches. For further discussion of behavioral assessment, see Chapters 2, 3, 4, 5, 11, 14, and 15.

## *Development of User-Friendly Sport Psychology Manuals for Athletes*

A book such as this is written for advanced college students and sport practitioners. What about easy-to-use, self-instructional manuals to guide athletes and/or coaches in the use of sport psychology techniques without the aid of a practitioner? That is an area that has also received some attention. Some of the early manuals (e.g., see Nideffer, 1976; Orlick, 1980, 1986; Tutko & Umberto, 1976), often with "sport psyching" or "mental training" in the title, were prepared by practitioners with a cognitive–behavioral orientation and were meant for athletes in general. More recent versions of such manuals include Goldberg (1998) and Orlick (2008). Other manuals have been prepared for athletes in individual sports, such as curling (Martin & Martin, 2006), dance (Taylor & Taylor, 1995), figure skating (Martin & Thomson, 2010), golfing (Martin & Ingram, 2001), and hockey (Martin, 2010). What is needed is research evaluating the effectiveness of such manuals.

## Summary

Behavioral sport psychology involves the use of behavioral analysis principles and techniques to enhance the performance and satisfaction of athletes and others associated with sports. Behavioral sport psychology developed a firm foundation in the 1970s with early leadership provided by Brent Rushall, Darryl Siedentop, Thom McKenzie, Ron Smith, and Frank Smoll. Prominent characteristics of behavioral sport psychology include the following: (a) it identifies target behaviors of athletes and/or coaches in a way that they can be reliably measured, and it uses changes in the behavioral measure as the best indicator of the extent to which the intervention has been successful; (b) its treatment procedures and techniques are grounded in the principles and procedures of Pavlovian and operant conditioning; (c) many of its interventions have been developed by practitioners who follow a cognitive–behavioral orientation; (d) many of its researchers have relied heavily on the use of single-subject research designs; and (e) it places high value on accountability for everyone involved in the design, implementation, and evaluation of an intervention. Major areas of application of behavioral sport psychology have included (a) motivating practice and fitness training, (b) teaching new sport skills, (c) decreasing persistent errors in sport skills, (d) decreasing problem behaviors of athletes in sport environments, (e) managing emotions to maximize athletic performance, (f) using self-talk and/or imagery to improve athletic performance, (g) maximizing confidence and concentration for peak performance during competitions, (h) developing user-friendly behavioral assessment tools for athletes, and (i) developing user-friendly sport psychology manuals for athletes.

## References

Allen, K. D. (1998). The use of an enhanced simplified habit-reversal procedure to reduce disruptive outbursts during athletic performance. *Journal of Applied Behavior Analysis, 31*, 489–492.

Allison, M. G., & Ayllon, T. (1980). Behavioral coaching in the development of skills in football, gymnastics, and tennis. *Journal of Applied Behavior Analysis, 13*, 297–314.

Anderson, G., & Kirkpatrick, M. A. (2002). Variable effects of a behavioral treatment package on the performance of inline roller speed skaters. *Journal of Applied Behavior Analysis, 35*, 195–198.

Bell, K. F. (1983). *Championship thinking: The athlete's guide to winning performance in all sports*. Englewood Cliffs, NJ: Prentice-Hall.

Brunelle, J. P., Janelle, C. M., & Tennant, L. K. (1999). Controlling competitive anger among male soccer players. *Journal of Applied Sport Psychology, 11*, 283–297.

Buzas, H. P., & Ayllon, T. (1981). Differential reinforcement in coaching tennis skills. *Behavior Modification, 5*, 372–385.

Connelly, D. (1988). Increasing intensity of play of nonassertive athletes. *The Sport Psychologist, 2*, 255–265.

Critchfield, T. S., & Vargas, E. A. (1991). Self-recording, instructions, and public self-graphing: Effects on swimming in the absence of coach verbal interaction. *Behavior Modification, 15*, 95–112.

Desiderato, O., & Miller, I. B. (1979). Improving tennis performance by cognitive behavior and modification techniques. In G. L. Martin & D. Hrycaiko (Eds.), *Behavior modification and coaching: Principle, procedures, and research* (pp. 293–295). Springfield, IL: C.C. Thomas.

Dickinson, J. (1977). *A behavior analysis of sport*. Princeton, NJ: Princeton Book Company.

Donohue, B., Miller, A., Crammer, L., Cross, C., & Covassin, T. (2007). A standardized method of assessing sport specific problems in the relationships of athletes with their coaches, teammates, family, and peers. *Journal of Sport Behavior, 30*, 375–397.

Galvan, Z. J., & Ward, P. (1998). Effects of public posting on inappropriate on-court behaviors by collegiate tennis players. *The Sport Psychologist, 12*, 419–426.

Goldberg, A. S. (1998). *Sport slump busting*. Champagne, IL: Human Kinetics.
Gravel, R., Lemieux, G., & Ladouceur, R. (1980). Effectiveness of a cognitive behavioral treatment package for cross-country ski racers. *Cognitive Therapy and Research, 4*, 83–89.
Hazen, A., Johnstone, C., Martin, G. L., & Skrikameswaran, S. (1990). A videotaping feedback package for improving skills of youth competitive swimmers. *The Sport Psychologist, 4*, 213–227.
Hrycaiko, D., & Martin, G. L. (1996). Applied research studies with single-subject designs: Why so few? *Journal of Applied Sport Psychology, 8*, 183–199.
Hume, K. M., & Crossman, J. (1992). Musical reinforcement of practice behaviors among competitive swimmers. *Journal of Applied Behavior Analysis, 25*, 665–670.
Hume, K. M., Martin, G. L., Gonzalez, P., Cracklen, C., & Genthon, S. (1985). A self-monitoring feedback package for improving freestyle figure skating practice. *Journal of Sport Psychology, 7*, 333–345.
Jones, C. (1993). The role of performance profiling in cognitive behavioral interventions in sport. *The Sport Psychologist, 7*, 160–172.
Kirchenbaum, D. S., Ordman, A. M., Tomarken, A. J., & Holtzbauer, R. (1982). Effects of differential self-monitoring and level of mastery of sports performance: Brain, power bowling. *Cognitive Therapy and Research, 6*, 335–342.
Kladopoulos, C. N., & McComas, J. J. (2001). The effects of form training on foul-shooting performance in members of a women's college basketball team. *Journal of Applied Behavior Analysis, 34*, 329–332.
Komaki, J., & Barnett, F. T. (1977). A behavioral approach to coaching football: Improving the play execution of the offensive backfield on a youth football team. *Journal of Applied Behavior Analysis, 10*, 657–664.
Koop, S., & Martin, G. L. (1983). Evaluation of a coaching strategy to reduce swimming stroke errors in beginning age-group swimmers. *Journal of Applied Behavior Analysis, 16*, 447–460.
Krane, V., & Williams, J. M. (2010). Psychological characteristics of peak performance. In J. M. Williams (Ed.), *Applied sport psychology: Personal growth and peak performance* (6th ed., pp. 169–188). New York: McGraw Hill.
Landers, D. M., & Arent, S. M. (2010). Arousal-performance relationships. In J. M. Williams (Ed.), *Applied sport psychology: Personal growth to peak performance* (6th ed., pp. 221–246). New York: McGraw Hill.
Landin, D., & Hebert, E. P. (1999). The influence of self-talk on the performance of skilled female tennis players. *Journal of Applied Sport Psychology, 11*, 263–282.
Leslie-Toogood, A., & Martin, G. (2003). Do coaches know the mental skills of their athletes? Assessments from volleyball and track. *Journal of Sport Behavior, 26*, 56–69.
Lines, J. B., Schwartzman, L., Tkachuk, G. A., Leslie-Toogood, S. A., & Martin, G. L. (1999). Behavioral assessment in sport psychology consulting: Applications to swimming and basketball. *Journal of Sport Behavior, 22*, 558–569.
Mahoney, M. J., Gabriel, P. J., & Perkins, T. S. I. (1987). Psychological skills and exceptional athletic performance. *The Sport Psychologist, 1*, 181–199.
Malott, R. W., & Whaley, D. L. (1983). *Psychology*. Holmes Beach, FL: Learning Publications.
Martin, G. L. (2010). *A sport psychology manual for hockey players*. Winnipeg, MB: Sport Science Press.
Martin, G. L. (2011). *Applied sport psychology: Practical guidelines from behavior analysis* (4th ed.). Winnipeg, MB: Sport Science Press.
Martin, G. L., & Hrycaiko, D. (1983). Effective behavioral coaching: What's it all about? *Journal of Sport Psychology, 5*, 8–20.
Martin, G. L., & Ingram, D. (2001). *Play golf in the zone: The psychology of golf made easy*. San Francisco: Van der Plas Publications.
Martin, G. L., & Martin, T. (2006). *Curl in the zone: The psychology of curling made easy*. Winnipeg, MB: Sport Science Press.

Martin, G. L., & Pear, J. J. (2011). *Behavior modification: What it is and how to do it* (9th ed.). Upper Saddle River, NJ: Pearson-Prentice Hall.

Martin, G. L., Thompson, K., & Regehr, K. (2004). Studies using single-subject designs in sport psychology: 30 years of research. *The Behavior Analyst, 27*, 123–140.

Martin, G. L., & Thomson, K. (2010). *A sport psychology self-instructional manual for figure skaters*. Winnipeg, MB: Sport Science Press.

Martin, G. L., & Tkachuk, G. A. (2000). Behavioral sport psychology. In J. Austin & J. E. Carr (Eds.), *Behavioral sport psychology: Handbook of applied behavior analysis* (pp. 399–422). Reno, NV: Context Press.

Martin, G. L., & Toogood, A. (1997). Cognitive and behavioral components of a seasonal psychological skills training program for competitive figure skaters. *Cognitive and Behavioral Practice, 4*, 383–404.

Martin, G. L., Toogood, A., & Tkachuk, G. A. (1997). *Behavioral assessment forms for sport psychology consulting*. Winnipeg, MB: Sport Science Press.

McKenzie, T. L., & Liskevych, T. N. (1983). Using the multi-element baseline design to examine motivation in volleyball training. In G. L. Martin & D. Hrycaiko (Eds.), *Behavior modification and coaching: Principles, procedures, and research* (pp. 187–202). Springfield, IL: Charles C. Thomas.

McKenzie, T. L., & Rushall, B. S. (1974). Effects of self-recording on attendance and performance in a competitive swimming training environment. *Journal of Applied Behavior Analysis, 7*, 199–206.

Ming, S., & Martin, G. L. (1996). Single-subject evaluation of a self-talk package for improving figure skating performance. *The Sport Psychologist, 10*, 227–238.

Nelson, R. O. (1983). Behavioral assessment: Past, present, and future. *Behavioral Assessment, 5*, 195–206.

Nelson, R. O., & Hayes, S. C. (1979). Some current dimensions of behavioral assessment. *Behavioral Assessment, 1*, 1–16.

Nicklaus, J. (1974). *Golf my way*. New York: Simon & Schuster.

Nideffer, R. M. (1976). *The inner athlete: Mind plus muscle for running*. New York: Crowell.

Nideffer, R. M., & Sagal, M. (2006). Concentration and attention control training. In J. M. Williams (Ed.), *Applied sport psychology: Personal growth to peak performance* (5th ed., pp. 382–403). New York: McGraw-Hill.

Orlick, T. (1980). *In pursuit of excellence*. Champaign, IL: Human Kinetics Publishers.

Orlick, T. (1986). *Psyching for sport: Mental training for athletes*. Champaign, IL: Human Kinetics Publishers.

Orlick, T. (1989). Reflections on sport psych consulting with individual and team sport athletes at summer and Olympic winter games. *The Sport Psychologist, 1*, 4–17.

Orlick, T. (1996). The wheel of excellence. *Journal of Performance Education, 1*, 3–18.

Orlick, T. (2008). *In pursuit of excellence* (4th ed.). Champaign, IL: Human Kinetics.

Orlick, T., & Partington, J. (1988). Mental links to excellence. *The Sport Psychologist, 2*, 105–130.

Pear, J. J. (2001). *The science of learning*. Philadelphia: Psychology Press.

Rush, D. B., & Ayllon, T. (1984). Peer behavioral coaching: Soccer. *Journal of Sport Psychology, 6*, 325–334.

Rushall, B. S. (1979). *Psyching in sport: The psychological preparation for serious competition in sport*. London: Pelham Books.

Rushall, B. S. (1992). *Mental skills training for sports: A manual for athletes, coaches, and sport psychologists*. Spring Valley, CA: Sport Science Associates.

Rushall, B. S., & Pettinger, J. (1969). An evaluation of the effects of various reinforcers used as motivators in swimming. *Research Quarterly, 40*, 540–545.

Rushall, B. S., & Siedentop, D. (1972). *The development and control of behavior in sport and physical education*. Philadelphia: Lea & Febiger.

Rushall, B. S., & Smith, K. C. (1979). Coaching effectiveness of the quality and quantity of behavior categories in a swimming coach. *Journal of Sport Psychology, 1*, 138–150.

Scott, D., & Scott, L. M. (1997). A performance improvement program for an international-level track and field athlete. *Journal of Applied Behavior Analysis, 30*, 573–575.

Scott, L. M., Scott, D., Bedic, S. P., & Dowd, J. (1999). The effects of associative and dissociative strategies on rowing ergometer performance. *The Sport Psychologist, 13*, 57–68.

Silva, J. M., III (1982). Competitive sport environments: Performance enhancement through cognitive intervention. *Behavior Modification, 6*, 443–463.

Simek, T. C., & O'Brien, R. M. (1981). *Total golf: A behavioral approach to lowering your score and getting more out of your game*. New York: Doubleday (Now available from B-Mod Associates, Suite 109, 4230 W. Hempstead Turnpike, Bethpage NY 11714).

Skinner, B. F. (1953). *Science and human behavior*. New York: McMillan.

Smith, R. E., & Little, L. M. (1998). A review of behavioral assessment forms for sport psychology consulting. *The Sport Psychologist, 12*, 104–105.

Smith, R. E., Schutz, R. W., Smoll, F. L., & Ptacek, J. T. (1995). Development and validation of a multi-dimensional measure of sport-specific psychological skills: The athletic coping skills inventory-28. *Journal of Sport and Exercise Psychology, 17*, 379–398.

Smith, R. E., Smoll, F. L., & Christensen, D. S. (1996). Behavioral assessment and intervention in youth sports. *Behavior Modification, 20*, 3–44.

Smith, R. E., Smoll, F. L., & Curtis, B. (1979). Coach effectiveness training: A cognitive-behavioral approach to enhancing relationship skills in youth coaches. *Journal of Sport Psychology, 1*, 59–75.

Smoll, F. L., & Smith, R. E. (2010). Conducting psychologically oriented coach-training programs: A social-cognitive approach. In J. M. Williams (Ed.), *Applied sport psychology: Personal growth to peak performance* (6th ed., pp. 417–440). New York: McGraw-Hill.

Smoll, F. L., Smith, R. E., & Curtis, B. (1978). Behavioral guidelines for youth sport coaches. *Journal of Physical Education and Recreation, 49*, 46–47.

Swain, A., & Jones, G. (1995). Effects of goal-setting interventions on selected basketball skills: A single-subject design. *Research Quarterly for Exercise and Sport, 66*, 51–63.

Taylor, J., & Taylor, C. (1995). *Psychology of dance*. Champaign, IL: Human Kinetics Publishers.

Thelwell, R. C., & Greenlees, I. A. (2003). Developing competitive endurance performance using mental skills training. *The Sport Psychologist, 17*, 318.

Tkachuk, G., Leslie-Toogood, A., & Martin, G. L. (2003). Behavioral assessment in sport psychology. *The Sport Psychologist, 17*, 104–117.

Tutko, T., & Umberto, T. (1976). *Sports psyching: Playing your best game all the time*. Los Angeles: J. D. Tarcher, Inc.

Vealey, R. S., & Greenleaf, C. A. (2010). Seeing is believing: Understanding and using imagery in sport. In J. M. Williams (Ed.), *Applied sport psychology: Personal growth to peak performance* (6th ed., pp. 267–304). New York: McGraw-Hill.

Virués-Ortega, J., & Martin, G. L. (2010). Guidelines for sport psychologists to evaluate their interventions in clinical cases using single-subject designs. *Journal of Behavioral Health and Medicine, 3*, 158–171.

Wanlin, C., Hrycaiko, D., Martin, G. L., & Mahon, M. (1997). The effects of a goal setting package on the performance of young female speed skaters. *Journal of Applied Sport Psychology, 9*, 212–228.

Ward, P., & Carnes, M. (2002). Effects of posting self-set goals on collegiate football players' skill execution during practice and games. *Journal of Applied Behavior Analysis, 35*, 1–12.

Weinberg, R. S., & Gould, D. (2007). *Foundations of sport and exercise psychology* (4th ed.). Champaign, IL: Human Kinetics.

Weinberg, R. S., Seabourne, T. G., & Jackson, A. (1981). Effects of visuo-motor behavior rehearsal, relaxation, and imagery on karate performance. *Journal of Sport Psychology, 3*, 228–238.

Williams, J. M. (2010). Relaxation and energizing techniques for regulation of arousal. In J. M. Williams (Ed.), *Applied sport psychology: Personal growth to peak performance* (6th ed., pp. 247–266). New York: McGraw-Hill.

Wilson, V. E., Peper, E., & Schmid, A. (2006). Strategies for training concentration. In J. M. Williams (Ed.), *Applied sport psychology: Personal growth to peak performance* (5th ed., pp. 333–348). New York: McGraw-Hill.

Ziegler, S. G. (1987). Effects of stimulus cueing on the acquisition of groundstrokes by beginning tennis players. *Journal of Applied Behavior Analysis, 20,* 405–411.

Zinsser, N., Bunker, L., & Williams, J. M. (2006). Cognitive techniques for building confidence and enhancing performance. In J. M. Williams (Ed.), *Applied sport psychology: Personal growth to peak performance* (5th ed., pp. 349–381). New York: McGraw-Hill.

# Part II
# Assessment and Measurement

# Chapter 2
# Actigraphy: The Ambulatory Measurement of Physical Activity

Warren W. Tryon

Measurement is as fundamental to modern sport as it is to science. The outcomes of Olympic trials and competitions are sometimes determined by tenths or hundredths of a second. Athletic training typically entails performance measurement in order to guide and enhance training methods. Better performance is often its own reward – that is, observing improvements may strongly motivate competitive athletes.

This chapter has several purposes, and correspondingly two major sections. The first purpose of this chapter is to introduce readers to actigraphy: what it is, available instruments, and basic methodological issues. This is accomplished in the first major section of this chapter. The second purpose of this chapter is to apply this information to sports. In the second section, I begin with circadian issues, since actigraphy can track activity level 24 h per day, seven days per week, 365 days per year. Subsequently, I will discuss nocturnal activity and sleep since athletes need to be properly rested. Following this, I will consider diurnal activity as training occurs during waking hours. This discussion will include high-resolution actigraphy to better understand behavioral topography in sports such as track and field, bowling, golf, skating, gymnastics, and skiing.

## Methods of Measuring Human Activity

### Indirect Methods

Devices such as sensitive touch pads installed in swimming pools or high-speed video cameras strategically mounted in stadiums and rinks capture human movements for subsequent reviewing, evaluating, informing choices regarding medals, and reviewing decisions made on the field by referees. While these methods enable athletes to move freely, measurement can occur only within the confines of a particular space. Our meaning of ambulatory extends beyond such boundaries. As such, these measurement methods will not be considered further in this chapter.

---

W.W. Tryon (✉)
Fordham University, Bronx, NY, USA
e-mail: wtryon@fordham.edu

## Heart Rate

Athletic performances increase heart rate. Montoye, Kemper, Saris, and Washburn (1996, pp. 98–105) discussed the use of heart rate monitoring to track physical activity. Searching for "ambulatory heart rate monitors" on the Internet yields a wide variety of ever-changing equipment models. While it is true that greater activity levels produce higher heart rates, factors other than activity level can also alter heart rate. For instance, the excitement of competition can increase heart rate while the athlete in question observes other athletes prior to their performance. One cannot separate heart rate increases caused by psychological factors from those due to increased exertion except by a carefully kept activity diary that identifies the times of day during which the athlete performed or trained. Because heart rate is an *indirect* measure of activity, I will not discuss it further in this chapter.

## Core Body Temperature

O'Brien, Hoyt, Buller, Castellani, and Young (1998) introduced a method of measuring core body temperature based on having participants swallow a pill-sized transducer/transmitter that sends core body temperature to a receiver worn by the person. Because core body temperature is an indirect measure of activity and because body temperature changes lag sufficiently behind activity level changes, I will not discuss it further in this chapter.

## Doubly Labeled Water

Montoye et al. (1996, pp. 17–25) discuss a method for measuring energy expenditure in free-living people; in this method, the people drink water laced with stable isotopes of hydrogen and oxygen. The loss of these isotopes over time as assessed from saliva, urine, or blood provides an estimate of energy expenditure, considered a gold standard, that is directly proportional to activity level. Because doubly labeled water is an indirect measure of activity and because it provides only crude temporal resolution, I will not discuss it further in this chapter.

## *Direct Methods*

### Pedometers/Digital Step Counters

One of the earliest documented forms of direct measurement of athletic-related behavior comes from Leonardi de Vinci (1452–1519), who invented the pedometer during the midpoint of his life (Gibbs-Smith, 1978). Thomas Jefferson encountered the pedometer during his tour as US ambassador to France between 1785 and 1789 and sent it back to America, along with other items (Wilson & Stanton, 1999). The Japanese introduced the first commercial pedometer under the name of manpo-meter, where "manpo" in Japanese means 10,000 steps. Heel-toe transitions involved in walking move the hips up and down. Putting one foot in front of the other displaces the hips left and right. Together, walking moves the attached sensor in a spiral trajectory. Old-style pedometers contained a pendulum that moved in response to hip movements associated with walking and related behaviors such as stooping to pick things up from the floor. A distance indicator was connected to the pendulum through a series of gears, one of which was a stride-length setting that could only be crudely set in an effort to make the unit of measure the mile. Stride length was estimated by counting steps while walking a measured distance and dividing. Hence, the unit of measure was crudely estimated. Running would entail a much larger stride than indicated – thus, seriously underestimating distance traversed. Bending to pick up items entails no forward movement, but is counted as a stride – thus, underestimating distance walked to an extent that is directly proportional to frequency of this behavior. Modern step counters digitally convert steps into distance. While a precise stride length can be registered and can be accurately multiplied by the steps registered, the problem of variable stride lengths remains.

*Units of measure.* The previous section refers to digital step counters since that is the primary mechanism of the modern pedometer. Vertical movements of a small weight increments a digital counter with each movement of the waist activate the counter. In this regard, the step is the unit of measure. Each person's step differs depending upon their height, which makes leg length an important covariate when comparing steps taken across persons of varying heights. However, I submit that such variation is a natural part of human activity and not something that one necessarily wants to control for. Consider the following situation where an adult and a small child cross a street holding hands. The adult strides easily while the child walks rapidly in an effort to keep up. Have they been equally active because they traversed the same curb-to-curb distance? Or has the child been much more active than the adult because their much shorter legs required many more steps to traverse the same distance? I submit that the latter conclusion is valid.

Entering "pedometers" or "step counters" into a search engine will identify many vendors selling a wide variety of instruments that range from high to low quality. One probably gets what one pays for. Assessment of instrument reliability and consistency among devices should be done under laboratory conditions, using some form of bench test (such as a shaker) on which several devices can be mounted simultaneously. Data from devices that over-count or under-count can be adjusted using a conversion factor derived from such a test. For example, if after 100 back and forth movements, Device A counts 115 and Device B counts 95, the conversion factor for Device A would be $100/115 = 0.8696$, with the conversion factor for Device B being $100/95 = 1.0526$.

We shall see below that studies frequently report steps per day. This metric does not control for waking hours and activities for which the pedometer cannot be worn such as swimming. Someone who sleeps late and goes to bed early may get a low step count that day despite being rather active. If that person also went swimming for an hour or two during such a day, their step count for that day would be even lower. However, dividing the steps per day by the minutes that the pedometer was worn might more correctly reflect the person's average activity level. The method I have been using for over 19 continuous years studying my own activity level is as follows. Upon dressing in the morning, I record the date and time I attached my waist-worn step counter on one line of a 3 × 5 index card. Upon undressing at night, I record the time I took my step counter off using military 24-h designation. I enter a one- or two-word note if I did something unusual that day and then record the step count. If I went swimming that day, then I would record the time off and back on as well. This enables me to record 10 days of data per card. At the time of this writing, I have been using this procedure for almost 24 years. Thus, my personal example demonstrates that longitudinal data collection is both possible and feasible. The point of recording time on and off is to determine the minutes of wearing time so that I can divide steps taken by minutes of wearing time in order to control for time worn as longer wearing times can lead to higher step counts even if activity level is lower. Montoye et al. (1996, pp. 72–75) also discussed the use of pedometers to measure activity level.

An important limitation of standard step counters is that someone must read and record the data at specified intervals. Several models of Actigraph LLC actigraphs have software that converts actigraph data into step counts to simulate pedometer functionality (www.theactigraph.com). This function enables one to change the unit of measure from milli-g to steps. New Lifestyles (http://new-lifestyles.com/) retails five models of accelerometer-based step counters with memories in addition to four models of coiled spring pedometers and two models of hair spring pedometers (http://www.thepedometercompany.com/pedometers.html).

## Actigraphs

Actigraphs are small lightweight computerized accelerometer-based devices worn typically at the waist, wrist, and/or ankle that rapidly and simultaneously digitize movement in one, two, or three dimensions every 15, 30, or 60 s continuously 24 h a day for as many days as memory allows (which typically spans 7–28 days). Further information regarding the term "actigraph" can be found at http://en.wikipedia.org/wiki/Actigraph. A list of actigraph vendors and links to most of their products is provided in Table 2.1.

*Units of measure.* There are no standard units of measurement across actigraphs by various vendors, despite the fact that all of these devices use accelerometers to measure activity level. Velocity, typically understood as speed, is defined as the distance covered per unit time (e.g., miles per hour or meters per second). Acceleration

Table 2.1 Actigraph vendors and devices

| Vendor | Device/URL |
| --- | --- |
| Actigraph LLC<br>http://www.theactigraph.com | GT1M series<br>http://www.theactigraph.com/productsGT1M.asp<br>ActiTrainer<br>http://www.theactigraph.com/index.php?option=com_virtuemart&page=shop.product_details&flypage=flypage.tpl&product_id=7&26Itemid=87 |

**Table 2.1** (continued)

| Vendor | Device/URL |
|---|---|
| Ambulatory Monitoring, Inc. http://www.ambulatory-monitoring.com/ | MotionLogger http://www.ambulatory-monitoring.com/motionlogger.html MicroMini-Motionlogger and family of sensors http://www.ambulatory-monitoring.com/micro_sensors.html Motionlogger Buzz Bee http://www.ambulatory-monitoring.com/buzz_bee.html |
| Body Media, Inc. SenseWear http://www.sensewear.com/ | SenseWear BMS http://www.sensewear.com/BMS/solutions_bms.php |
| Cambridge neurotechology limited http://www.camntech.com/ | Actiwatch http://www.camntech.com/ |
| IM Systems http://www.imsystems.net/ | ActiTrac http://www.imsystems.net/actitrac/actitrac.htm DigiTrac (12 bit A/D Triaxial, 40 Hz) http://www.imsystems.net/actitrac/actitrac.htm BioTrainer-Pro http://www.imsystems.net/btpro/btpro.htm BioTrainer II http://www.imsystems.net/bt2/bt2.htm BedMate http://www.imsystems.net/bedmate/bedmate.htm SleepCheck http://www.imsystems.net/sleepcheck/sleepcheck.htm |
| Mini mitter http://www.minimitter.com/ | Actiwatch http://ribn.respironics.com/ |
| New Lifestyles http://new-lifestyles.com/ | Pedometers http://new-lifestyles.com/content.php?_p_=100 http://www.thepedometercompany.com/pedometers.html |
| Nokia http://www.nokiausa.com/ Cellphone actigraphy | N95, N95 8GB, N82, N93i, 6210, N79, N85, N96 Phones http://betalabs.nokia.com/apps/nokia-step-counter |
| PAL Technologies Ltd http://www.paltechnologies.com/ | ActivPAL http://www.paltech.plus.com/products.htm#activpal |
| Philips directlife activity monitor http://exercise.about.com/od/productreviews/fr/philipsactivitymonitor.htm | Activity monitor http://exercise.about.com/gi/o.htm?zi=1/XJ&zTi=1&sdn=exercise&cdn=health&tm=91&gps=123_265_1020_517&f=10&su=p284.9.336.ip_p674.7.336.ip_&tt=6&bt=1&bts=1&st=24&zu=http%3A//www.directlife.philips.com/how_it_works/advanced_activity_monitor/ |
| Polar http://www.polarusa.com/us-en | Activity monitors http://www.polarusa.com/us-en/products/get_active Polar AW200 activity monitor http://www.dickssportinggoods.com/product/index.jsp?productId=2715949&CAWELAID=110638143 |
| Stayhealthy http://www.stayhealthy.com/en_us/main/ | RT3 http://www.stayhealthy.com/en_us/main/research_activity_monitor |

is defined as the change in velocity per unit time; typically meters/second/second. Acceleration is frequently measured in units of "g" for gravity, where 1 g equals the rate with which bodies freely fall to Earth, which is 9.80616 m/s/second at sea level at 45° latitude and mean sea level.

The problem begins with the material used to make the accelerometer. Piezoceramic accelerometers emit a voltage only while they are undergoing positive or negative acceleration. The charge bleeds off to zero when acceleration is constant, which includes the absence of movement. This is understandable as no movement should be measured as zero, and the fact that limbs are jointed and attached to the torso means that they cannot accelerate at a constant rate in a single direction for very long. All changes in direction produce acceleration. This rate of angular movement, measured in Hertz, modifies the actual acceleration value. Because actigraphs do not measure these frequencies, it is impossible to accurately report in units of g. However, because most actigraphs bandpass filter movement frequency from approximately 0.1–3.6 Hz in order to preclude artifact from being recorded as human movement, one could use the midpoint of this frequency range to convert accelerometer voltages to g units. The technical specifications of each vendor should be consulted regarding this issue.

Some actigraphs contain analog-to-digital (A/D) converters that divide a g-force range into parts. For example, one actigraph used an 8-bot A/D converter to divide a –2.13 g to +2.13 g maximum range into $2^8 = 256$ levels of acceleration (cf. Tryon & Williams, 1996). Dividing 4.26 g by 256 gives 0.01664 g/s/count on the A/D converter. This actigraph makes 10 measurements per second resulting in a sampling period of 0.1 s. Integrating over this interval corresponds to multiplying 0.01664 g/s/count by 0.1 s resulting in 0.001664 g/count = 1.664 milli-g/count. Other actigraphs integrate the area under the curve created by the time varying voltage from the accelerometer. The resulting volt-second units are not standard.

## *Methodological Issues*

The reader should be aware of the following four methodological issues when considering actigraphy: (1) site of attachment, (2) instrument reliability, (3) clinical repeatability, and (4) instrument validity. The following three sections address these issues.

### Site of Attachment

Activity level is commonly considered to be something akin to a personality trait (i.e., a rather stable feature of the person). This conceptualization is incorrect in two major ways. First, activity is measured by placing a sensor on a body part such as the wrist, waist, or ankle. The instrument actually responds to its own movement, which corresponds to movements of the site of attachment only. Placing instruments at multiple body sites provides information about those sites, but only about those sites. While walking and running move all body sites, these behaviors move them differently. Sitting in a chair reading a magazine immobilizes the waist and ankles, but not the arms and hands, which are involved in turning pages and perhaps writing notes. Securely attaching actigraphs to a belt or waist band places it relatively close to the body's center of gravity. Vertical movements of this site are directly proportional to energy expenditure.

One should therefore think in terms of the site of attachment that most reflects the behavior of interest. For example, the wrist is the most active site in waking people and, therefore, the site of interest when assessing sleep. All computer sleep-scoring algorithms assume that the data are from the wrist. It does not seem to matter whether one measures the left or right wrist in left- or right-handed people.

The second problem is that activity level is not constant over time, but varies in two substantial and important ways. Autocorrelation is the first characteristic of how activity level varies over time when behavior is measured in one-min or 30-s epochs. If one is walking through a given minute, it is rather probable that one will also be walking during the next minute as it usually takes more than one min to walk anywhere. If one is sitting through a given minute, it is rather probable that one will be sitting during the next minute also. Autocorrelation violates the common assumption of independence made by most statistical methods such as t-tests and analysis of variance (ANOVA), thus precluding their use. Aggregating activity level over sufficiently long blocks of time such as 15, 30, 45, or 60 min tends to reduce autocorrelation. The second characteristic of repeated activity measurements is that at the one-min epoch of temporal resolution, activity level tends to form a Poisson distribution where the standard deviation equals the mean. Most observations lie within 1 standard deviation of the Poisson mean versus $\pm 3$ standard deviations in a normal distribution. A graph of activity vs. time using one-min epochs reveals that the magnitude of activity level changes radically from one min to the next, thereby creating enormous variability. Attempting to normalize this integral feature of activity level is *not* recommended for at least two reasons. The first, and perhaps the most persuasive, reason is that one is ignoring a central feature of activity level. The second reason is that all transformations complicate interpretation. For example, how should one interpret the square root or the logarithm (natural or base 10) of activity level or, worse yet, the square root of the logarithm of activity level?

**Instrument Reliability**

Physical instruments and psychological tests differ in fundamental ways that influence how one assesses their reliability and validity. Psychological tests must be given to people in order to obtain data from which to compute reliability and validity coefficients. The sample studied can markedly influence the obtained results, which is why informed psychometricians understand that tests are reliable and valid only for some samples and some purposes, but not others. In short, reliability and validity are not entirely about the test, per se. This limitation does not pertain to instruments whose functional properties can be studied in the laboratory with machines capable of accurately reproducing specific movements.

The concept of reliability requires that the same phenomenon be measured at least twice, and preferably multiple times, to see if the same value is returned. The source of movement used to study the reliability of an instrument should vary as little as possible; preferably variation should be negligible so that it can be assumed to be effectively zero. Then, all observed variation over repeated measurements can be entirely attributed to the unreliability of the device. However, more commonly, investigators have people repeatedly perform the same behavior and attribute all observed variability to the unreliability of the device. This assumes that the people have precisely repeated the requested behaviors – I submit that this is rarely, if ever, true. For example, participants are asked to repeatedly walk a measured distance or repeatedly climb a set of stairs, or repeatedly perform a task such as hammering a nail. Attributing all observed variation to measurement unreliability assumes that human variability is negligible, when in fact it is both measurable and substantial. Hence, the variability of instruments should always be established under laboratory conditions, and never with people performing specific behaviors as this concerns clinical repeatability, which is discussed below.

The standard methods by which psychometricians calculate the reliability of psychological tests are inappropriate when measuring the reliability of instruments for methodological and statistical reasons. The typical method for psychological tests is to administer them to a group of people on one occasion and to compute Cronbach's alpha using commercially available software to determine the test's reliability, which is a measure of internal consistency. When possible, psychologists administer the test to a group of people on two occasions to determine test–retest temporal stability. Here the reliability coefficient is the correlation coefficient between the test and retest scores. The time interval must be carefully chosen: long enough so that participants do not clearly recall their prior answers but short enough so that real change does not occur. Both methods assume substantial variation across people.

Instruments are typically constructed to a physical standard to minimize interdevice variability and then calibrated to remove as much remaining interdevice variability as possible. The resulting homogeneity artificially reduces traditional psychometric indices of reliability in direct proportion to the extent to which devices perform the same way. This is the reverse of what one wants. A solution I have recommended is to compute the coefficient of variation (CV) on a set of repeated measurements taken from a machine such as a pendulum or shaker (cf. Tryon & Williams, 1996; Tryon, 2005). This is done by dividing the standard deviation (SD) of the repeated measurements for a single device by the mean of those measurements and multiplying by 100 to yield a percentage. The more close one measurement is to another, the smaller is its SD and CV. This method enables one to determine a reliability coefficient for each device.

When an investigator has multiple devices, they may observe that the means used to compute the CAs are not identical. One can compute a correction coefficient for each device as follows. Compute the grand mean, the mean of all the means across devices. The correction coefficient for each device is the difference between its mean and grand mean, i.e., the number that must be added to or subtracted from the instrument's mean in order to obtain the grand mean; i.e., some correction values are negative and others positive. This correction constant is then added to every measurement made with that instrument. This will minimize any systematic differences across instruments. This issue is avoided for individuals when the same instrument is used at the same body site for the same person across time. However, this issue occurs when two or more instruments are used to compare the behavior of two or more individuals.

*Pedometers.* Bassett et al. (1996) reported that the "manpo" pedometers initially introduced by the Japanese were subject to large measurement errors, but that the next generation of electronic pedometers (i.e., step counters) is reasonably accurate for assessing walking-related activities. Modern pedometers, especially those using the "KS10 and JW200 pedometer engines, are quite accurate. Vincent and Sidman (2003) tested 24 Yamax MLS-2000 digital pedometers using a shake test. The average deviation over 100 shakes was 0.39 steps ± 0.29, before what they characterize as heavy use in a large study, and 0.60 ± 0.62 steps after the study was completed. All pedometers were within 5% of nominal values, i.e., within 5 steps of the programmed 100 shakes. The authors also reported results for a standard walking where the mean was 2.26 and the standard deviation was 0.80 before the study. The walking test was repeated after the study ended, when the mean was 1.71 and the standard deviation was 0.88. The authors reported that the walking test produced significantly more error ($F(1, 46) = 109.04, p < 0.01$). Note that the walking test mean of 2.26 is 5.79 times as large as the shake test mean of 0.39 before the study began, and the mean of 1.71 was 2.85 times as large as the shake test of 0.60 after the study ended. Hence, we can conclude that walking tests overestimate pedometer error from approximately 300 to 600% – thus supporting the recommendation made above to restrict assessments of the reliability of activity monitors to laboratory studies.

*Actigraphs.* The reliability and validity of actigraphs has also been studied under laboratory conditions where known physical forces can be repeatedly applied with considerable precision. Tryon and Williams (1996) studied the reliability and validity of 40 CSA Model 7164 actigraphs using a spinner and a 5 feet 7 inch pendulum. They reported reliability coefficients between 97.5 and 99.4%. Validity was established by comparing the observed performance with expectation during pendulum decay and spinning. Tryon (2005) repeatedly tests four MotionLogger$^{TM}$ and four BuzzBee$^{TM}$ actigraphs 10 times on a precision pendulum. He reported reliability coefficients of 0.98 and validity coefficients of 0.99.

**Clinical Repeatability**

It is important to know how much variability is associated with efforts that people make to reproduce behaviors in the same way, because this level of variability limits our ability to detect change such as improvements due to training. All instrumented measures of human activity level in applied contexts such as sports necessarily confound instrument unreliability with human biomechanical, neural, and psychological limits and will necessarily be more variable than instrument reliability suggests. It is important for trainers and athletes to repeatedly measure performances that they feel are the same and compare them with measurements of behaviors that they feel are different.

Aggregates of behavior are more repeatable than are single measurements of behavior. Hourly measures are more repeatable than are minute-by-minute measures. Weekly measures are more repeatable than are daily measures. Epstein (1979, 1980, 1983, 1986) clearly demonstrated that aggregation improves test–retest reliability including good agreement. He also demonstrated that the Spearman–Brown prophecy formula enables one to accurately estimate reliability from the number of repeated measurements taken.

**Instrument Validity**

Instruments are designed and constructed to measure specific quantities. For example, the accelerometers in modern actigraphs measure acceleration, and little else, as long as they are operated within specified temperature extremes and not dropped, i.e., exposed to extreme accelerations that might damage them. Nevertheless, it is important to establish their operating characteristics, which is best done under laboratory conditions for all of the reasons discussed above concerning reliability. Tryon and Williams (1996) used both a large 5 foot 7 inch pendulum and a spinner device to assess both reliability and validity.

## Application to Sports

I now turn to the question of what can be done to enhance sport performance with pedometers and actigraphs. I separate this discussion into two parts because the possible applications differ by virtue of the different technical capabilities of pedometers and actigraphs.

### *Pedometers*

#### General Fitness Using Pedometers

Athletes must be generally fit in order to benefit from specialized training. The President's Council on Physical Fitness and Sports (2001) identified physical inactivity as important to a healthy life style and made recommendations for using pedometers to improve general fitness.

*Normative data.* Bohannon (2007) reported a meta-analysis of the average and 95% confidence interval for the number of steps taken by 6,199 participants in 42 studies. The overall average was 9,448 with a 95% confidence interval of 8,899–9,996 steps. Participants below the age of 65 took an average of 9,797 steps per day with a 95% confidence interval of 9,216–10,377 steps. Participants 65 and older took an average of 6,565 steps per day with a 95% confidence interval of 4,897–8,233 steps.

Tudor-Locke and Myers (2001) compiled normative results from 32 studies and reported that activity level decreases with age; they also noted a sex effect. Healthy 8–10-year-old children take between 12,000 and 16,000 steps per day, boys being more active than girls. Vincent and Pangrazi (2002) studied more than 700 children aged 6–12 years old and reported that boys took between 12,300 and 13,989 steps per day whereas girls took between 10,479 and 11,274 steps per day. Wilde (2002) studied more than 600 adolescents aged 14–16 years old and reported between 11,000 and 12,000 steps per day, boys being more active than girls. Rowlands, Eston, and Ingledew (1999) reported that 8–10-year-old UK children take between 12,000 and 16,000 steps per day.

Tudor-Locke and Myers (2001) reported that healthy young adults take between 7,000 and 13,000 steps per day, men being more active than women, whereas healthy older adults take between 6,000 and 8,500 steps per day with men again being more active than women. Individuals living with disabilities and chronic diseases can be expected to take between 3,500 and 5,500 steps per day.

Suzuki et al. (1991) reported that children and adults aged 3–22 years took an average of 14,500 steps per day if they were intellectually disabled, 12,700 steps per day if blind, 17,400 steps per day if deaf, and 8,050 steps per day if physically handicapped.

*How active should we be?* Initial recommendations by Japanese investigators were for 10,000 steps per day to achieve general fitness (Hatano, 1993; Yamanouchi et al., 1995), which corresponds to approximately 300–400 calories per day (Hatano, 1997) depending upon walking speed, sex, age, and body size. This is at least double the amount of activity (150 kcal/day) recommended by the U.S. Surgeon General (U.S. Department of Health and Human Services, 1996). The American College of Sports Medicine (ACSM: www.acsm.org) has endorsed the following categorization of activity levels. Taking less than 5,000 steps per day is termed "Sedentary." Taking between 5,000 and 7,499 steps per day is termed "Low Active." Taking between 7,500 and 9,999 steps per day is termed "Somewhat Active." Taking between 10,000 and 12,500 steps per day is termed "Active." Taking more than 12,500 steps per day is termed "Highly Active." The President's Council on Physical Fitness and Sports (2001) recommended that children take at least 11,000 steps per day, at least five days per week, as a standard healthy base. The more recent ACSM recommended daily activity level for children is between 12,000 and 16,000 steps per day. Leermakers, Dunn, and Blair (2000) suggested that at least 15,000 steps per day may be necessary to achieve weight loss goals.

*Effects of body composition.* Overweight adults take fewer steps than do normal-weight adults (McClung, Zahiri, Higa, Amstutz, & Schmalzried, 2000; Tryon, Pinto, & Morrison, 1991; Tudor-Locke & Myers, 2001; Tudor-Locke, Jones, Myers, Paterson, & Ecclestone, 2002). The same relationship holds for children (Rowlands et al., 1999). Tudor-Locke and Myers (2001) have shown that people who take more than 9,000 steps per day frequently have a normal body mass index (BMI), whereas individuals who take less than 5,000 steps per day frequently are considered obese by BMI standards. However, physicists define work as mass times distance. Multiplying body weight by steps taken frequently reveals that overweight people expend more energy than do normal weight people (Tudor-Locke & Myers, 2001).

*Using pedometers to promote activity.* Sidman (2002) has reported at book length about promoting activity in sedentary women using pedometers. However, I am aware of no studies that used pedometers to enhance athletic performance in healthy people even in such likely journals as *Sports Medicine, Research Quarterly for Exercise and Sport,* and *Medicine and Science in Sports and Exercise.* The focus of research with pedometers is on sedentary people and/or sedentary people with health issues such as obesity, diabetes, and hypertension.

Richardson et al. (2008) reported a meta-analysis of studies designed to promote activity level. Their inclusion criteria were extensive. Each study had to use pedometers as a motivational tool including setting a step-count goal. The study was a controlled trial or had a pre-post design. The study did not use concurrent dietary intervention. Participants were both sedentary at baseline and overweight or obese. Intervention lasted at least four weeks. The following databases were searched: CINAHL, EMBASE, MEDLINE, PsycINFO, SportDiscus, and the Web of Science. The authors identified 9 studies covering 307 participants in programs lasting from four weeks to one year. Results indicated that participants' average activity level increased by 3,656 steps.

Bravata et al. (2007) also conducted a meta-analysis of pedometer-based activity promoting programs. They searched for all English-language articles in the MEDLINE, EMBASE, Sport Discus, PsychINFO, Cochrane Library, Thompson Scientific (previously known as Thompson ISI), and ERIC databases from 1966 through 2007, and retrieved 2,246 citations. Of these 26 studies, 8 randomized controlled trials (RCTs) and 18 observational studies met the following inclusion criteria. Studies had to include more than five participants; studied participants in naturalistic settings; counseled participants relative to activity goals; measured BMI, glycemic control, serum lipid levels, and blood pressure; and expressed baseline activity as steps per day using a pedometer. As noted above, the steps per day metric fails to control for length of waking day and for activities such as swimming during which the pedometer would be removed. Participants were 49 years old on average (SD = 9), although five studies concerned people whose age was greater than 60 years on average. Nine studies exclusively enrolled women. Overall, men accounted for just 15% of the samples. When race and ethnicity were reported, 93% were white, on average. Most participants were obese by BMI standards, but had relatively normal serum lipid levels.

Interventions took from 3 to 104 weeks, with an average and standard deviation of 18 and 24, respectively. Five of the interventions took place at work. Counseling sessions ranged from 0 to 104 with a mean and standard deviation of 7 and 19, respectively. The average steps per day during baseline were 7,473 with a standard deviation of 1,385 and a range of 2,140–12,371 steps per day. The 155 participants across the 8 RCTs that actively used pedometers to increase activity took an average of 2,491 more steps per day than did the 122 control participants. The 95% confidence interval ranged from 1,098 to 3,885 steps per day. Participants in the 18 observational studies who used pedometers to increase activity level took an average of 2,183 more steps per day. The 95% confidence interval ranged from 1,571 to 2,796 steps per day. When combined, using a pedometer with an activity goal such as 10,000 steps per day resulted in an average activity increase of 26.9%. This change was associated with an average BMI reduction of 0.38 with a 95%

confidence interval ranging from −0.05 to −0.72. Systolic blood pressure decreased by 3.8 mmHg with the 95% confidence interval ranging from −1.7 to −5.9 mmHg. These changes were more pronounced in participants who had a higher initial blood pressure and who took more steps per day suggesting a dose–response relationship between activity and health benefits.

*Conclusions.* Pedometers provide numerical evidence of activity level that can be incorporated into a planned regimen favoring greater activity and corresponding improvements in fitness. The existing literature shows that even unathletic people can increase their activity level and improve fitness. It therefore seems reasonable that athletes should be able to do as well or better at achieving similar goals. However, pedometers cannot be used to measure activity while swimming, and while pedometers can be worn while bike riding and weight training, they will not accurately measure caloric expenditure during these activities. Hence, pedometers pertain to general fitness that derives from ambulation.

## *Actigraphs*

Actigraphs offer two important advantages over even the best accelerometer-based pedometers: (1) proportionality and (2) time-locked repeated measurements. Whereas the earliest actigraphs registered presence of movement but not intensity, modern actigraphs respond in direct proportion to the intensity of activity. While this information can be reduced to "steps," much information is lost in doing so because actigraphs measure activity level at least 10 times per second, and then average over a user-defined epoch (typically one min, i.e., 600 measurements/min). Measuring activity level so intensively and reporting and storing results at one-min time slices provide a much more detailed record of activity level – this therefore enables more applications than pedometers.

### Sleep

It is important that athletes get proper sleep in order to give their best performance. Polysomnography (PSG) is the gold standard for measuring sleep, but requires one to sleep in a sleep lab, which would be prohibitively expensive for continuous use. Home PSG is possible, but its use is also restricted to diagnosing sleep disorders rather than as a training resource for athletes. Actigraphy provides an alternative instrumented method for studying sleep. The American Academy of Sleep Medicine updated its Practice Parameters for the use of actigraphy to assess sleep (Morgenthaler et al., 2007). These Practice Parameters are also available on the American Academy of Sleep Medicine Web page (http://www.aasmnet.org/PracticeParameters.aspx?cid=-1) and on the National guideline Clearinghouse Web page (http://www.ngc.gov/summary/summary.aspx?doc_id=10779). A PubMed search for "actigraphy, sleep" returned 720 articles on April 18, 2010, indicating that a substantial body of research supports these guidelines.

Actigraphy and PSG differ with regard to sleep measures for primarily two reasons (cf. Tryon, 2004): (1) PSG is a multichannel physiological (e.g., EEG, EMG, respiration) monitoring system; actigraphy is a single-channel behavior-monitoring system, and (2) PSG and actigraphy key on different parts of the sleep-onset spectrum. PSG sleep scoring continues to be based on the Rechtschaffen and Kales (1968) sleep scoring criteria for humans that score wake and then various stages of sleep. However, it is now clear that sleep onset entails several systematic changes and is not a discrete event. Tryon (2004) described the following three phases of sleep onset: (1) People become inactive for a period of time that actigraphy considers characteristic of sleep onset. People with insomnia are noted for their ability to remain awake but motionless. Good sleepers complete this phase of sleep onset much more rapidly. (2) The beginning of the second stage of sleep onset is marked by muscle relaxation resulting in dropping handheld objects. This was the gold standard criterion of sleep onset that was used to validate the onset of PSG-based sleep and consequently continues to mark the point when PSG marks sleep onset. An empty spool of thread held between the thumb and the forefinger was typically used to determine this point of muscle relaxation. (3) The beginning of the third stage of sleep onset is marked by an elevation of the auditory threshold, i.e., when awareness of one's surroundings is lost. This is the point of subjective sleep onset and corresponds to sleep onset times recorded in sleep logs. Waking up rapidly reverses the three stages of sleep onset. Actigraphy cannot measure all that PSG can, but Tryon (1996) has shown that actigraphic measures of four sleep parameters are highly correlated with PSG measures of the same parameters. For example, validity correlations for total sleep time ranged from $r(19) = 0.72$ to $r(3) = 0.98$. Validity correlations for percent sleep ranged from $r(19) = 0.82$ to $r(2) = 0.96$. Validity correlations for sleep efficiency ranged from $r(23) = 0.63$ to $r(11) = 0.91$. Validity correlations for wake after sleep onset ranged from $r(37) = 0.56$ to $r(67) = 0.87$.

Athletes sometimes fly long distances before competing, and that can result in jet lag, which can interfere with athletic performance. Montaruli, Roveda, Calogiuri, La Torre, and Carandente (2009) reported results from an actigraph-based study demonstrating how jet lag can be minimized and sleep can be improved. They used actigraphs to measure the sleep of 18 athletes who flew from Milan to New York, where 12 of them ran the 2007 New York City Marathon. They divided these 12 athletes into two groups of six: a morning training group (MTG) who trained in Milan from 7 a.m. until 9 a.m. for one month and an evening training group (ETG) who trained in Milan from 7 p.m. to 9 p.m. for one month. The remaining six athletes served as a control group (CG); they did not train and did not run the marathon. In New York, the MTG and ETG groups both trained in the morning from 7 a.m. to 9 a.m. Their results showed that the transatlantic flight fragmented the sleep of the ETG and CG significantly more than that of the MTG and that morning workouts repaired this problem.

## Circadian Applications

Circadian rhythms are those biological functions that wax and wane over an approximately 24-h period. Fit individuals typically have robust circadian rhythms. Activity level is normally characterized by a circadian rhythm in that it should be much higher during waking hours than during sleep. While it is possible to assess circadian rhythm over a single 24-h period, a much more accurate assessment results when evaluated over a week or month. The average activity level over a 24-h period or multiple periods is called the *measor*. The time at which peak activity level occurs is called *acrophase*. Cosinor software can be used to determine the best-fitting cosine wave and deduce acrophase from its peak. Amplitude refers to the height of the fitted cosine function. The suprachiasmatic nucleus (SCN) is believed to be the biological clock in mammals that regulates circadian rhythms. Zeitgebers are environmental cues that entrain, i.e., regulate, circadian rhythms. The solar light/dark cycle is a prominent zeitgeber that can be disrupted by long jet flights where the light/dark cycle of the destination differs substantially from that of the point of departure. The study reviewed above by Montaruli et al. (2009) shows how physical training during morning hours can help return circadian rhythms to normal.

**Improving Sleep**

Monitoring sleep during training is practical and feasible using sleep logs and actigraphy. Sleep logs provide a rough estimate of sleep as they primarily contain the time the person started trying to sleep and the time that they awoke. Actigraphy can provide additional objective information, such as the time that the person went to sleep and the time that they awoke with an accuracy of one-min. The athlete needs to wear only a wristwatch-size actigraph to bed every night. Data need to be downloaded only once each week and sleep scoring has been simplified to a menu selection. The Zeo is a new sleep-monitoring system that can be used to monitor sleep (http://www.myzeo.com/). Data are archived on a website in order to keep track of sleep quality over time. Bedtime, alcohol consumption, and diet can all be modified as necessary to keep sleep scores up.

**Diurnal Activity**

*Low resolution.* Actigraphs normally measure from 10 to 30 times per second and average over one-min epochs. This level of temporal resolution is much more detailed than pedometer data and frequently adequately characterizes the duration and intensity of ambulation-based workouts that include running or walking. The Fitbit system (http://www.fitbit.com/) uses a triaxial accelerometer to track activity level throughout the day. The Nike+ system (http://www.apple.com/ipod/nike/, http://nikerunning.nike.com/nikeos/p/nikeplus/en_US/) creates a personal fitness trainer by wirelessly connecting a sensor placed in the heel of running shoes with an iPhone or iPod to collect data while exercising that is then sent to a server for further processing.

*High resolution.* Sometimes greater temporal resolution is helpful in quantifying athletic performance. The RT3 sold by StayHealthy has a one-second recording epoch, which gives 60 times better temporal resolution than a one-min recording epoch. The ActiTrainer Solution Package sold by Actigraph LLC measures and records activity level at 30 Hz (30 times per second), and their GT3X model can sample and record at 80 Hz, which should be sufficient to track a golf swing or a bowling approach. I could not find published applications of high-resolution actigraphs for these purposes.

## References

Bassett, D. R., Ainsworth, B. E., Leggett, S. R., Mathien, C. A., Main, J. A., Hunter, D. C., et al. (1996). Accuracy of five electronic pedometers for measuring distance walked. *Medicine and Science in Sports and Exercise, 28*, 1071–1077.

Bohannon, R. W. (2007). Number of pedometer-assisted steps taken per day by adults: A descriptive meta-analysis. *Physical Therapy, 12*, 1642–1650.

Bravata, D. M., Smith-Spangler, C., Sundaram, V., Geinger, A. L., Line, N., Lewis, R., et al. (2007). Using pedometers to increase physical activity and improve health: A systematic Review. *Journal of the American Medical Association, 298*, 2296–2304.

Epstein, S. (1979). The stability of behavior; I. On predicting most of the people much of the time. *Journal of Personality and Social Psychology, 37*, 1097–1126.

Epstein, S. (1980). The stability of behavior, II. Implications for psychological research. *American Psychologist, 35*, 790–806.

Epstein, S. (1983). Aggregation and beyond: Some basic issues on the prediction of behavior. *Journal of Personality, 51*, 360–392.

Epstein, S. (1986). Does aggregation produce spuriously high estimates of behavior stability? *Journal of Personality and Social Psychology, 50*, 1199–1210.

Gibbs-Smith, C. (1978). *The inventions of Leonardo da Vinci.* London: Phaidon Press.

Hatano, Y. (1993). Use of the pedometer for promoting daily walking exercise. *International Council for Health, Physical Education, and Recreation, 29*, 4–8.

Hatano, Y. (1997). Prevalence and use of pedometer. *Research Journal of Walking, 1*, 45–54.

Leermakers, E. A., Dunn, A. L., & Blair, S. N. (2000). Exercise management of obesity. *Medical Clinics of North America, 84*(2), 419–440.

McClung, C. D., Zahiri, C. A., Higa, J. K., Amstutz, H. C., & Schmalzried, T. P. (2000). Relationship between body mass index and activity in hip or knee arthroplasty patients. *Journal of Orthopaedic Research, 18*, 35–39.

Montaruli, A., Roveda, E., Calogiuri, G., La Torre, A., & Carandente, F. (2009). The sportsman readjustment after transcontinental flight: A study on marathon runners. *Journal of Sports Medicine and Physical Fitness, 49*(4), 372–381.

Montoye, H. J., Kemper, H. C. G., Saris, W. H. M., & Washburn, R. A. (1996). *Measuring physical activity and energy expenditure.* Champaign, IL: Human Kinetics.

Morgenthaler, T., Alessi, C., Friedman, L., Owens, J., Kapur, V., Boehlecke, B., et al. (2007). Practice parameters for the use of actigraphy in the assessment of sleep and sleep disorders: An update for 2007. *Sleep, 30*, 519–529.

O'Brien, C., Hoyt, R. W., Buller, M. J., Castellani, J. W., & Young, A. J. (1998). Telemetry pill measurement of core temperature in humans during active heating and cooling. *Medicine & Science in Sports & Exercise, 30*, 468–472.

President's Council on Physical Fitness and Sports. (2001). *The President's challenge physical activity and fitness awards program.* Washington, DC: President's Council on Physical Fitness and Sports, U.S. Department of Health and Human Services. http://www.fitness.gov/Reading_Room/Digests/pcpfsdigestjune2002.pdf

Rechtschaffen, A., & Kales, A. (Eds.). (1968). *A manual of standardized terminology, techniques, and scoring system for sleep stages of human subjects.* Los Angeles: Brain Information Service/Brain Research Institute, UCLA.

Richardson, C. R., Newton, T. L., Abraham, J. J., Sens, A., Jimbo, M., & Swartz, A. M. (2008). A meta-analysis of pedometer-based walking interventions and weight loss. *Annals of Family Medicine, 6*, 69–77.

Rowlands, A. V., Eston, R. G., & Ingledew, D. K. (1999). Relationship between activity levels, aerobic fitness, and body fat in 8- to 10-yr-old children. *Journal of Applied Physiology, 86*, 1428–1435.

Sidman, C. L. (2002). *Promoting physical activity among sedentary women using pedometers.* Mesa, AZ: Arizona State University.

Suzuki, M., Saitoh, S., Taskaki, Y., Shimonmura, Y., Makishima, R., & Hosoya, N. (1991). Nutritional status and daily physical activity of handicapped students in Tokyo metropolitan schools for deaf, blind, mentally retarded, and physically handicapped individuals. *American Journal of Clinical Nutrition, 54*, 1101–1111.

Tryon, W. W. (1996). Nocturnal activity and sleep assessment. *Clinical Psychology Review, 16*, 197–213.

Tryon, W. W. (2004). Issues of validity in actigraphic sleep assessment. *Sleep, 27*, 158–165.

Tryon, W. W. (2005). The reliability and validity of two ambulatory monitoring actigraphs. *Behavior Research Methods Instruments & Computers, 37*, 492–497.

Tryon, W. W., Pinto, L. P., & Morrison, D. F. (1991). Reliability assessment of pedometer activity measurements. *Journal of Psychopathology and Behavioral Assessment, 13*, 27–44.

Tryon, W. W., & Williams, R. (1996). Fully proportional actigraphy: A new instrument. *Behavior Research Methods Instruments & Computers, 28*, 392–403.

Tudor-Locke, C., Jones, G. R., Myers, A. M., Paterson, D. H., & Ecclestone, N. A. (2002). Contribution of structured exercise class participation and informal walking for exercise to daily physical activity in community-dwelling older adults. *Research Quarterly for Exercise and Sport, 73*, 350–356.

Tudor-Locke, C. E., & Myers, A. M. (2001). Methodological considerations for researchers and practitioners using pedometers to measure physical (ambulatory) activity. *Research Quarterly for Exercise and Sport, 72*, 1–12.

U.S. Department of Health and Human Services. (1996). *Physical activity and health: A report of the surgeon general.* Atlanta, GA: U.S. Department of Health and Human Services, Centers for Disease Control and Prevention, National Center for Chronic Disease Prevention and Promotion.

Vincent, S. D., & Pangrazi, R. P. (2002). An examination of the activity patterns of elementary school children. *Pediatric Exercise Science, 14*, 432–441.

Vincent, S. D., & Sidman, C. L. (2003). Determining measurement error in digital pedometers. *Measurement in Physical Education and Exercise Science, 7*(1), 19–24.

Wilde, B. E. (2002). *Activity patterns of high school students assessed by a pedometer and a national activity questionnaire.* Mesa, AZ: Arizona State University.

Wilson, D. L., & Stanton, L. (1999). *Jefferson abroad.* New York: Modern Library.

Yamanouchi, K., Takashi, T., Chikada, K., Nishikawa, T., Ito, K., Shimizu, S., et al. (1995). Daily walking combined with diet therapy is a useful means for obese NIDDM patients not only to reduce body weight but also to improve insulin sensitivity. *Diabetes Care, 18*, 775–778.

# Chapter 3
# Quantitative Analysis of Sports

Derek D. Reed

In 2003, Michael C. Lewis published the book *Moneyball: The Art of Winning an Unfair Game*, detailing Billy Beane's (the general manager of the Oakland Athletics Major League Baseball [MLB] team) contemporary use of advanced statistical methods to draft or select players and to devise strategic approaches to game play in hope of launching the team into the competitive echelon of the MLB, despite the numerous odds against them. To the novice reader or sports enthusiast, this simple description seems an endearing tale of an underdog's success, and rightly so – the Oakland Athletic's, with a salary budget of only $41 million, competed against teams with much higher salaries, such as the New York Yankees with $200 million to spend on its players. Transcending beyond this "triumph over adversity" tale, however, Lewis's *Moneyball* has become a panacea for analytically maximizing outcomes from an economic approach. Perhaps more importantly, *Moneyball* has both glamorized and popularized the previously obscure and seemingly excessively academic use of advanced statistics of *sabermetrics* in measuring within-game/season performance to judge success to predict future outcomes. As David Grabiner (n.d.) describes in *The Sabermetric Manifesto*,

> The most common uses of statistics are to evaluate past performance (such as to determine who should win the MVP award) and to predict future performance (such as to evaluate a trade that was just made). In both cases, [sabermetricians] are interested in measuring contribution to games won and lost.

Since the publication of *Moneyball*, this use of sabermetrics – termed after the Society for American Baseball Research (see http://www.sabr.org) – has been adopted by many MLB teams, who now employ full-time sabermetricians or statisticians as part of their staff (Heller, 2010).

The argument to abandon simple statistics and to utilize advanced quantitative measures in elite sports was first publicly and seriously advanced with Cook's 1964 publication of *Percentage Baseball* (Schwarz, 2005). Cook, a metallurgist and

---

D.D. Reed (✉)
Department of Applied Behavioral Science, University of Kansas, Lawrence, KS 66045, USA
e-mail: dreed@ku.edu

consultant on the Manhattan Project whose only real baseball experience was in college, embarked on his pursuit to refine baseball analyses using probability theory simply in an effort to prove that Ty Cobb was indeed a better batter than Babe Ruth (Schwarz, 2005). What resulted from Cook's analyses of professional baseball was a litany of findings, suggesting gross overuse of the sacrifice bunt, inadequate utilization of relief pitchers, problems with traditional batter order arrangements, and many other findings shaking the foundation of baseball lore concerning strategy and play. As such, in a review of Cook's findings, Frank Deford of *Sports Illustrated* (1964) titled his editorial piece "Baseball Is Played All Wrong."

Despite the fact that contemporary quantitative analyses of athletics emerged from the sport of baseball, interesting findings abound away from the ballpark. In 2010, Kevin Kelley, the head coach of the Pulaski Academy High School American-rules football team (hereafter, American-rules football will be simply termed "football") in Little Rock, Arkansas, was a panel presenter at the MIT Sloan Sports Analytics Conference (Baxamusa, 2010). How a high school football coach found himself presenting at an elitist sports conference is explained through his novel approach to offensive play calling – he does not punt on fourth down. After reading statistical accounts akin to those employed in sabermetrics, Kelley learned that, statistically, the offense converts over 75% of fourth down plays to first down (see Easterbrook, 2007). Moreover, with a 33% chance of an offensive play series resulting in scoring, calling a rush or pass on fourth down increases scoring opportunities and subsequently decreases opportunities for the opposing team to score. Since Kelley has adopted this offensive strategy, he has led his varsity football team to multiple state titles.

Like the example of Kevin Kelley and football, the translation of sabermetrics to basketball also has its success stories. Mark Cuban, a brash entrepreneur, worked his way up from selling garbage bags door-to-door in New Jersey to starting and selling companies that yielded enough profit to finance his purchase of the Dallas Mavericks organization of the National Basketball Association (NBA) in 2000 (D'Angelo, 2006). Prior to Cuban's purchase and management of the Mavericks, the team's average winning percentage during the 1990s barely broke 30%. During his first year of ownership, Cuban, customarily sitting in the seats among fans during Mavericks games, encountered Wayne Winston, Cuban's former statistics teacher (Hruby, 2004). Cuban and Winston subsequently discussed ways to improve the team and, in doing so, decided to follow the lessons from the pages of *Moneyball* and employ more precise and analytic quantitative approaches to management. Consequently, Winston became a statistical consultant for the Mavericks and has since written a widely acclaimed book on quantitative approaches to sports (see Winston, 2009). Similar to Beane's transformation of the Oakland Athletics, following Cuban and Winston's statistical approach guiding player and play selections, the Mavericks have become a competitive organization in the NBA, with nearly 70% winning record under their tutelage.

With sabermetrics gaining national press and serious consideration in baseball (Neyer, 2002), and the sports of basketball and football slowly translating this science to practice in their respective arenas[1], a group of sabermetricians banded together to form the *Journal of Quantitative Analysis in Sports* (http://www.bepress.com/jqas/) to provide a singular outlet for researchers interested in the subject – previous to this, such researchers had to find publication homes in multidisciplinary academic journals or had to simply compile their findings and thoughts for books and book chapters (see Alamar, 2005). Given the aforementioned examples, it is evident that quantitative analyses of sport are (a) gaining interest in pop culture (e.g., *Moneyball*, 2003), (b) becoming increasingly used in sports management (e.g., Mark Cuban), and (c) growing as a legitimized subfield of science and sport (e.g., *Journal of Quantitative Analysis in Sports*). As such, the behavioral approach to sport psychology may benefit from adopting and expanding upon these techniques. Moreover, given the success of quantitative analyses of operant behaviors in the lab and field (e.g., Marr, 1989; Mazur, 2006; McDowell, 1988; Nevin, 2008; Shull, 1991), behavioral sport psychology researchers may offer the traditional sabermetricians additional variables to consider in their practice.

The difference between a behavior analytic approach and quantitative analysis from the sports examples provided above, however, lies in the derivation and application of the mathematical models themselves. In particular, when sabermetricians report on a quantitative model of behavior, what they are actually reporting is novel means of data analysis. To quote J. C. Bradbury, the author of *The Baseball Economist: The Real Game Exposed* (2007), sabermetrics is a science that "[evaluates] players based on a few readily available statistics" (p. 150). To be more specific, such quantitative analyses typically rely upon multiple regression models where a smorgasbord of variables are entered into a program to see which are most related to a sport statistic (e.g., batting average in baseball) of interest. While this quantification of sport is useful for scouting reports and managerial decisions, it does little in describing processes underlying sport behavior. The quantitative analyses employed by behavior analysts, however, are used to evaluate whether a particular hypothesis of a behavioral phenomenon – one based upon repeated measures of steady-state responding in well-controlled experiments and organized into an equation – better accounts for both laboratory and field observations of behavior than other hypotheses (i.e., other quantitative models of behavior). To quote James Mazur (2006), quantitative models of behavior are advantageous in that "[t]ranslating a verbal hypothesis into a mathematical model forces a theorist to be precise and unambiguous, and this can point to ways of testing competing theories that sound as if they make similar predictions when they are stated in words" (p. 287). In essence, quantitative analyses of behavior are used to both describe and predict patterns of behavior, with the goal to elucidate a behavioral process central to the observations. These models then compete in the peer-reviewed literature to

---

[1] The application of advanced statistical analyses in basketball has been termed APBRmetrics, after the Association for Professional Basketball Researcher (see http://www.apbr.org). In football, analysts simply borrow the term *sabermetrics* (e.g., Campos & Chait, 2004), despite its origin from baseball.

find one quantitative model that best accounts for the observations shared among behavior analytic labs. Thus, while the application of quantitative analysis differs substantially between sabermetricians and behavior analysts, both parties agree that much may be gained through the use of equations to describe a behavior of interest, not just relying on verbal accounts by savvy commentators or well-versed academic writers.

## Quantitative Analyses of Behavior

In order to understand sport performance within the auspices of a quantitative model of behavior, one must accept the notion that sport performance is indeed under the control of the environment and, thus, susceptible to operant principles. Undoubtedly, the chapters of the present volume provide an abundance of support for this conception. Nevertheless, recall Grabiner's (n.d.) quote from *The Sabermetric Manifesto* in the opening paragraph of this chapter, which states the focus of sabermetrics is in understanding past data to predict future performance in an effort to improve sport behaviors (e.g., batting orders in baseball). Compare this notion with B. F. Skinner's (the father of operant behaviorism) quote from his 1953 treatise on what it means to have a behavioral analytic science of behavior:

> Science not only describes, it predicts. It deals not only with the past but with the future. Nor is prediction the last word: to the extent that relevant conditions can be altered, or otherwise controlled, the future can be controlled. If we are to use the methods of science in the field of human affairs, we must assume that behavior is lawful and determined. (p. 6)

Given the similar interests driving sabermetricians and behavior analysts, it is of no surprise that behavioral researchers have recently begun applying their quantitative analyses to athletic performance. That behavior analysts turn to quantitative models should be expected, given the benefits of doing so described above and in the literature (see Critchfield & Mazur, 2006; Reed, 2009). For example, framing behavior within a quantitative model provides the most parsimonious explanation for how and why the behavior is controlled by the environment. Second, the quantitative model itself provides a succinct description of a behavioral phenomenon for prediction by organizing the phenomenon into a core functional relation in the form of an equation. Third, the equation itself organizes the environment-behavior relations using parameters – both constant and free – as predictors and descriptors of behavior. Finally, the model is tolerant to deviations from the core relation and factors in modulating variables that govern these behavioral variants.

Numerous applications of quantitative models have been made in behavioral approaches to human behavior (e.g., Davison & McCarthy, 1988; Herrnstein, Rachlin, & Laibson, 1996; Hull, 1943; Hursh, Raslear, Shurtleff, Bauman, & Simmons, 1988; Madden & Bickel, 2010; Nevin, 1988, 2008). However, the two quantitative models most relevant and directly translatable to the study of sport behavior are the matching law and discounting. Thus, the remainder of this chapter will specifically focus on (a) the research behind these models, (b) how these models fit into the framework of quantitative analysis of behavior as outlined above, and

(c) specific research questions related to sport that have been addressed, or may be addressed, by these behavioral models.

## Matching

Arguably the most influential quantitative model of behavior, the matching law (Herrnstein, 1961), originates from the basic experimental analysis of pigeons' key pecking in a well-controlled experimental study. Herrnstein's seminal study describes a simple concurrent operants arrangement in which pigeons could earn access to grain by pecking on one of two keys. Both keys featured concurrent variable interval schedules of reinforcement, such that pecking on a key after a specific amount of time had passed since the previous peck would result in access to reinforcement. Since both keys were concurrently available, pecking one key did not influence the schedule on its alternative. What Herrnstein found was that when he manipulated the schedules, the pigeon's rate of pecking on the keys proportionally "matched" the reinforcement schedule. As such, Herrnstein's matching equation simply states that relative rates of behavior will "match" relative rates of reinforcement. In mathematical form,

$$\frac{B_1}{(B_1 + B_2)} = \frac{R_1}{(R_1 + R_2)} \quad (1)$$

the matching law equation states that the proportion of a particular behavior ($B_1$) to the total amount of behavior emitted ($B_1 + B_2$) is equivalent to the proportion of reinforcement obtained for that behavior ($R_1$) to the total amount of reinforcement obtained ($R_1 + R_2$). This relatively simple equation dramatically shifted the analysis of basic operant principles and has become a mainstay in experimental analyses of behavior. Moreover, this basic notion of matching has accounted for many real-world behaviors such as teen pregnancy (Bulow & Meller, 1998), academic behaviors (Billington & DiTommaso, 2003; Reed & Martens, 2008), and attending to conversational peers (Borrero et al., 2007; Conger & Killeen, 1974). Most germane to this discussion, however, is the recent translation of the matching law to sports (e.g., Alferink, Critchfield, Hitt, & Higgins, 2009; Reed, Critchfield, & Martens, 2006; Romanowich, Bourret, & Vollmer, 2007; Stilling & Critchfield, 2010; Vollmer & Bourret, 2000).

In the aforementioned extensions of the matching law to real-world behaviors, these translational researchers utilized a derivation of Herrnstein's 1961 equation, which permits and quantifies deviation away from strict matching using the generalized matching equation (Baum, 1974). The generalized matching equation states,

$$\log \frac{B_1}{B_2} = a \frac{R_1}{R_2} + \log b \quad (2)$$

where the logarithmically transformed behavior ($B_1/B_2$) and reinforcement ($R_1/R_2$) ratios derive from Equation (1), such that unit changes in one ratio are proportional to unit changes in the other. The *a* parameter represents the slope of the best-fit line of the correlation between the two ratios, with log *b* representing the *y*-intercept of that line. In a behavior analytic sense, *a* represents the sensitivity of an organism's behavior to changes in the reinforcement ratio. Moreover, log *b* may be considered the bias that the organism has for some response alternative (i.e., preference for an alternative that cannot be accounted for by the reinforcement ratio alone).

In the graphic format, the core relation is viewed by behavior analysts as how close the best-fit line resembles strict matching in the sense of the line's slope near 1 and bias of zero (see left panel of bottom row of Fig. 3.1). Strict conformance would translate to a perfect relation between the behavior and reinforcement ratios,

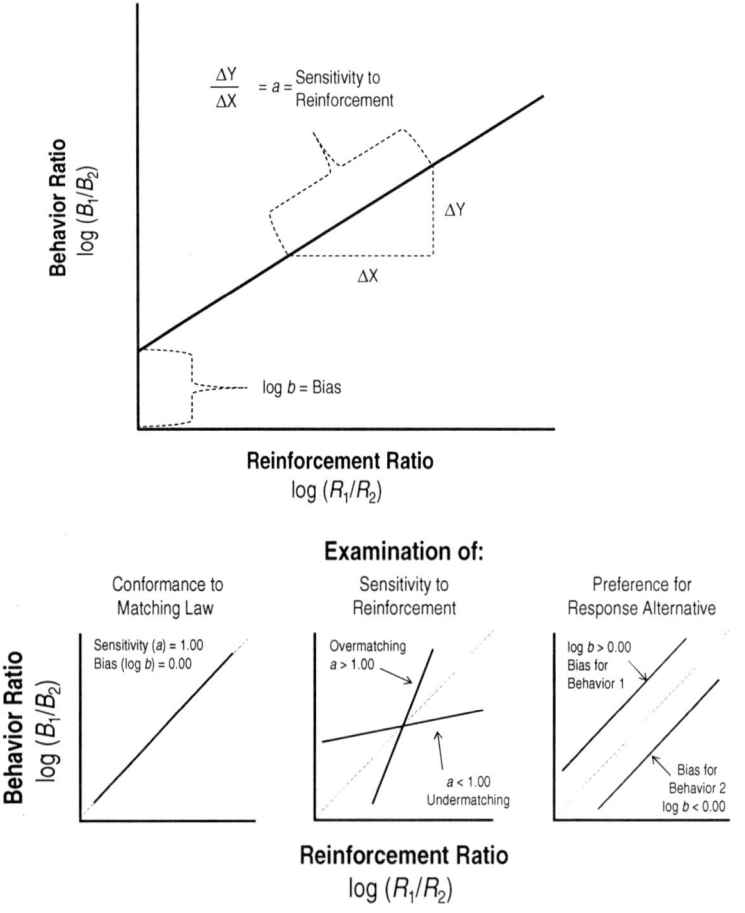

**Fig. 3.1** *Top panel* depicts how a matching analysis is plotted on a coordinate plane, with specification of how the matching analysis is derived from the slope and *y*-intercept of the least-squares linear regression best-fit line. *Bottom panel* depicts three analyses that can be done using the generalized matching equation (Equation 2), with associated examples of data and their interpretation

as is expected in Equation (1). When behavior analysts look to understand the influence of an environmental event (i.e., a modulating factor) on an organism's sensitivity to reinforcement, they examine how deviant the slope of the best-fit line is away from 1 (see middle panel of bottom row of Fig. 3.1). In examining sensitivity modulation, when the observed slope is greater than 1, the organism's behavior is termed as "overmatching," as the organism's behavior has overmatched proportional changes in reinforcement – undermatching thus implies insensitivity in the organism's behavior to changes in reinforcement. Finally, bias modulation (see right panel of bottom row in Fig. 3.1) is understood by behavior analysts through examination of the $y$-intercept's relation to the scatter plot's origin. Positive $y$-intercepts imply a bias for Behavior 1, with negative $y$-intercepts implying a bias for Behavior 2.

In the first translation of the matching law to sport behavior, Vollmer and Bourret (2000) analyzed the allocation of two- and three-point shots by 13 male and 13 female National Collegiate Athletic Association (NCAA) Division I basketball players. In NCAA basketball, an arc designated with a painted line extends from the center of the hoop with a radius of 6.02 m (19 ft 9 in). When a player makes a shot from beyond this line (i.e., greater than 6.02 m from the hoop), that player's team is awarded three points. Shots (not counting free throws) made within the line are rewarded only with two points. Thus, at any given point during game play, a player with the ball has the choice to take a three-point shot, or advance closer to the basket for a two-point shot. Vollmer and Bourret viewed this arrangement as a natural extension of Herrnstein's (1961) choice paradigm with pigeons. As such, these researchers sought to examine a real-world sports example of matching by analyzing the proportion of two- and three-point shots and comparing this against the proportion of the number of points obtained for each shot type using Equation (2). As predicted by the matching law, the proportion of shots taken nearly perfectly matched the proportion of reinforcement the players obtained for making those shots (see top panel of Fig. 3.2).

In addition to simply capturing molar shot selection–reinforcement relations (that is, summarizing large amounts of data collectively, rather than looking at game-to-game performance), Vollmer and Bourret (2000) also sought to determine whether they could predict future shot selections. Toward this end, Vollmer and Bourret calculated the running aggregate allocation of shots from all previous games following each game to make a prediction about the allocation of shots for the next game (see bottom panel of Fig. 3.2). These researchers found their predictions became more and more accurate across the course of the season. Thus, not only does analyzing data at the molar level (i.e., analyzing data at the end of the season) within a matching framework describe shot selection as an operant behavior, but this analytic approach may also be translated to game-by-game data to predict *future* behaviors.

Following Vollmer and Bourret's (2000) lead, Reed et al. (2006) sought to replicate the finding that sport behavior is explainable using quantitative models of operant learning. In traditional football, the offense (the team with the ball) has four chances (i.e., downs) to advance the ball 10 yards. Upon advancement of 10 (or more) yards, the offense is allotted an additional four down to advance 10 additional yards. The goal of advancing the ball down the field is to cross the ball over the

**Fig. 3.2** *Top panel* depicts two generalized matching equation analyses (Equation 2) of Vollmer and Bourret's (2000) study on 2 vs. 3 point shots as operant choice. *Bottom panel* depicts Vollmer and Bourret's concatenated analyses to examine the ability of the matching relations to predict future allocations to 2 vs. 3 point shots

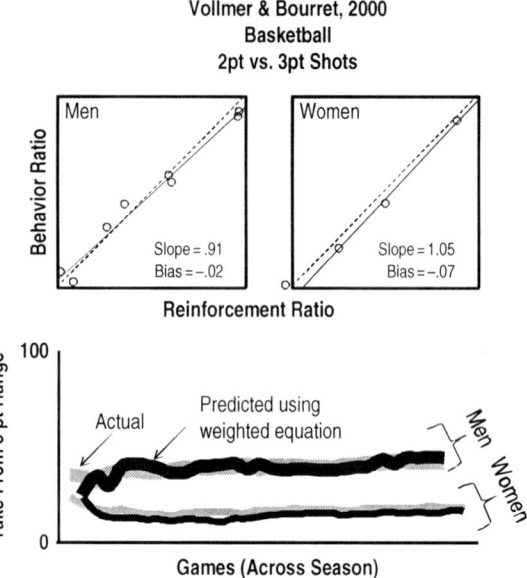

threshold of the opposing team's end zone. Doing so awards the offense six points and an extra point opportunity. To advance the ball, the offense has two options: (1) pass the ball (throwing to a receiving player) or (2) rush the ball (handing the ball to a player to run upfield). Given this simple two-choice arrangement, as well as the clear identification and quantification of reinforcement (i.e., yards gained), Reed and colleagues posited that offensive play calling could be explained using Equation (2). In particular, Reed et al. examined the offensive play calling of elite football teams to determine if the relative proportion of passing to rushing plays approximated the relative proportion of yards gained passing to yards gained rushing. Indeed, these researchers found that Equation (2) did an excellent job in explaining offensive play calling across numerous elite football leagues (e.g., National Football League [NFL], Arena Football League, National Women's Football Association [NWFA], several large NCAA conferences, etc.; see top panel of Fig. 3.3).

Similar to Vollmer and Bourret's (2000) analysis, Reed et al.'s (2006) analyses went beyond simply describing the relationship between responses and reinforcement. In one analysis, Reed and colleagues posited that the bias parameter (log $b$) of Equation (2) could be used to analyze preferences for play types across downs during game play in the NFL. Specifically, Equation (2) was applied to passes and rushes as described above and was analyzed across first, second, and third down play situations. As armchair quarterbacks are aware, traditional football lore suggests that teams run the ball on first down and throw the ball on third down. The findings from Reed et al.'s study suggest that this belief is supported using matching law analyses (see bottom panel of Fig. 3.3). In their interpretation of these data, these researchers put forth the notion that the risk of turning over the ball in either

**Fig. 3.3** *Top panel* depicts two generalized matching equation analyses (Equation 2) of Reed et al.'s (2006) study on passing versus rushing as operant choice. *Bottom panel* depicts Reed et al.'s analysis of teams' bias for passing versus rushing as a function of down, using the bias parameter (log $b$) of the generalized matching equation (Equation 2)

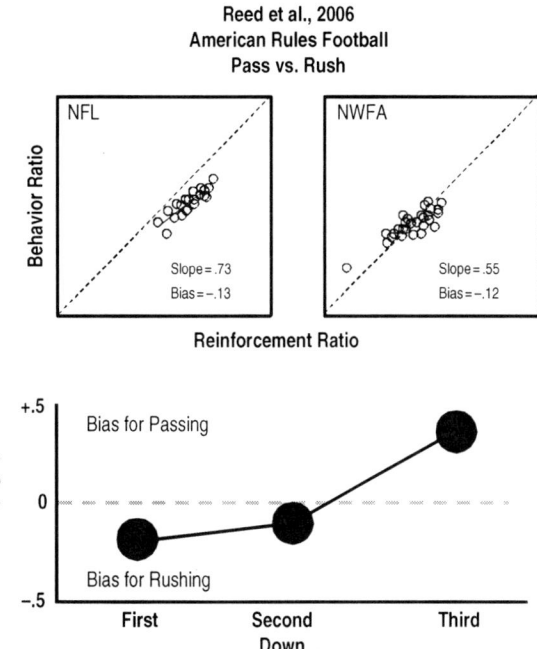

play call would increase the bias toward the alternative. To examine this, Reed and colleagues created a turnover rate index for NFL teams, which was derived via logarithmic transformation of the ratio of fumbles per rushing play to interceptions per passing play. The researchers found a significant correlation between turnover rate and the bias parameter from the matching analyses (obtained using Equation 2), corroborating their hypothesis. Finally, in an effort to provide external validity to the operant account of offensive play calling, the researchers correlated the variance accounted for by Equation (2) with winning percentage across all NFL teams. Data indicated that the degree to which NFL teams conformed to the matching law (i.e., variance accounted for by Equation (2)) was significantly correlated with winning percentage – that is, teams that "matched" relatively better according to the matching law won more games than teams that did not.

Following the field sabermetrics' example of progressing from simple quantitative descriptions of sport phenomena, contemporary matching law research in sports has shifted its focus to explaining and predicting factors affecting play. Such progression is noteworthy, as understanding such data advances the field's ability to apply this science to inform coaches and athletes of the kinds of variables and statistics they should consider when making decisions affecting strategy. This level of scientific translation echoes the notion put forth by Baer, Wolf, and Risley (1968), as well as Van Houten et al. (1988), that behavior analytic services should provide the consumer with the most conceptually systematic and effective means of changing socially important behaviors.

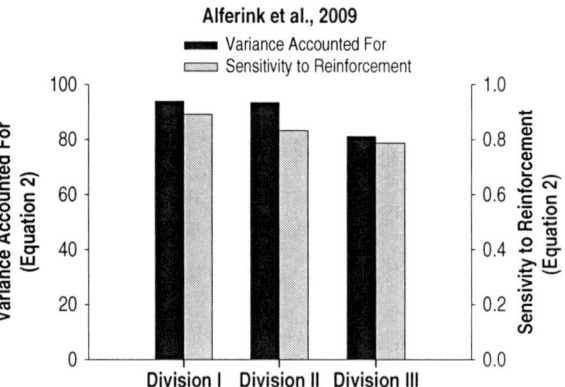

**Fig. 3.4** Bar graph depicting Alferink et al. (2009) data on generalized matching equation (Equation 2) variables across Division I, II, and III college basketball teams

In a major extension of matching theory to understand factors affecting shot selection in basketball, Alferink et al. (2009) sought to determine the extent to which matching law (using Equation (2)) accounted for the variance in 320 Division I college basketball teams. From these results, Alferink et al. demonstrated that their large sample resembled shot selection patterns similar to those reported by Vollmer and Bourret (2000) and Hitt, Alferink, Critchfield, & Wagman (2007), further suggesting that matching theory is a robust phenomenon in basketball. Alferink and colleagues then investigated the difference in matching between Division I, II, and III teams. As Fig. 3.4 indicates, more elite teams (i.e., Division I or II) conformed to matching theory to a greater extent than less elite teams (i.e., Division III). Moreover, Alferink and colleagues then compared regulars and substitutes from these teams, and found that regulars better conformed to matching theory than did substitutes. In these examples, Alferink et al. demonstrate that a relationship between matching and success exists – that is, there appears to be advantages to conforming to matching expectations. Nevertheless, it remains unclear whether better teams select players who conform to matching, or whether matching itself makes a team successful.

In an effort to better explain football offensive play calling, Stilling and Critchfield (2010) provide a plethora of analyses to complement those utilized by Reed et al.'s (2006) study. Specifically, Stilling and Critchfield examined sensitivity to reinforcement, bias, and variance accounted for across numerous NFL play-calling situations. Generally speaking, their analyses indicate that sensitivity to reinforcement remains stable across downs, yards to the goal line, and score (i.e., whether winning, losing, or tied). However, their analyses revealed that teams became more sensitive to reinforcement as the end of the half approached and decreased as the number of yards needed for a first down decreased. Note that none of these differences were statistically significant, although they suggested that a team's sensitivity to reinforcement remains relatively constant across game situations.

In addition to evaluating how sensitivity to reinforcement changed throughout differing situations, Stilling and Critchfield (2010) also examined teams' preferences for play types using the bias parameter of Equation (2) (the $y$-intercept of the best-fit line). In each game situation evaluated, the change in bias parameter was statistically significant ($p \leq .0002$). In particular, bias increased toward passing across downs (first to third), as the half came closer to a close, as the chances of losing increased, and as the number of yards needed for both a first down and a goal increased. While any armchair quarterback would predict these data, the fact that the matching equation lends some validity to football lore provides evidence beyond Reed et al.'s (2006) assertion that football play calling is an operant behavior.

## Other Quantitative Models of Behavior

Apart from matching analyses, the extent to which quantitative models from the experimental analysis of behavior can account for sports remains unknown. In fact, the only other quantitative model from behavior analysis that has been researched for sports is the behavioral momentum principle (see Chapter 9; Nevin, 1988). However, these sports applications have focused only on theoretical accounts of momentum – they have failed to actually fit sports data to the quantitative model of momentum (Mace, Lalli, Shea, & Nevin, 1992; Roane, Kelley, Trosclair, & Hauer, 2004). A third quantitative model – with no applications to sport, to date – comes from the basic experimental literature on self-control. In particular, the notion of discounting (i.e., the relative devaluation of rewards as a function of increasing effort, risk, or delay) has a rich history of successfully quantifying organisms' impulsive and irrational decision-making (see Madden & Bickel, 2010). It is logical, then, that this robust quantitative model would also account for decision-making in sports. For example, consider the reasoning that coaches make as the probability of a successful play decreases, as the distance from a goal increases, or as the time left in a game decreases. In each of these circumstances, a coach's decision to execute a particular play or utilize some strategy will change as a function of such variables. Moreover, it is likely the case that a quantitative model of discounting would account for these behaviors and decisions. For a discussion of such models, see Madden and Johnson (2010), Myerson and Green (1995), as well as Myerson, Green, and Warusawitharana (2001).

## Translating Quantitative Analyses to Sports Applications

Given the evidence above for the matching law's relevance to sports, as well as the suppositions regarding momentum and discounting, the utility of quantitative models seems relevant for improving performance. Unfortunately, the research on these subjects has not yet been extended beyond the ivory tower – that is, what we know is purely academic. What is lacking in the extant literature on quantitative models of sport behavior is evidence of its utility on the playing field. This is difficult for several reasons. First, teams are reluctant, for likely good reasons, to share non-public data on strategies and statistics. Thus, the extent of our analyses is limited to basic statistics that do not factor in situational factors (an exception, of course, is to approach analyses in a manner such as that described by Stilling and Critchfield (2010); nevertheless, this is labor intensive and requires an extensive database). Second, when researchers find relations between behavioral phenomena and athletic success, the logical next phase of translation is to examine functional relations between the operant process and success. This requires, however, directly intervening on play calling. As one might expect, it is incredibly hard to recruit actual athletes/teams/coaches to change their strategies for experimental purposes. Thus, the external validity of our scholarly pursuits remains untested. If researchers remain on the sidelines (no pun intended) with their findings, athletes and coaches will remain skeptical of what these analyses have to offer.

Despite the bleak outlook conveyed in the preceding paragraph regarding barriers to translation, there are numerous ways in which behavior analytic quantitative models may contribute to improved performance. First, given that these models seem to correlate with positive outcomes, it is possible that simply educating coaches and athletes about these findings will prompt them to hone in on the relevant statistics that comprise the quantitative analyses. For instance, showing a coach the team's sensitivity to reinforcement (and explaining what this metric means and how it is calculated) may clue him/her into how efficiently their play calls yield successful outcomes. Providing this feedback and reviewing these statistics after every game may improve subsequent play-calling profiles; this will hopefully result in more points/goals/wins/etc. Second, the mere demonstration that sport behavior conforms to a quantitative model of the same operant principles that govern other human behavior lends credibility to the notion that a behavioral approach to sports performance improvement is a worthwhile venture.

## Data Considerations

The premise of this chapter is to introduce the quantitative analysis of behavior as a precise means to assess the relevancy of behavioral processes to sport, while remaining conceptually systematic to the behavioral orientation to sports psychology. As discussed throughout this chapter, quantitative models provide an efficient means to organizing one's research questions while objectively and quantitatively assessing differing behavioral models' abilities to explain the sport phenomena of interest. Prior to such investigations, interested researchers – however novice or experienced – should take precautions to retain the fidelity of their quantitative analyses.

Like many translational approaches to science, behavior analytic data collection outside of the laboratory is fraught with possible confounds. Sport is no different. Analyses of sport, however, are somewhat more direct as the data of interest are typically readily available on team websites or can be easily gleaned from published records and statistics. Moreover, the sport variables of interest to behavior analytic researchers are often directly assessed within the game or sporting event itself (e.g., field goals attempted and made in basketball, passing plays called in football, home runs in baseball). Fortunately, the *third-variable* confounds (i.e., some existing variable that moderates the relation between two variables of interest) are often just as easily accessible. Having these kinds of data also in hand permits more interesting – and perhaps more meaningful – analyses of behavior. Controlling for these kinds of variables is paramount for assuring that one is truly examining the model's ability to explain the relation between the variables of interest.

## Sources of Data

Once the researcher has finalized his/her research question – and has hypothesized ways to analyze the research question while best reducing confounds – he/she must find a data source to complete the analysis. As described above, the logical first step in this process is to simply consult team or league websites (e.g., http://www.nba.com, http://www.nfl.com, http://mlb.com). Most team or league websites publish the kinds of statistics that are reported in box scores or described in game/event summaries (i.e., the data most recognized and understood by novice sports fans and the lay public). Moreover, television channels devoted to sports often post statistics on their sites (e.g., http://espn.com, http://msn.foxsports.com). While many basic analyses can be appropriately conducted using these kinds of data, situational data are often much more meaningful to the research questions of interest to teams or academic communities. Situational data are those that are parsed by sport situations – that is, sport behavior in context (e.g., football play calling on fourth down in the red zone, baseball pitch selection on a 3–0 count against a power hitter when no runners are on base, probability of calling a full-court press on an in-bounds pass following a goal when the score is tied in basketball).

Obtaining situational sport data may be difficult if one does not have proprietary rights to the data sets – unless, of course, one wishes to watch and score a sporting event in real time, coding for situational variables along the way time left in the game, score, location on the court/field, etc. Fortunately, many useful data sets are available online for basic situational analyses. For example, the website http://82games.com offers detailed NBA statistics, such as teams' shot selections, shooting data by position, shot clock usage, and others. For MLB enthusiasts, the website http://www.retrosheet.org offers play-by-play and box score data for most MLB games since 1952 (box score data are available for games since 1920). Unfortunately, few free access sites exist for researchers interested in NFL data – perhaps due to the rising popularity of fantasy football leagues. However, for serious researchers, premium websites such as http://www.twominutewarning.com or http://www.footballoutsiders.com offer advanced statistics and detailed play summaries for a fee. Perhaps more important, many of these premium websites – particularly the two referenced – are maintained by expert sabermetricians.

Researchers, coaches, or devoted sport aficionados interested in coding their own sporting events for eventual quantitative analysis have several options available to assist such pursuits. For the reader with an interest in football, CompuSports, Inc. (http://www.compusports.com) offers several products that aid in data organization and analysis. For instance, both Easy-Scout XP Plus© and Easy-Scout XP Professional© offer a data entry system in which all aspects (e.g., hash side, down, distance, field position, yards gained) of an offensive or defensive play can be entered. With such data, the user can create reports that generate statistics categorized by variable (e.g., percentage of passing plays with a gain in yards when the game situation is a third down with more than seven yards to go). Moreover, the Easy-Scout XP Professional© software integrates video coding and editing so that the user needs only to use videos of games or plays to generate data. Reducing the need for real-time data coding during the live game permits more time for actual coaching or spectating. Also available from CompuSports© are statistical software packages that integrate with Personal Desktop Assistants [PDAs] to allow for real-time recording of player statistics that synchronize with the statistics database for eventual data analyses.

Similar to the football software described above, TurboStats Software Company© (http://www.turbostats.com) offers the ScoreKeeper© program for baseball/softball and basketball that uses PDAs to record real-time events into a statistics database. This company also offers a TurboStats© program, which uses these data to generate advanced analyses based upon situational events. For example, interested users can generate baseball reports that delineate batting statistics by pitch count, pitch type, or pitch location. Basketball reports can provide the percentage of shots made by location on the court or statistics broken down by home/away games.

## Analyzing Data

Quantitative analyses of behavior (i.e., sport or otherwise) necessitate the use of advanced software to statistically analyze data and to fit quantitative models to the data sets. While Microsoft Office Excel® is the spreadsheet program perhaps the most widely used by the lay public, many of the relevant analyses cannot be handled with this software alone. Nevertheless, for those readers with access to Excel®, rest assured that some of the basic quantitative analyses could indeed be conducted within this program. For example, to conduct matching law analyses, one need only to use the regression function available in the Analysis ToolPak add-in, which comes standard in Excel®. For more information on using Excel® for matching analyses, the reader should consult Reed (2009). Moreover, if one is interested in obtaining area-under-the-curve estimates for discounting plots, Excel® can easily be programmed to compute this metric using the trapezoidal rule (a simple Web search of the term "trapezoidal rule in Excel" [without quotation marks] will yield a plethora of examples of how to do this). With relatively simple programming, Excel® can aid in many quantitative research pursuits. Such programming requires extensive knowledge of Excel® functions and codes, as well as an intimate understanding of the quantitative models relevant to the research question. However, with other software packages available that require little to no additional programming for quantitative models, the serious researcher might invest in products such as IBM SPSS Statistics Base® (http://www-01.ibm.com/software/analytics/spss/products/statistics/base/), SigmaPlot® (http://www.sigmaplot.com), and/or GraphPad Prism® (http://www.graphpad.com/prism/prism.htm). These advanced programs are much more user friendly concerning nonlinear regression models, as well as selecting appropriate statistical tests. Moreover, these products generate professional-quality graphs and data displays, which require much less postanalysis editing than Excel.

## Summary

In many ways, the current state of the behavior analytic approach to the quantitative analysis of sport is akin to that of the sabermetrician's in the mid-1960s when Cook first published *Percentage Baseball* (1964). That is, similar to Cook's analyses published in 1964, behavior analysts have translated quantitative analyses to sport, and have happened upon interesting findings. Moreover, much like early sabermetrics, behavior analysis has yet to apply these findings to promote meaningful improvements in sport performance. As further refinement of sabermetrics enhances sport, more athletes and coaches will begin to take notice of and adopt these analyses into everyday practice.

Through volumes such as this book, coaches and athletes may begin to understand the value of behavior analysis in sport. Recognition of both the analytical approach and the utility of behavioral principles by coaches and athletes may be guided by the practice of behavioral researchers. For instance, a common complaint regarding behavioral studies is the extensive use of jargon. As Lindsley proposes (1991), behavioral researchers – in the present case, those interested in sport – should write to the lay public to better translate their wares to the needs of their athletic consumers. Another way to broaden the impact of quantitative analyses on actual coaches and athletes is to present findings from such quantitative analyses at sports conferences or through submission to sports psychology journals. Far too often, laboratory-based quantitative analyses are marketed to *researchers*, not consumers likely to benefit from understanding these findings. Finally, it is important for quantitative researchers to acknowledge that when their studies are reported, it would benefit the consumer to hear the researchers' thoughts about how these analyses may be applied in the "real world" of sport psychology. And also, researchers should offer direct suggestions for how to test these models in either simulated or actual sporting events.

## References

Alamar, B. (2005). A first step. *Journal of quantitative analysis in sports, 1*, 1–3.
Alferink, L. A., Critchfield, T. S., Hitt, J. L., & Higgins, W. J. (2009). Generality of the matching law as a descriptor of shot selection in basketball. *Journal of Applied Behavior Analysis, 42*, 595–608.

Baer, D. M., Wolf, M. M., & Risley, T. R. (1968). Some current dimensions of applied behavior analysis. *Journal of Applied Behavior Analysis, 1*, 91–97.

Baum, W. M. (1974). On two types of deviation from the matching law: Bias and undermatching. *Journal of the Experimental Analysis of Behavior, 22*, 231–242.

Baxamusa, S. (2010, March 11). State of sabermetrics: Insights from the 2010 Sloan Sports Analytics Conference. *The Hardball Times*. Retrieved from http://www.hardballtimes.com/

Billington, E., & DiTommaso, N. M. (2003). Demonstrations and applications of the matching law in education. *Journal of Behavioral Education, 12*, 91–104.

Borrero, J. C., Crisolo, S. S., Tu, Q., Rieland, W. A., Ross, N. A., Francisco, M. T., et al. (2007). An application of the matching law to social dynamics. *Journal of Applied Behavior Analysis, 40*, 589–601.

Bradbury, J. C. (2007). *The baseball economist: The real game exposed*. New York: Plume.

Bulow, P. J., & Meller, P. J. (1998). Predicting teenage girls' sexual activity and contraception use: An application of the matching law. *Journal of Community Psychology, 26*, 581–596.

Campos, P., & Chait, J. (2004, December 12). Sabermetrics for football. *The New York Times Magazine*. Retrieved from http://www.nytimes.com

Conger, R., & Killeen, P. (1974). Use of concurrent operants in small group research: A demonstration. *Pacific Sociological Review, 17*, 399–416.

Cook, E. (1964). *Percentage baseball*. Cambridge, MA: MIT Press.

Davison, M., & McCarthy, D. (1988). *The matching law: A research review*. Hillsdale, NJ: Erlbaum.

Deford, F. (1964, March 23). Baseball is played all wrong. *Sports Illustrated, 20*(12), 14–17.

D'Angelo, T. (2006, June 8). Cuban a unique NBA owner. *The Palm Beach Post*. Retrieved from http://www.palmbeachpost.com.

Easterbrook, G. (2007, November 15). New annual feature! State of high school nation [Internet posting]. Retrieved from http://www.espn.com.

Grabiner, D. (n.d.). *The sabermetric manifesto*. Retrieved from http://www.baseball1.com/bb-data/grabiner/manifesto.html

Heller, O. (2010, January 20). Sabermetrics and new statistics in baseball: Moneyball, Billy Beane and using statistical analysis to find talent [Web log post]. Retrieved from fttp://baseball.suite101.com/article.cfm/sabermetrics

Herrnstein, R. J. (1961). Relative and absolute strength of response as a function of frequency of reinforcement. *Journal of the Experimental Analysis of Behavior, 4*, 267–272.

Herrnstein, R. J., Rachlin, R., & Laibson, D. I. (1996). *The matching law: Papers in psychology and economics*. New York: Russell Sage Foundation.

Hitt, J. L., Alferink, L. A., Critchfield, T. S., & Wagman, J. B. (2007). Choice behavior expressed in elite sport competition: Predicting shot selection and game outcomes in college basketball. In L. A. Chiang (Ed.), *Motivation of exercise and physical activity* (pp. 79–91). Hauppauge, NY: Nova Science.

Hruby, P. (2004, April 13). Numbers game. *The Washington Times*. Retrieved from http://www.washingtontimes.com.

Hull, C. L. (1943). *Principles of behavior: An introduction to behavior theory*. Oxford: Appleton-Century.

Hursh, S. R., Raslear, T. G., Shurtleff, D., Bauman, R., & Simmons, L. (1988). A cost-benefit analysis of demand for food. *Journal of the Experimental Analysis of Behavior, 50*, 419–440.

Lewis, M. (2003). *Moneyball: The art of winning an unfair game*. New York: W. W. Norton & Company, Inc.

Lindsley, O. R. (1991). From technological jargon to plain English for application. *Journal of Applied Behavior Analysis, 24*, 449–458.

Mace, F. C., Lalli, J. S., Shea, M. C., & Nevin, J. A. (1992). Behavioral momentum in college basketball. *Journal of Applied Behavior Analysis, 25*, 657–663.

Madden, G. J., & Bickel, W. K. (Eds.) (2010). *Impulsivity: The behavioral and neurological science of discounting*. Washington, DC: American Psychological Association.

Madden, G. J., & Johnson, P. S. (2010). A delay-discounting primer. In G. J. Madden & W. K. Bickel (Eds.), *Impulsivity: The behavioral and neurological science of discounting* (pp. 11–37). Washington, DC: American Psychological Association.

Marr, M. J. (1989). Some remarks on the quantitative analysis of behavior. *The Behavior Analyst, 12*, 143–151.

Mazur, J. E. (2006). Mathematical models and the experimental analysis of behavior. *Journal of the Experimental Analysis of Behavior, 85*, 275–291.

McDowell, J. J. (1988). Matching theory in natural human environments. *The Behavior Analyst, 11*, 95–109.

Myerson, J., & Green, L. (1995). Discounting of delayed rewards: Models of individual choice. *Journal of the Experimental Analysis of Behavior, 64*, 263–276.

Myerson, J., Green, L., & Warusawitharana, M. (2001). Area under the curve as a measure of discounting. *Journal of the Experimental Analysis of Behavior, 76*, 235–243.

Nevin, J. A. (1988). Behavioral momentum and the partial reinforcement effect. *Psychological Bulletin, 103*, 44–56.

Nevin, J. A. (2008). Control, prediction, order, and the joys of research. *Journal of the Experimental Analysis of Behavior, 89*, 119–123.

Neyer, R. (2002, November 6). Sabermetricians slowly being added to the inner circle. [Internet posting]. Retrieved from http://www.espn.com.

Reed, D. D. (2009). Using Microsoft Office Excel® 2007 to conduct generalized matching analyses. *Journal of Applied Behavior Analysis, 42*, 867–875.

Reed, D. D., Critchfield, T. S., & Martens, B. K. (2006). The generalized matching law in elite sport competition: Football play calling as operant choice. *Journal of Applied Behavior Analysis, 39*, 281–297.

Reed, D. D., & Martens, B. K. (2008). Effects of task difficulty on children's relative problem completion rates according to the generalized matching law. *Journal of Applied Behavior Analysis, 41*, 39–52.

Roane, H. S., Kelley, M. E., Trosclair, N. M., & Hauer, L. S. (2004). Behavioral momentum in sports: A partial replication with women's basketball. *Journal of Applied Behavior Analysis, 37*, 385–390.

Romanowich, P., Bourret, J., & Vollmer, T. R. (2007). Further analysis of the matching law to describe two- and three-point shot selection by professional basketball players. *Journal of Applied Behavior Analysis, 40*, 311–315.

Schwarz, A. (2005). *The numbers game: Baseball's lifelong fascination with statistics*. New York: Thomas Dunne Books.

Shull, R. L. (1991). Mathematical description of operant behavior: An introduction. In I. H. Iversen & K. A. Lattal (Eds.), *Experimental analysis of behavior, Part 2* (pp. 243–282). Amsterdam: Elsevier.

Skinner, B. F. (1953). *Science and human behavior*. New York: Macmillan.

Stilling, S. T., & Critchfield, T. S. (2010). The matching relation and situation specific bias modulation in professional football play selection. *Journal of the Experimental Analysis of Behavior, 93*, 435–452.

Van Houten, R., Axelrod, S., Bailey, J. S., Favell, J. E., Foxx, R. M., Iwata, B. A., et al. (1988). The right to effective behavioral treatment. *Journal of Applied Behavior Analysis, 21*, 381–384.

Vollmer, T. R., & Bourret, J. (2000). An application of the matching law to evaluate the allocation of two- and three-point shots by college basketball players. *Journal of Applied Behavior Analysis, 33*, 137–150.

Winston, W. L. (2009). *Mathletics: How gamblers, managers, and sports enthusiasts use mathematics in baseball, basketball, and football*. Princeton, NJ: Princeton University Press.

# Chapter 4
# Single-Case Evaluation of Behavioral Coaching Interventions

James K. Luiselli

Behavioral coaching involves intervening with athletes to improve their skills and competitive success. As presented in this book, intervention procedures are most effective when they are evidence based and empirically supported. Whatever the coaching venue, behavioral sport psychology professionals such as clinicians and consultants should be responsible for not only implementing the most potentially effective procedures but also carefully evaluating the effects of those procedures.

This chapter concerns the application of single-case evaluation designs within behavioral coaching. Specifically, my intent is to show how behavioral sport psychology professionals can incorporate single-case methodology for assessing the impact of instructional and training interventions on athletic performance. The chapter briefly considers principles of single-case evaluation designs and then describes four designs that have practical application within behavioral coaching. I also review research studies that illustrate design adaptations within several sports.

Single-case evaluation designs are sometimes referred to as *single-case research designs* and $N = 1$ research, but neither label is precise. For example, although single-case designs have a rich tradition in clinical and applied research (Kazdin, 2011), they have utility beyond a formal research investigation. As indicated, the premise of this chapter is that behavioral sport psychology professionals should incorporate single-case methodology to evaluate their coaching and training recommendations. Note, too, that "single-case" does not mean that only one person is evaluated at a time or that groups of individuals are excluded. In actuality, single-case research designs can examine an intervention across several people and have included large groups. Accordingly, for this chapter I chose the term single-case evaluation designs (a) to highlight the emphasis on person-specific performance and (b) to avoid the perception that the designs are used solely for research.

Before describing basic principles of single-case evaluation designs, it is instructive to contrast them with more traditional group, or "large N," methods. Typically, group research recruits multiple participants (subjects) from either normative or

J.K. Luiselli (✉)
May Institute, Randolph, MA 023681, USA
e-mail: jluiselli@mayinstitute.org

clinical samples, or the population at large. Participants are matched on inclusion criteria and then assigned to control and treatment groups. Most often, the dependent variables in group research are measures acquired from standardized tests and rating instruments. These data are averaged per group, and treatment efficacy and effectiveness are determined by between-group statistical analyses (e.g., chi-square, t-tests, ANOVA).

With single-case evaluation designs, each person serves as her/his control. The effects of a treatment or intervention are ascertained by repeatedly measuring one or more relevant behaviors. Measurement is usually conducted through direct observation in real time or from video recordings. Visual inspection of measurement data determines whether a person's behavior changes in response to the presence or absence of intervention.

Keeping with the practitioner focus of this chapter, single-case evaluation designs enable a behavioral sport psychology professional to target performance-specific measures vital to the success of an individual athlete. In essence, these measures are the skills needed for peak performance during practice and competitive events. Stated succinctly by Freeman and Lim (2010), single-case methodology is "an idiographic approach for describing, examining, and comparing the performance of an individual against his or her own performance at different points in time or in different settings" (p. 397).

## Principles and Operations

Although this chapter is not an exhaustive and detailed presentation of single-case evaluation designs, it is, nevertheless, important to grasp basic operational logic and underlying principles. Readers seeking more in-depth coverage of single-case methodology should consult exemplary texts by Kazdin (2011) and Barlow, Nock, and Hersen (2008).

*Measurement.* Direct measurement of critical behaviors is at the heart of single-case evaluation designs. In the realm of sport psychology, athletic performance represents desirable behaviors that should occur frequently and undesirable behaviors that should occur infrequently or not at all. To illustrate, the measure of improved free-throw shooting by a basketball player would be percentage of successful shots. A behavior-reduction measure would be fewer penalties incurred by an ice hockey team. Importantly, performance measures must be defined in behavior-specific terms so that they can be recorded accurately and are not influenced by observer bias.

Many single-case evaluations rely on *event recording*, either behavior frequency or rate. Frequency data are obtained by counting the number of times a behavior occurs; dividing the frequency count by some unit of time yields a rate measure. Other measurement methods are *duration*, the length of time that behavior is exhibited, and *interval recording*, documenting whether behavior did or did not occur during a specific period of time. There are many considerations when selecting a measurement method, including, but not limited to, the physical characteristics (topography) of behavior, the performance setting, and the expected outcome from intervention. A comprehensive review of behavioral assessment and measurement specific to sport psychology can be found in Tkachuk, Leslie-Toogood, and Martin (2003). Readers interested in more information about behavioral measurement theory and general application should consult Cooper, Heron, and Heward (2007) and Martin and Pear (2011).

*Baseline evaluation.* All single-case evaluation designs begin with a baseline phase. One purpose of conducting baseline measurement is to document a person's behavior in the absence of intervention. Furthermore, the data recorded at baseline provide a standard by which intervention effectiveness can be judged. Some single-case evaluation designs as described subsequently, include not only an initial baseline phase but also one or more replications of baseline conditions.

The length of a baseline phase depends on the trend and stability of the behaviors being recorded. The top graph in Fig. 4.1 shows a stable trend across five hypothetical baseline data points. These results would mean that it is reasonable to introduce intervention because a positive or negative effect from it could be isolated (i.e., behaviors during intervention improve or worsen relative to the steady-state responding in baseline). Conversely, the second and third graphs shown in Fig. 4.1 illustrate unstable trends at baseline. In the second graph, the hypothetical data represent a behavior to be *increased* with intervention. The five data points labeled "decreasing trend" would justify intervention because the person's performance is worsening overtime. The five data points labeled "increasing trend" argue against intervention because the person's performance is improving. The same concerns about baseline trends also apply to the third graph. Here, the behavior to be *reduced* is increasing and intervention would be needed. When an undesirable behavior is decreasing during baseline, intervention should be delayed.

*Intervention.* The type of trend analysis through visual inspection of graphed data in a baseline phase also extends to intervention. Behaviors selected for intervention also must change in a desirable direction, with minimal variability, and at a level that is clinically significant. One of the standard guidelines when conducting a single-case evaluation design is to change only one independent variable at a time per intervention phase. This convention enables the evaluator to isolate the controlling influence of single procedures. Of course, there are many situations in which intervention is comprised of more than one procedure. In such cases, it is acceptable to evaluate the intervention relative to baseline and, if warranted, strategically withdraw and reintroduce procedures to determine which ones are required.

*Internal and external validity.* Kazdin (2011) has written extensively about internal and external validity in the context of single-case evaluation designs. Briefly, *internal validity* refers to changes in behavior that can be attributed to the independent variable and not extraneous (uncontrolled) influences or alternative explanations. Major threats to internal validity include maturation, history, and features of the measurement methods. *External validity* refers to the extent that the results of a single-case evaluation can be generalized to other people and conditions. Some of the major threats to external validity are person-specific attributes, the

**Fig. 4.1** Examples of behavior trends during baseline measurement

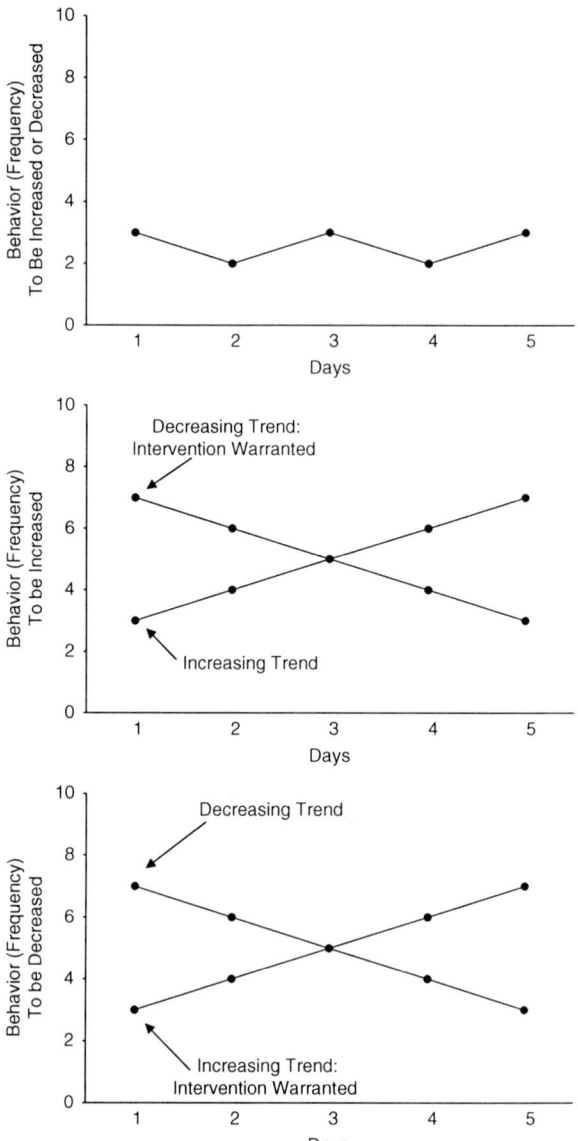

situations that constituted the evaluation, and reactivity to measurement. For behavioral sport psychology professionals, internal and external validity have practical significance, most notably (a) the ability to judge confidently that a coaching intervention improved an athlete's performance (internal validity) and (b) that the coaching intervention should be recommended for other athletes in the same sport (external validity).

## Description of Single-Case Evaluation Designs

In this section I describe four single-case evaluation designs, how they are implemented, and methodological variations that are sometimes indicated. Where applicable, I highlight behavioral sport psychology research examples of each design.

### A-B-A-B Design

The A-B-A-B design, sometimes called a *reversal* design, begins with a baseline (A) phase. During baseline, intervention is not in effect. Once baseline data are stable, intervention (B) is introduced, followed by a second baseline (A) phase and then a second intervention (B) phase. This systematic alteration of phases is intended to show that a person's performance improves with intervention and is less proficient when intervention is not implemented.

Figure 4.2 plots hypothetical data in an A-B-A-B design. For the purpose of illustration, imagine that the performance measure is the number of steps in a 10-step skill sequence that an athlete executes accurately. These data demonstrate that intervention effectively increased the number of accurate steps relative to the baseline phases. Because the desired effect was replicated convincingly, the results would predict future levels of performance if intervention was maintained.

Sometimes an A-B-A-B design verifies a modest change in behavior and the need for additional intervention. Figure 4.3 shows an A-B-A-B evaluation where a second intervention procedure, "C," was added to "B." When this combined intervention boosted performance, it was removed briefly during a reversal-to-baseline

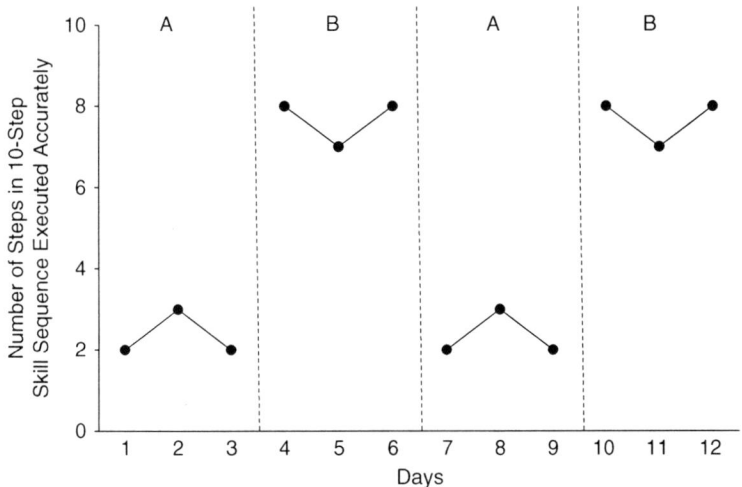

**Fig. 4.2** Example of the A-B-A-B single-case evaluation design

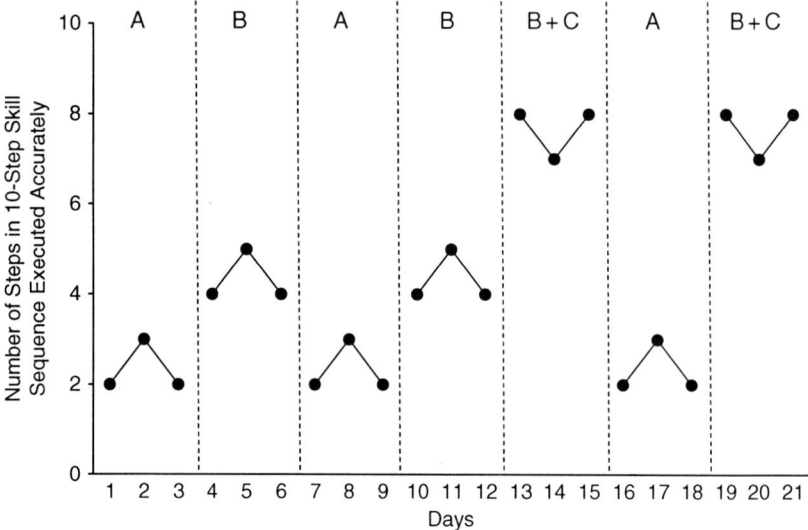

**Fig. 4.3** Example of the A-B-A-B-B+C-A-B+C single-case evaluation design

(A) phase in which the athlete performed less accurately. The "B+C" intervention was implemented again with good success. So conducted, this sequence would be labeled an A-B-A-B-B+C-A-B+C design.

The logic of the A-B-A-B design can also be applied for evaluating questions about the intensity of intervention. Referencing Fig. 4.4, the hypothetical data

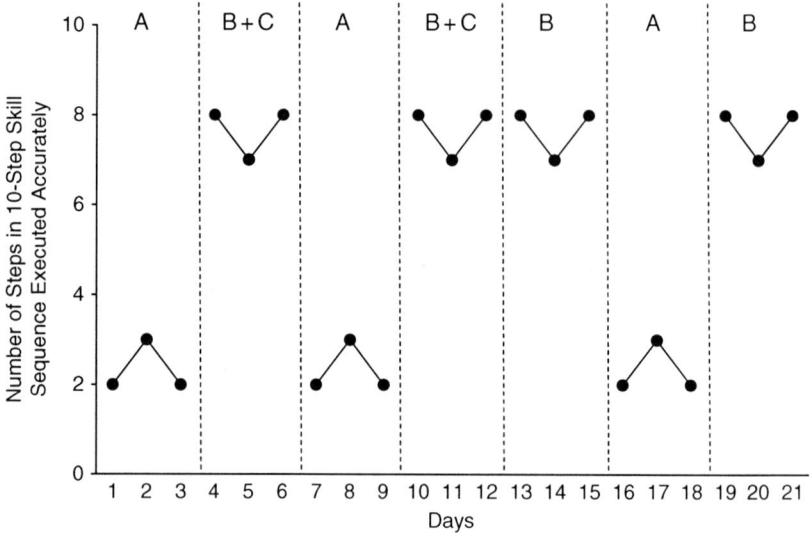

**Fig. 4.4** Example of the A-B+C-A-B+C-B-A-B single-case evaluation design

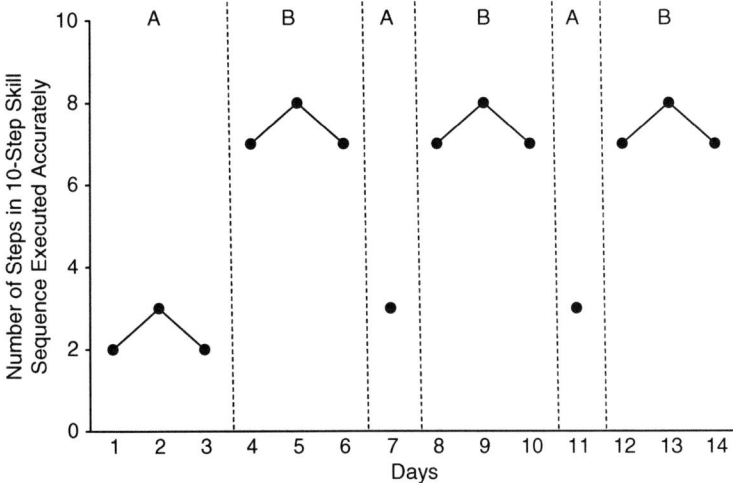

**Fig. 4.5** Example of one-day reversal "probes" within the A-B-A-B single-case evaluation design

are plotted in an A-B+C-A-B+C-B-A-B design. The "B+C" intervention clearly improved performance. Whether both "B" and "C" procedures of intervention were required was addressed by withdrawing "C," reversing to baseline (A), and reinstating "C." The interpretation of these data would be that the "B" procedure alone was as effective as implementing it with "C."

Finally, one-day reversal "probes," depicted in Fig. 4.5, are an A-B-A-B design variant for practical application. With this design, the reversal-to-baseline phases last a single day, inserted between more lengthy intervention phases. Although a solitary, one-day reversal effect by itself is not convincing, demonstrating the effect several times is a quick way to make confident recommendations about an intervention.

*Research examples.* Allison and Ayllon (1980) used A-B-A-B designs to study a behavioral coaching intervention with athletes (ages 11–35 years) participating in football, gymnastics, and tennis. The performance measures were blocking (football), backward walkovers, front hand-springs, reverse hips (gymnastics), and forehand, backhand, and service strokes (tennis). During baseline phases for each sport, the respective coaches carried out their usual procedures with the athletes. The behavioral coaching intervention was comprised of systematic verbal instructions, performance feedback, positive and negative reinforcement, modeling, and imitation. Compared to the baseline phases, all of the athletes had a higher percentage of skill execution when the coaches implemented the behavioral protocols. Keep in mind that as conducted, the A-B-A-B design in Allison and Ayllon (1980) could not isolate the controlling effects from the different procedures comprising the superior behavioral coaching intervention.

As noted previously, the prototype A-B-A-B design has many variations. In a study with three wide receivers (ages not specified) on a Division II college football team, Smith and Ward (2006) evaluated several coaching procedures in what would be described as an A-B-A-C-A-B+C design. The performance measures were the percentage of blocks, pass routes, and releases from the line of scrimmage, each wide receiver executed correctly during practices and games. In baseline (A), the coach reviewed expectations with the players, gave them verbal feedback, and corrected errors. The three intervention phases were public posting of performance (B), goal setting (C), and public posting of performance with goal setting (B+C). The three coaching interventions were equally effective with the players and better than baseline. Note, however, that although the baseline phase in the study was replicated twice, the three coaching interventions were not repeated beyond a single application.

*Summary.* The A-B-A-B design and its options are adaptable to many behavioral coaching contexts. Yet the design has two constraints. One limiting factor is having to temporarily withdraw a seemingly effective intervention. That is, if a performance deficit is revealed during an initial baseline evaluation and subsequent intervention is implemented with positive result, is it reasonable (some would argue ethical) to stop the intervention in a reversal-to-baseline phase? Remember that the baseline reversal phase does not need to be lengthy when conducting an A-B-A-B single-case evaluation design. Nevertheless, selecting this design must be tempered by the possible negative outcome of briefly terminating an intervention on both an athlete's performance and his/her attitude.

The second concern about the A-B-A-B design is that some behaviors are not "reversible." Think of a baseball pitcher who has been taught a cognitive control strategy that helps him prepare to face batters and throw more strikes. It is unlikely that the pitcher would abandon the strategy when he is told to do so during a reversal-to-baseline phase. Another reason that a behavior may not reverse is that with intervention, the behavior possibly contacts other reinforcing consequences. For example, visual markers such as colorful tape sometimes are applied to the sticks of beginning hockey players to teach them proper hand position. After learning to pass and shoot the puck more accurately through many hours of practice, we should not expect players to perform less fluently when the markers are removed. In effect, their skills are no longer dependent on the intervention–as such, withdrawing it would not be associated with lesser performance.

## *Multiple Baseline Design*

The multiple baseline design (MBD) comes in three forms. In a *MBD across behaviors*, two or more performance measures are targeted for one person. With a *MBD across settings*, a performance measure is recorded for one person in two or more locations. The third MBD format, the *MBD across individuals*, focuses on the same or similar performance measures in two or more people.

Figures 4.6, 4.7, and 4.8 show hypothetical data for the three MBDs. Each figure has two panels, the minimal number required to demonstrate an intervention effect. Figure 4.6 is a MBD across behaviors, showing an athlete's execution of

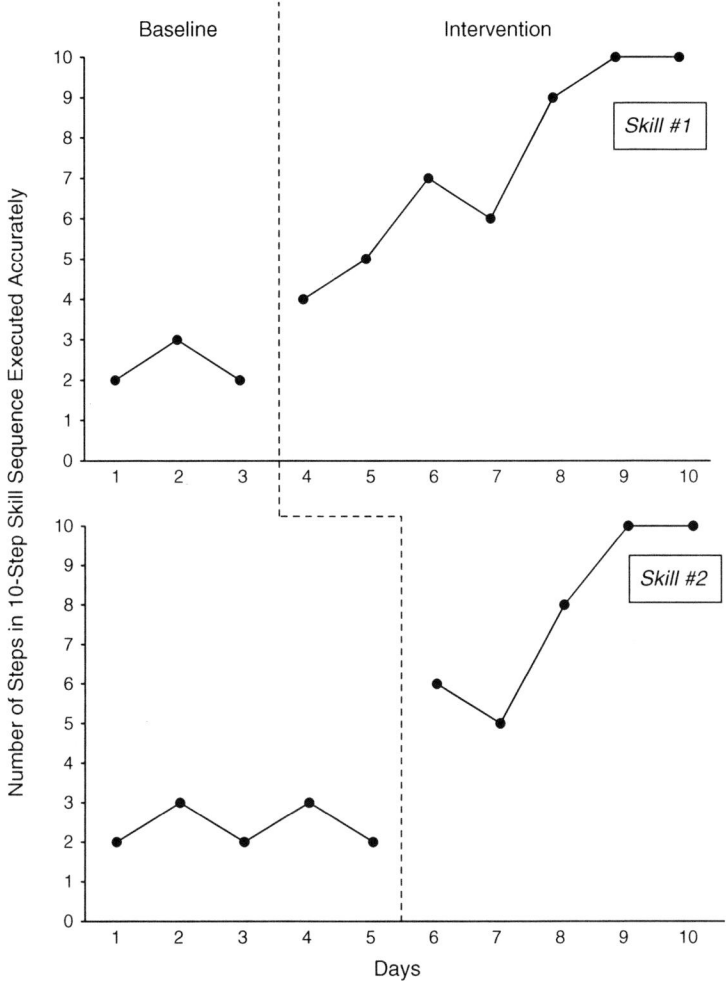

**Fig. 4.6** Example of the multiple baseline across behaviors single-case evaluation design

two, 10-step skill sequences. Figure 4.7, a MBD across settings, is the skill sequence performance of one athlete during practice sessions and games. In Fig. 4.8, the performance measure is plotted for two athletes. Each of these MBDs is intended to demonstrate desirable changes in baseline performance following the sequential introduction of intervention. That is, the designs simultaneously monitor multiple performance measures under baseline conditions so that the effect of intervention can be confirmed each time it is applied to them.

*Research examples.* The MBD across individuals has been the most popular MBD in behavioral sport psychology research. Ziegler (1987) conducted a study with 24 beginning tennis players (19–31 years old), establishing three groups, each comprised of eight participants. The performance measures were executing

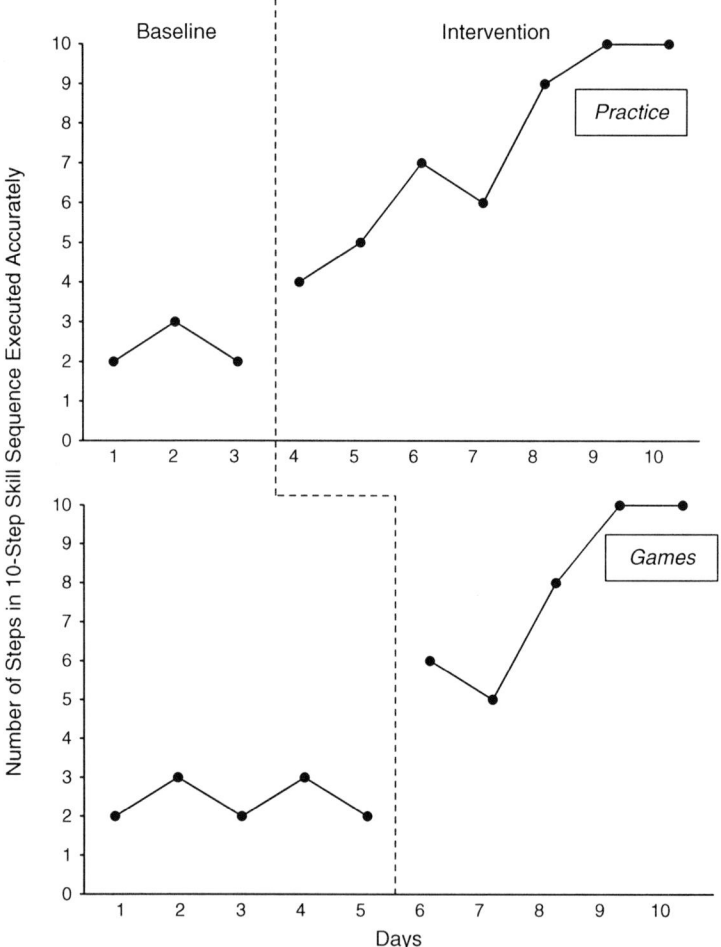

**Fig. 4.7** Example of the multiple baseline across settings single-case evaluation design

forehand and backhand return strokes during weekly lessons. Intervention consisted of a stimulus cueing technique: having the players focus on and quietly vocalize "ball tracking" responses for each stroke. The intervention was evaluated by introducing it sequentially across the three groups of players. Of note, the study by Ziegler (1987) is a good example of adapting single-case evaluation designs, in this case an MBD, to groups of athletes and not just one person.

Another example of the MBD across individuals is a study by Kladopoulos and McComas (2001). Three players (ages 19–20 years) on a women's NCAA Division II basketball team participated in the study. The intervention, termed "form training," was intended to increase the percentage of successful foul shots and the percentage of foul shots taken with correct form. Following customary baseline

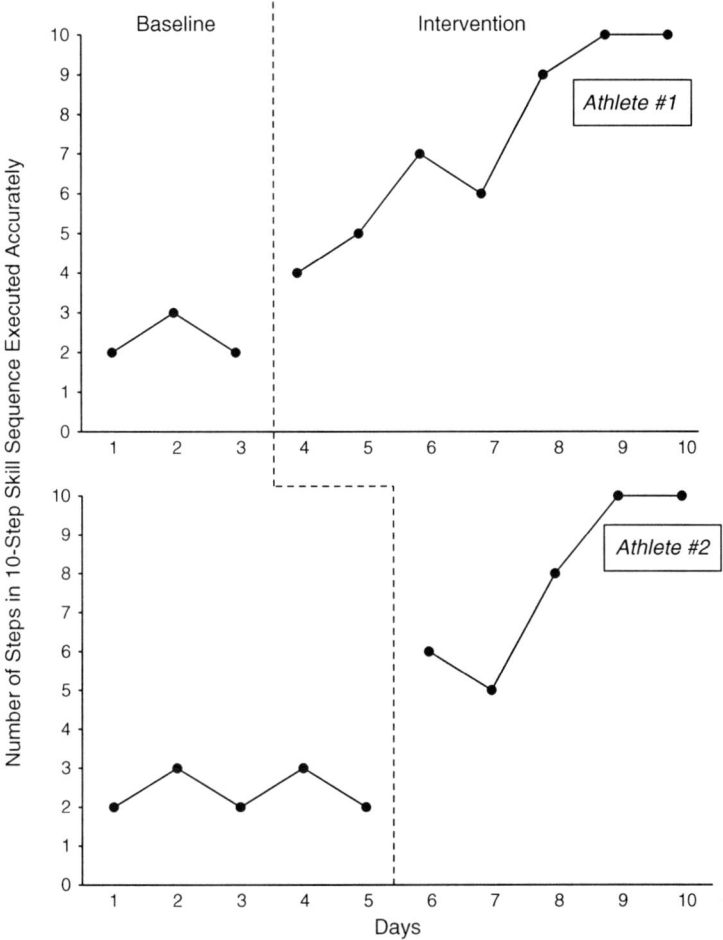

**Fig. 4.8** Example of the multiple baseline across individuals single-case evaluation design

measurement, intervention comprised of pre-practice review, social reinforcement (praise), and performance feedback was implemented successfully with each player. This MBD illustrates another design option in that two performance measures, foul shooting success and form, were recorded within baseline and intervention phases. Be aware that the capacity to collect data on more than one performance measure is not exclusive to MBDs but is a feature of all of the single-case evaluation designs described in this chapter.

Finally, Stokes, Luiselli, Reed, and Fleming (2010) designed a study that evaluated three behavioral coaching interventions within a MBD across individuals. The participants were five offensive linemen (ages 15–17 years) on a varsity high school football team. The offensive line coach recorded the percentage of steps the players executed correctly according to a 10-step, task analyzed blocking sequence.

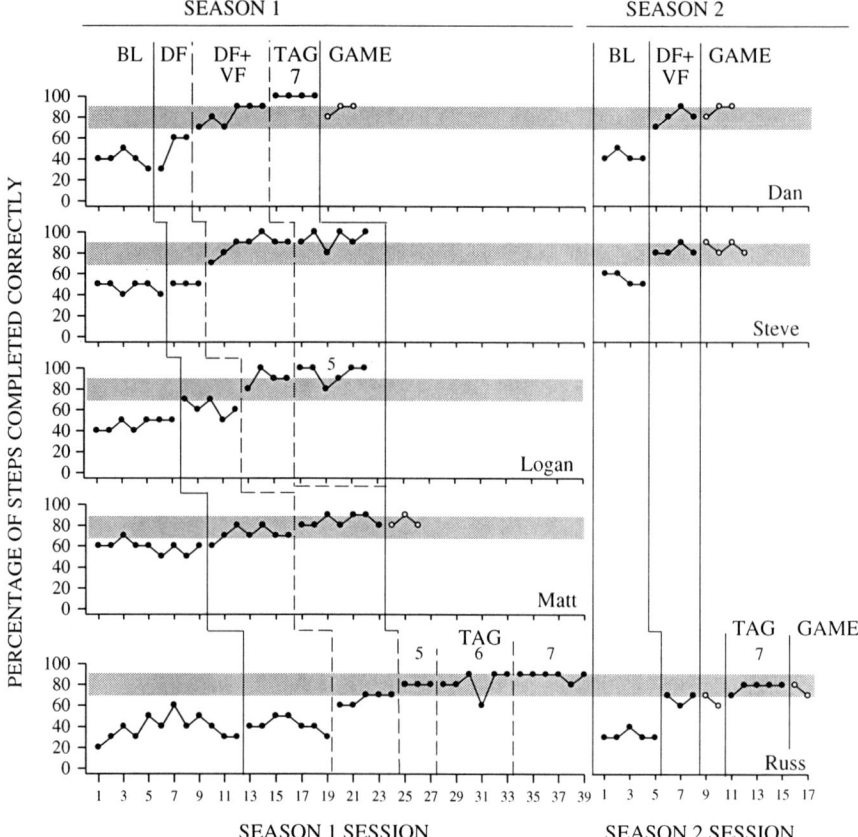

**Fig. 4.9** Evaluation of three coaching interventions in a multiple baseline design across individuals. The shaded horizontal lines represent the normative pass blocking performance of starting varsity linemen. From Stokes et al. (2010)

Figure 4.9 shows that the different interventions were implemented in staggered fashion with each player: (a) descriptive (nonverbal) feedback (DF), (b) descriptive and verbal feedback (DF + VF), and (c) teaching with acoustical guidance (TAG). The results revealed that the players responded similarly to the intervention procedures, that in-game performance improved following intervention, and that the intervention procedures had to be reinstated to support performance during a second season.

The MBD across behaviors has also been represented in behavioral sport psychology research. Brobst and Ward (2002) evaluated a combined intervention of public posting, goal setting, and verbal feedback with three high school soccer players (ages 15–17 years). The same performance measures were selected for each player: (a) keeping and maintaining ball possession, (b) moving to an open position during a game restart, and (c) moving to an open position after passing the ball. For each player, the multi-procedural intervention was implemented sequentially with each of the performance measures. Another example of the MBD across behaviors is a study by Boyer, Miltenberger, Batsche, and Fogel (2009) on the effects of video modeling and video feedback with four competitive youth gymnasts (ages 7–10 years). The intervention was implemented first for performing a backward giant circle to hand stand, then a kip cast, and then a clear hip circle (all uneven bar maneuvers). The controlling effects of intervention were demonstrated when each performance measure improved in response to intervention. Finally, Harding, Wacker, Berg, Rick, and Lee (2004) conducted a MBD across behaviors with two adults (ages 33 and 40 years) participating in martial arts training. The objective of intervention was to improve their punching and kicking techniques during drill and sparring sessions. Differential reinforcement of technique execution was implemented first for punching, followed by kicking, and was effective with both adults.

*Summary.* Compared to the A-B-A-B single-case evaluation design, the MBD does not require a reversal-to-baseline phase in order to verify intervention-induced changes in behavior. Another advantage of the MBD is that it enables the behavioral sport psychology professional to address "real world" questions about generalization. For example, the MBD across behaviors can answer the question, "Does a coaching intervention implemented for one performance measure extend to measures not selected for intervention?" Similarly, the MBD across settings could discern whether intervention conducted in practice changes performance favorably during competition.

A relative disadvantage of the MBD is that at least two performance measures, be they the same behavior of several people or one person's behavior in more than one setting, may be difficult to arrange in some situations. However, behavioral coaching usually considers more than a single athletic skill. As for team sports, the MBD across individuals would be a reasonable choice for evaluating intervention with several players.

## *Changing Criterion Design*

After the baseline phase, intervention in a changing criterion design is introduced at a predetermined standard (the "criterion"), usually a performance measure that results in positive reinforcement. When the performance measure consistently matches the criterion, thereby showing improvement, the criterion is increased slightly, and so on, until a terminal performance indicator is achieved. The influence of intervention is demonstrated by showing that the performance measure changes desirably with each step-wise increase in the criterion.

Figure 4.10 presents hypothetical data in a changing criterion design. The baseline phase reveals below 30% accurate execution of a 10-step skill sequence. With intervention, the athlete gains access to something desirable when she/he matches or exceeds each advanced criterion three times consecutively (denoted by "C" in the figure). Such results would confirm that the athlete performed better as a function of intervention.

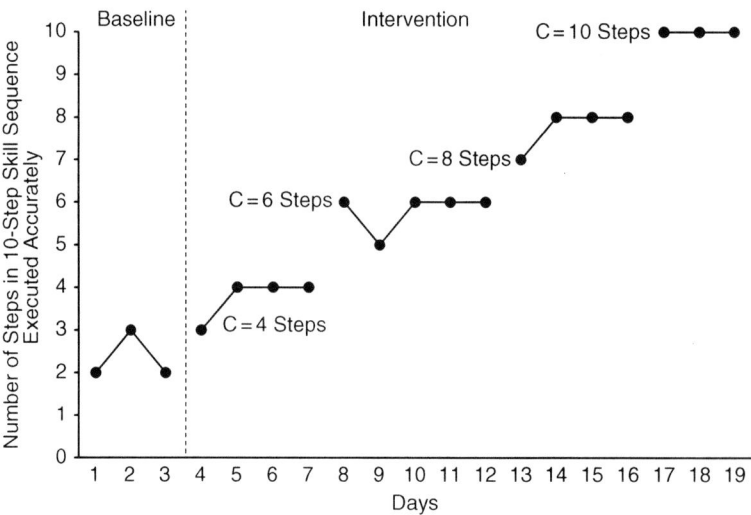

**Fig. 4.10** Example of the changing criterion single-case evaluation design

There are no hard-and-fast rules for adjusting criterion in a changing criterion design. Most behavioral sport psychology professionals would agree that the best approach is to advance criteria in steps small enough to ensure success. This guideline is especially important when many steps make up the skill sequence. An additional stipulation for evaluating a potentially effective intervention is that a criterion should increase following several successful (usually consecutive) performance opportunities at that criterion.

*Research examples.* Fitterling, Martin, Gramling, Cole, and Milan (1988) used a changing criterion design to evaluate a behavioral intervention for aerobic exercise training with five adults (ages 33–56 years) who suffered from vascular headache. Although the participants in this study were not athletes and the focus was not sport psychology, exercise is certainly a performance measure consistent with the theme of this book (see Chapter 8). In Fitterling et al. (1988), the adults were given a personalized exercise program based on their age and activity preferences. The program was based on Cooper (1977) in which "points" are awarded for exercise adherence. Following baseline, the adults set performance goals, starting low, and then increased the goals gradually in criterion steps. Contingent on meeting their goals, the adults earned back portions of a $100 deposit, received positive performance feedback, and were praised. Results indicated that exercise frequency and fitness increased progressively as the intervention "demands," the imposed criteria, became more stringent.

In a changing criterion design study specifically centered on sport psychology, Scott, Scott, and Goldwater (1997) evaluated a prompting and shaping intervention with a 21-year-old university pole vaulter. The performance concern preceding intervention was that on planting his pole, the vaulter did not extend his arms completely prior to take-off. His average hand height during baseline measurement was 2.25 m relative to a maximum arm extension height of 2.54 m. During intervention the desired height started at 2.30 m, the vaulter was prompted to "reach" as he ran down the runway, and an audible tone (a conditioned positive reinforcer) sounded when he broke a photoelectric beam that had been set at the height marker. Contingent on his success, the specified height was increased in 0.5 m steps to a terminal height of 2.52 m. The changing criterion design revealed that the vaulter extended his arms correctly each time the desired height was advanced. As illustrated in the previous research example, the changing criterion design used by Scott et al. (1997) made it possible to measure performance in direct relation to gradual intervention changes.

*Summary.* Like the MBD, intervention evaluation in a changing criterion design does not require a reversal-to-baseline phase. The design is also well suited to the types of coaching interventions designed by behavioral sport psychology professionals. For example, many interventions have the objective of breaking down a performance skill into its composite steps, teaching each step until it is perfected, and tying the steps together so that the athlete performs them fluently (see Chapter 10, this volume). The steps correspond to progressively increasing criteria that are linked to the intervention.

The changing criterion design usually targets positive reinforcement interventions such as "rewarding" an athlete when she/he achieves a performance standard. However, the intervention can be relatively simple as teaching a beginning track and field runner to clear hurdles. In such a case, the intervention could begin by setting the height of the hurdles low to the ground, reinforcing the runner upon clearing each hurdle with proper form, and then making the hurdles higher through gradual height adjustments. Another example would be building physical endurance of athletes in any number of sports by systematically increasing training demands (e.g., more weight training repetitions, running longer distances). Of course, it would be expected that some type of positive reinforcement and feedback would be given to the athletes for meeting the performance objectives. Whatever the intervention, the basis for the changing criterion design is evaluating procedures that incrementally shape skills.

## *Alternating Treatments Design*

The alternating treatments design (ATD) is used principally to compare the behavior-altering effects of two or more interventions. After baseline data are collected, the interventions are introduced at different times in the same day or one time on randomly selected, consecutive days. This comparative evaluation continues until performance differentiates between or among the interventions. Keeping with the examples presented throughout the chapter, Fig. 4.11 is an ATD in which an athlete's accurate execution of a 10-step skill sequence is measured in response to two interventions. Compared to baseline performance, the athlete improved slightly with intervention #1. By contrast, performance was better on days in which intervention #2 was implemented. The third phase of Fig. 4.11, customary when conducting an ATD, verifies the performance-enhancing effect of the most successful intervention.

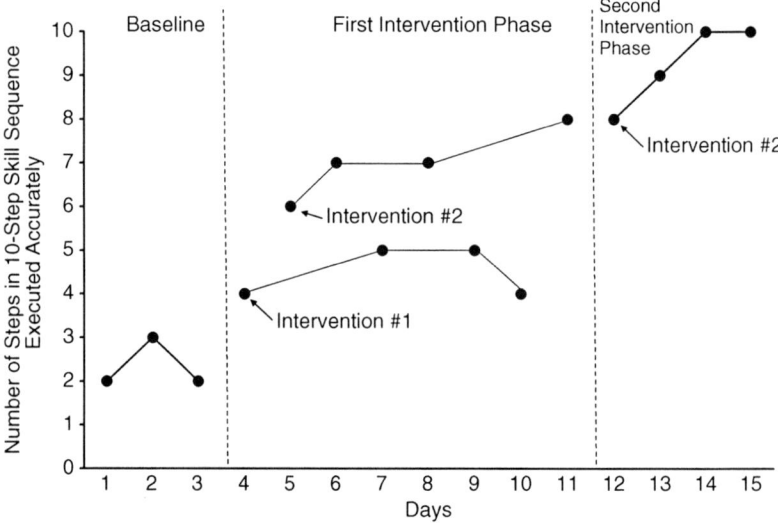

**Fig. 4.11** Example of the alternating treatments single-case evaluation design

One reason the ATD can reasonably compare two or more interventions is that it controls for sequence effects (Barlow & Hayes, 1979). Using an A-B-A-B design, for example, a behavioral sport psychology professional might try to compare two interventions by implementing one intervention during the first "B" phase and the second intervention during the second "B" phase. If an athlete performed more skillfully in the second intervention phase, the result could have occurred because she/he was exposed to an earlier intervention, not necessarily because the second intervention was superior to the first intervention. In an ATD, the influence of intervention sequence is minimized by rapidly and randomly altering conditions.

*Research examples.* Osborne, Rudrud, and Zezoney (1990) studied curveball hitting proficiency of five college baseball players (ages not specified) under baseline and two intervention conditions in an ATD. Before intervention, the players practiced hitting against a pitching machine that was adjusted to simulate a curveball thrown at a standard speed. The interventions consisted of marking the seams of baseballs with either ¼ inch or 1/8 inch orange stripes. Each of these marked-ball conditions was compared to the unmarked-baseball condition during two batting practice sessions each day. The ATD showed that curveball hitting proficiency improved with the marked-ball interventions. This study is a good example of how "treatments" in an ATD can actually be any number of conditions, contexts, or procedures that can be manipulated to compare the one(s) that is/are optimal.

*Summary.* The ATD gives the behavioral sport psychology professional an evaluation tactic that addresses a common coaching objective, namely comparing different methods with individual athletes. The design does not require a reversal-to-baseline phase and, as noted, is the only single-case evaluation design that controls for sequence effects. From a research perspective, there is concern about *multiple treatment interference* – whether the results of intervention in an ATD would be the same if they were the only intervention that was evaluated (Kazdin, 2011). From an applied perspective, the possibility of multiple treatment interference is a minor limitation when considering how rapidly two or more interventions can be evaluated using an ATD.

## Summary and Conclusions

Single-case evaluation designs are useful for measuring the effects of behavioral coaching interventions on athletic performance objectives. This chapter reviewed four designs, the principles of each design, and research examples within behavioral sport psychology. Some professionals may conclude that single-case evaluation designs are not practical and do not translate easily to practice and competitive settings. However, as I have emphasized, single-case evaluation of behavioral coaching interventions are desirable because they (a) concentrate on the individual athlete, (b) include direct measurement of performance, (c) are intended to isolate the most effective procedures, and (d) can be implemented in a relatively brief period of time. Thus, the designs are compatible with best practices in applied sport psychology intervention and consultation (Martin, 2011).

What can behavioral sport psychology professionals do to learn more about single-case evaluation designs? One recommendation is to read noteworthy texts by Kazdin (2011), Barlow et al. (2008), and Cooper et al. (2007). Peer-reviewed journals such as the *Journal of Applied Behavior Analysis, Journal of Clinical Sport Psychology,* and *Journal of Sport Behavior* also feature single-case research publications. Attending annual conferences sponsored by organizations such as the Association for Applied Sport Psychology is another way to gain knowledge. And seeking advice and direction from an experienced colleague can advance one's understanding of single-case design methodologies and their application to the athletic arena.

## References

Allison, M. G., & Ayllon, T. (1980). Behavioral coaching in the development of skills in football, gymnastics, and tennis. *Journal of Applied Behavior Analysis, 13,* 297–314.

Barlow, D. H., & Hayes, S. C. (1979). Alternating treatments design: One strategy for comparing the effects of two treatments in a single subject. *Journal of Applied Behavior Analysis, 12,* 199–210.

Barlow, D. H., Nock, M. K., & Hersen, M. (2008). *Single-case experimental designs: Strategies for studying behavior change* (3rd ed.). Boston: Allyn & Bacon.

Boyer, E., Miltenberger, R. G., Batsche, C., & Fogel, V. (2009). Video modeling by experts with video feedback to enhance gymnastics skills. *Journal of Applied Behavior Analysis, 42,* 855–860.

Brobst, B., & Ward, P. (2002). Effects of public posting, goal setting, and oral feedback on the skills of female soccer players. *Journal of Applied Behavior Analysis, 35,* 247–257.

Cooper, K. H. (1977). *The aerobics way.* New York: Bantam Books.

Cooper, J. O., Heron, T. E., & Heward, W. L. (2007). *Applied behavior analysis* (2nd ed.). Upper Saddle River, NJ: Merrill Prentice Hall.

Fitterling, J. M., Martin, J. E., Gramling, S., Cole, P., & Milan, M. A. (1988). Behavioral management of exercise training in vascular headache patients: An investigation of exercise adherence and headache activity. *Journal of Applied Behavior Analysis, 21*, 9–19.

Freeman, K. A., & Lim, M. (2010). Single subject research. In J. Thomas & M. Hersen (Eds.), *Handbook of clinical psychology competencies* (pp. 397–423). New York: Springer.

Harding, J. W., Wacker, D. P., Berg, W. K., Rick, G., & Lee, J. F. (2004). Promoting response variability and stimulus generalization in martial arts training. *Journal of Applied Behavior Analysis, 37*, 185–195.

Kazdin, A. E. (2011). *Single-case research designs: Methods for clinical and applied settings* (2nd ed.). New York: Oxford University Press.

Kladopoulos, C. N., & McComas, J. J. (2001). The effects of form training on foul-shooting performance in members of a women's college basketball team. *Journal of Applied Behavior Analysis, 34*, 329–332.

Martin, G. L. (2011). *Applied sport psychology: Practical guidelines from behavior analysis* (4th ed.). Winnipeg, MB: Sport Science Press.

Martin, G. L., & Pear, J. J. (2011). *Behavior modification: What it is and how to do it* (9th ed.). Upper Saddle River, NJ: Pearson-Prentice Hall.

Osborne, K., Rudrud, E., & Zezoney, F. (1990). Improved curveball hitting through the enhancement of visual cues. *Journal of Applied Behavior Analysis, 23*, 371–377.

Scott, D., Scott, L. M., & Goldwater, B. (1997). A performance improvement program for an international-level track and field athlete. *Journal of Applied Behavior Analysis, 30*, 573–575.

Smith, S.L., & Ward, P. (2006). Behavioral interventions to improve performance in collegiate football. *Journal of Applied Behavior Analysis, 39*, 385–391.

Stokes, J. V., Luiselli, J. K., Reed, D. D., & Fleming, R. K. (2010). Behavioral coaching to improve offensive line pass blocking skills of high school football athletes. *Journal of Applied Behavior Analysis, 43*, 463–472.

Tkachuk, G., Leslie-Toogood, A., & Martin, G. L. (2003). Behavioral assessment in sport psychology. *The Sport Psychologist, 17*, 104–117.

Ziegler, S. G. (1987). Effects of stimulus cueing on the acquisition of ground strokes by beginning tennis players. *Journal of Applied Behavior Analysis, 20*, 405–411.

# Chapter 5
# Cognitive Assessment in Behavioral Sport Psychology

Bradley Donohue, Yani L. Dickens, and Philip D. Del Vecchio III

The contribution of thoughts, emotions, and images to athletic training and competition has long been acknowledged. As Yogi Berra once said about baseball, "90% of this game is half mental" (Baseball Almanac, 2010). Less understood is the manner by which these processes can be formally assessed to guide optimum implementation of evidence-based behavioral intervention. Indeed, as emphasized throughout this book, evidence-based interventions are becoming increasingly utilized by sport psychologists. However, there is often a poor fit between cognitive assessment strategies and performance-enhancing behavioral interventions (Meyers, Whelan, & Murphy, 1996). It is important that students and professionals practicing within the field of sport psychology are familiar with the psychometric support and conceptual basis underlying cognitive assessment methods. Indeed, one of the challenges for professionals who work with athletes and performers is to develop an efficient and evidence-supported method for assessing cognitive constructs that have been historically difficult to fully understand. This chapter, therefore, provides a practical and evidence-based guide that may be used when conducting cognitive assessment in sport psychology consultation. We begin by underscoring commonly used cognitive strategies that have been identified to facilitate optimum sport performance, such as self-talk, imagery, and arousal management. We then review environmental factors that have been found to influence the attitudes and motivational sets of athletes. Lastly, we review our evidence-based approach to cognitive assessment in athletes.

## Common Factors Affecting Cognitive Assessment

### Self-Talk

Almost three decades ago, Albert Ellis (1982) acknowledged the pervasiveness of irrational thinking in sports. He reported that irrational negative thoughts lead to performance difficulties and suggested that thoughts could be restructured to enhance

B. Donohue (✉)
University of Nevada, Las Vegas, NV, USA
e-mail: bradley.donohue@gmail.com

performance. About this time, positive self-talk in sports was thought to improve physiological preparation (Rushall, 1982, 1984), motivation (Kirschenbaum & Bale, 1980; Weinberg, Jackson, & Smith, 1984), and instructional support (Rushall, 1975) in competitive situations. These processes were later demonstrated in outcome studies to enhance performance (e.g., Bunker, Williams, & Zinsser, 1993; Theodorakis, Weinberg, Natsis, Douma, & Kazakas, 2000; Zinnser, Bunker, & Williams, 1998).

When used within the context of sport psychology, self-talk usually refers to thoughts, beliefs, and attributions that are internally reviewed by athletes during practice and competition. Interestingly, however, self-talk contributes to sport performance outside athletic activities, as well. For instance, athletes may talk themselves into attending a late-night party the night before a championship game, or may perform poorly in a game due to self-deprecating thoughts that are influenced by a depressive disorder. Therefore, it is important to assess nonverbal speech in both athletic and non-athletic contexts.

Assessing the specific content of self-talk is important. Indeed, one word can have dire implications to performance in sport exercises (Van Raalte et al., 1995). Along these lines, instructions and ongoing self-assessments are best stated neutrally and without bias (e.g., "I'm running with my hands relaxed and open," "My split times are 2 s slower than usual"), whereas motivationally based thoughts should be positive, uplifting, and self-serving (e.g., "I feel like I can run all day today"). Attributional statements usually occur after sport-related behaviors are performed to assist athletes in understanding performance. We emphasize that the literature on attribution-related thinking patterns is complicated and must be interpreted with caution. As Hardy and colleagues (1996) point out, "precisely what constitutes self-talk" (p. 37) is problematic because "past researchers have been too 'loose' in their operationalization of self-talk" (pp. 37, 38). For example, it may be appropriate for novice athletes with poor self-efficacy to initially attribute poor performance to external factors. Such attributions are likely to protect against problems associated with embarrassment, shame, or threats to self-esteem. However, accurate performance attributions facilitate improvement in sports, particularly as athletes become more experienced (Gordon, 2008).

There is some evidence to suggest athletes should avoid self-statements that indicate they "need" or "should" do certain behaviors, as these thought patterns set up comparisons with others rather than facilitate accurate self-evaluation. Comparisons with others, whether downward (comparison with athletes who demonstrate lower skill) or upward (comparison with athletes who demonstrate higher skill), restrict opportunities to accurately become aware of one's true ability or skill level (Hewitt, 2009). As an alternative, athletes are more likely to do well when they get excited about the competition, preparing themselves with thoughts about opportunities they are looking forward to taking, and to focus on their own motivational and instructional sets (Donohue et al., 2006).

The timing of self-statements is critical for enhancing sport performance. For example, Donohue, Barnhart, Covassin, Carpin, and Corb (2001) found cross-country runners often voiced derogatory and self-defeating statements immediately prior to their competitions (e.g., "what if I fall in the loose sand"), but not during practice or hours before their competitions. When these athletes were provided task-relevant instructions immediately prior to running, however, their performance was enhanced relative to control conditions and equally effective as being told motivational statements. We have also found derogatory self-talk in athletes can manifest itself differently in training and competitive situations (Donohue, Covassin, et al., 2004). Therefore, sport psychologists need to assess self-talk within both of these contexts.

## *Imagery*

Imagery is another cognitive skill set that is often overlooked in the assessment of athletes. Specifically, imagery involves the ability of athletes and performers to imagine themselves in performance-related tasks. Athletes often utilize imagery prior to performance as a preparatory skill. It is common for athletes to watch themselves in a sport activity much like a movie (external imagery), or view themselves in a participatory manner as if they are performing the athletic endeavor in real time (internal imagery; Orlick & Partington, 1988; Williams & Krane, 2006). The literature indicates it is probably better to utilize participatory imagery, as the image can be experienced as if the event is happening with full utilization of all senses and emotions, including kinesthetic movement (Callow & Hardy, 1997; Louis, Guillot, Maton, Doyon, & Collet, 2008). The latter imagery strategy permits memory of important associations that are likely to occur during actual sport-related tasks. Although all senses may be imagined, it is appropriate for some senses (i.e., vision, touch) to be imagined more so than others (Gregg, Hall, & Nederhof, 2005). Moreover, images should focus on positive experiences that approximate optimum performance (Anderson, 2000). Positive images are also incompatible with anxiety and are thus likely to assist in arousal management during participation in athletic activities (Maddux, 2009). Other important facilitating factors associated with imagery include making the task simple, optimizing the timing of events, and being intellectually capable of vividly imagining the events with appropriate perspective (see Wright & Smith, 2009).

## *Arousal Management*

A thorough understanding of arousal management is essential in cognitive assessment, as this skill set is strongly associated with optimum sport performance (Meyers et al., 1996; Parfitt & Hardy, 1994; Patrick & Hrycaiko, 1998; Robazza, Bortoli & Nougier, 1998). As first hypothesized by Yerkes and Dodson (see Taylor & Wilson, 2002; Weinberg, 1990), task performance is typically poor when physiological arousal is low and improves as arousal increases to some relative extent. However, performance gets worse when arousal is relatively high. Of course, this relationship is grossly influenced by various factors, including the type of task, task difficulty, task familiarity, past experience, confidence with the task, and so on (see Gould & Udry, 1994). Optimum arousal is often associated with "flow state," which is a psycho-emotional state of mind in which athletes are completely engaged and intrinsically motivated, and often reference a distorted sense of time during peak performance (Nakamura & Csikszentmihalyi, 2009). During the flow experience, performers often report their perceived skill sets are capable of meeting task-relevant challenges that are perceived to be important (Abuhamdeh & Csikszentmihalyi, 2009).

Several studies have demonstrated relationships between anxiety, arousal, and self-confidence (Hardy, 1996; Hardy, Woodman, & Carrington, 2004). Bois, Sarrazin, Southon, and Boiché (2009) compared golfers who made a qualifying cut to those who did not. They found the golfers who made the cut demonstrated more cognitive and somatic anxiety, but also utilized relatively more relaxation strategies and emotional control. This supports Meyer's notion that how athletes respond to anxiety is probably more important than whether or not they experience anxiety. Interventions have been empirically developed to help athletes manage anxiety and arousal (Chapter 7, this volume; Donohue et al., 2006; Miller & Donohue, 2003). These interventions are generally aimed at modifying irrational and negative thoughts to be more neutral with perhaps a positive bent (Gould & Udry, 1994). Therefore, researchers appear to recognize the importance of cognitive assessment in arousal management and emphasize that employment of validated measures of anxiety are a necessary first step of intervention planning (Raglin & Hanin, 2000).

## Cognitions and Relationships

A primary focus of cognitive assessment is understanding how people influence athletes to think in sport-related activities. This can become quite complicated because these factors are dynamic and highly interactive in determining sport performance (see Zourbanos, Theodorakis, & Hatzigeorgiadis, 2006). There does, however, appear to be substantial evidence that frequent rewarding, social support, and democratic style in decision making lead to greater satisfaction in athletes (Weiss & Friedrichs, 1986) and professional performers (Quested & Duda, 2010). Team cohesion and sport performance appear to be interwoven (Carron, Colman, Wheeler, & Stevens, 2002). Of course, these findings suggest professionals who practice sport psychology need to assess the extent to which athletes perceive they are being supported by both their coaches and teammates. However, they also need to assess athletes' perceptions of familial relationships. Stress appears to exacerbate interactions between athletes and their parents (Brustad & Partridge, 2002; Weiss & Fretwell, 2005) and may limit support and encouragement from family (Brustad, 1993; Hellstedt, 1988; Martin & Dodder, 1991; Woolger & Power, 1993). Along these lines, athletes have reported that their family members contribute most to their sport performance, as compared with their coaches, teammates, and friends (Donohue, Miller, Crammer, Cross, & Covassin, 2007).

## Attitudes Toward Sport Psychology

Even when athletes experience cognitive, emotional, and environmental problems that interfere with sport performance, they may be unmotivated to pursue assistance from sport psychology consultants due to negative stigma associated with sport psychology (Donohue, Dickens, et al., 2004; Martin, 1998; Martin, Wrisberg, Beitel, & Lounsbury, 1997). Upon visiting sport psychologists, these beliefs may continue to exist, leading to skepticism about perceived effectiveness of consultation (Martin et al., 1997). Thus, in addition to assessment of cognitive factors that may interfere with sport performance, attitudes about help-seeking and help follow-through should be assessed prior to intervention planning and implementation.

## Description of an Empirically Guided Method in Cognitive Assessment

In the following sections, we highlight our method of understanding cognitive functioning in athletes and performers. We begin by describing the basic structure and format of our cognitive assessment sessions and progress to "hands-on" methods involved in this evidence-supported process, such as behavioral interviewing, utilization of psychometrically validated self-report measures, behavioral observation, and self-monitoring (see Gardner & Moore, 2006).

*Setting.* We typically conduct our initial assessment in the office with the identified client and subsequently examine our functional hypotheses in field settings. The office facilitates a quiet environment and assures privacy. This setting also permits us to quickly locate cognitive assessment measures that are often spontaneously administered during the interview process. Case information gathered during the initial meeting is utilized to determine when it is optimal to conduct on-site cognitive assessments during practice and competition, which offers distinct advantages, such as timely queries about cognitions that may have occurred when behaviors were observed during key activities. Indeed, we sometimes conduct our preliminary meetings in places where clients practice or compete, but do so only during off-hours when others are likely to be absent. In vivo cognitive assessment may be particularly useful in reducing stigma associated with the referral and often makes it easier for clients to be comfortable and better remember cognitions that may be triggered in specific locations where performance is expected to occur (i.e., state-dependent memory; Anderson, 2000). In vivo assessment also permits ongoing examination of cognitive restructuring exercises that are often assigned during intervention phases. When in vivo cognitive assessment is not possible, we encourage clients to bring videos of their performance to the office and subsequently instruct them to report cognitions they remember having during key events and activities. Note that it is important to review videos soon after they are recorded to minimize distortions in memory that occur with the passage of time.

*Collateral informants.* Clients are the chief source in assessing their own cognitions. However, collateral sources of information can be helpful in substantiating self-report data and offering unique insights relevant to the presenting problem. Informants often include coaches, teammates, trainers, team doctors, and family members. When the identified client is a minor, we always include legal guardians in the initial process of assessment, whereas adult clients are encouraged to invite one or two persons to the initial assessment meetings who they feel could shed light on the presenting problem. Later, others are involved in the assessment process as appropriate.

*Psychometrically validated scales to guide interviewing.* Our initial meeting begins with a general discussion of the presenting problem, including the reasons that led to the referral and perspectives of the presenting problem. We use a semi-structured behavioral interview format (Grills-Taquechel & Ollendick, 2008). The general areas of focus in the interview adjust based on our initial discussion of the presenting problem and the athlete's responses to standardized measures that are administered immediately prior to the behavioral interview. In general, however, we emphasize cognitive domains that have been empirically identified to influence performance in athletic activities (see review by Donohue, Silver, Dickens, Covassin, & Lancer, 2007). Potential cognitive domains include the following: (1) motivation to obtain professional assistance, (2) motivation to pursue the respective sport activities, (3) injury management, (4) relationships, (5) academic and professional issues, (6) dysfunctional thoughts, (7) stress, and (8) attitude (i.e., confidence, support from others).

To assist in determining which domains to emphasize in our cognitive assessment, we always first administer the Sport Interference Checklist (SIC; Donohue, Silver, et al., 2007) and the Student–Athlete Relationship Instrument (SARI; Donohue et al., 2007) at the start of our first meeting. The SIC was developed to assess a wide range of problems that have been identified to interfere with sport performance, including cognitive, emotional, motivational, and environmentally based problems. Developed with 141 NCAA and high school athletes, the SIC is unique to other measures in its ability to assess cognitive and behavioral problems that have been identified to commonly occur during both training (Problems in Sport Training Scale, PSTS) and competition (Problems in Sport Competition Scale, PSCS). In completing these scales, athletes are asked to indicate how often each of the 26 problem cognitions and behaviors interferes with their training, and separately competition, utilizing a seven-point frequency scale (see Table 5.1). For each of the cognitive or behavioral stems, athletes are asked to indicate whether they would go to a sport psychologist if possible (Desire for Sport Psychology Scale, DSPS). Factor analysis of PSCS items indicate six factors (Dysfunctional Thoughts and Stress, Academic and Adjustment Problems, Injury Concerns, Lack of Motivation, Overly Confident/Critical, and Pain Intolerance), whereas PSTS and DSPS items evidenced four factors (Dysfunctional Thoughts and Stress, Academic Problems, Injury Concerns, and Poor Team Relationships). The psychometric properties of this instrument, including its face validity, internal consistency, convergent and discriminative validity, are excellent (see Donohue, Silver, et al., 2007).

We prefer the SIC for use in cognitive assessment because many of its scales are specific to a wide range of commonly identified thought processes that have been

**Table 5.1** Sport Interference Checklist (SIC) Sample Items. Sample directions: "Below is a list of things that sometimes occur with athletes during their training or during their competition. Please circle the number that represents how often each of these things interfere with your performance during training, and separately, your performance during competition (1 = Never, 2 = Very Seldom, 3 = Seldom, 4 = Sometimes, 5 = Often, 6 = Very Often, 7 = Always). Then circle either "yes" or "no" to indicate if you would see a sport psychologist if this happened to you, and if a good sport psychologist were available to you."

| | | How often does this *interfere with* your performance during *training*? | How often does this *interfere with* your performance during *competition*? | Would you *go to a sport psychologist for this*, if possible? |
|---|---|---|---|---|
| 1 | Negative thoughts about personal performance | 1 2 3 4 5 6 7 | 1 2 3 4 5 6 7 | Yes No |
| 2 | Being too critical of myself | 1 2 3 4 5 6 7 | 1 2 3 4 5 6 7 | Yes No |
| 3 | Being too critical of teammates | 1 2 3 4 5 6 7 | 1 2 3 4 5 6 7 | Yes No |
| 4 | Distracted (or upset) by people who observe me | 1 2 3 4 5 6 7 | 1 2 3 4 5 6 7 | Yes No |

*Note.* The Sport Interference Checklist is freely available in Donohue, Silver, et al. (2007).

indicated to contribute to poor performance in both athletic competition and training. Moreover, its format permits rapid assessment of cognitive interpretations for problem circumstances that are environmentally determined (e.g., Injury Concerns). That is, we query how each of the items that were endorsed as having occurred at a frequency of "4" (sometimes) or higher within the elevated scales interferes with training and/or competition, as appropriate. For instance, if the Dysfunctional Thoughts and Stress scale was elevated, and an athlete indicated that she often was too critical of herself during competition, she would subsequently be asked how being too critical of herself interferes with her performance in competition. The SIC is also unique in that athletes can be asked to explain how the material reflected in the item stems is problematic for competition but not training, and vice versa. For instance, it may be that an athlete reports that she is critical of teammates during training, but not during competition, because during competition she is "focused on the task at hand," whereas training permits her greater "dead time" in which she has time to notice flaws in others. Of course, such queries assist in gathering valuable information that is directly relevant to intervention planning. Moreover, a quick glance at the corresponding DSPS item provides an indicator of the informant's willingness to obtain professional assistance in the respective problem area. Naturally, we praise informants when they indicate they are interested in receiving professional assistance and query what obstacles make assistance difficult to accomplish so solutions can be generated.

After the SIC interview, we administer the SARI to better understand the extent to which relationships may influence sport performance. This instrument was developed with 198 high school and collegiate athletes, and its psychometric support is very good (Donohue, Miller, et al., 2007). The SARI includes four inventories, each assessing a relationship constellation (i.e., Family, 23 items; Coaches, 25 items; Teammates, 23 items; Peers, 10 items). For each item, a prompt is read (i.e., "It's a problem for me in my sport that ...") prior to a problem stem (e.g., "I feel isolated from at least one of my coaches."). Participants respond according to a 7-point Likert-scale measuring the extent to which the respondent agrees with the problem statement. Subscales across the four inventories include pressure to perform, lack of support, pressure to use illicit substances, pressure to quit or continue unsafely, experiencing embarrassing comments and negative attitude, lack of concern for teamwork and safety, lack of involvement and high expectations, too demanding, not a team player, and too non-competitive (Table 5.2).

For each subscale that is elevated, we query how items endorsed "five" (somewhat agree) or higher are problematic (e.g., "How's being isolated from your coach a problem for you?"). These queries often lead to rich discussion about the underlying, and potentially erroneous, belief systems that athletes may adopt to interpret the qualitative aspects of their relationships. For instance, if a coach was reported to "expect too much," the athlete could be queried to report how this conclusion was determined, and how it could be resolved. Such questions are directly relevant to intervention planning. The SARI format also permits the assessor to compare cognitive problem sets across relationships to some extent. To illustrate, it may be that the Family Inventory indicates a parent is putting pressure on her daughter to participate in a sport, whereas coaches, peers, and teammates are not. In the latter example, the athlete could be queried to explain how the parents were contributing pressure, whereas the others were not. Lastly, the SARI may assist in determining intervention outcomes across time, particularly when interventions are designed to enhance relationships in team sports where negative and erroneous thinking patterns sometimes occur (e.g., feelings of isolation, jealousy).

To assist in the economy of our cognitive assessment, the remaining cognitive measures in our battery are selected based on our initial interviewing. We believe the Athletic Achievement Motivation Scale (Elbe, Wenhold, & Muller, 2005) is a great tool to employ when it is important to understand the different aspects of motivation.

**Table 5.2** Student–Athlete Relationship Instrument (SARI) Sample Items. Sample directions: "Please indicate the extent to which you agree or disagree with the following statements (1 = "extremely disagree," 7 = "extremely agree")."

It's a problem for me in my sport that ...
At least one of my family members needs to praise me more often. 1 2 3 4 5 6 7
At least one of my family members pressures me to participate in a sport when I don't want to participate. 1 2 3 4 5 6 7
At least one of my family members has me do things that could result in me being injured or worsen existing injuries. 1 2 3 4 5 6 7
At least one of my family members makes rude or embarrassing comments about me. 1 2 3 4 5 6 7

*Note.* The Student–Athlete Relationship Instrument is freely available in Donohue, Miller, et al. (2007).

For instance, this scale provides an assessment of situationally based intrinsic and extrinsic motivation, as well as poor motivation in athletes. Certainly, understanding motives is important to treatment planning, and the results of this scale complement information gained from the SIC in regard to the interest of athletes in pursuing sport psychology consultation for specific problem areas.

When "mental toughness" appears to be relevant to the presenting problem, the Sports Mental Toughness Questionnaire (SMTQ; Sheard, Golby, & van Wersch, 2009) is highly recommended for administration. The SMTQ is relatively brief (i.e., 14 items) and has strong psychometric support. Respondents are queried about the extent to which problems occur in sport performance-related domains (4-point Likert scale; not at all true, very true) that are specific to Constancy (e.g., "I get distracted easily and lose my concentration," "I give up on difficult situations"), Control (e.g., "I am overcome with self-doubt," "I worry about performing poorly"), and Confidence (e.g., "I have what it takes to perform well while I'm under pressure," "I interpret positive threats as positive opportunities"). The format for the SMTQ is similar to that for the SIC and SARI; thus we query respondents to report how endorsed items in elevated scales affect their sport performance as previously described. Other potentially useful psychometrically validated cognitive measures include (1) the short form of the Competitive State Anxiety Inventory-2 (Cox, Russell, & Robb, 1998), which measures cognitive and somatic anxiety, and state confidence with sport performance; (2) the Symptoms Check-List-90-Revised (Derogatis, 1994; Vallejo, Jordán, Díaz, Comeche, & Ortega, 2007), which has been used to identify psychiatric symptoms, including psychological distress, in athletes (Donohue, Covassin, et al., 2004); (3) the Flow State Scale (FSS; see Jackson & Eklund, 2002; Jackson & Marsh, 1996; Martin & Jackson, 2008), measuring nine factors that are relevant to perceptions of being fully engaged in their sport; (4) the Dispositional Flow Scale (Jackson & Eklund, 2002) to assess concentration in sport-relevant tasks; (5) the Self-Efficacy in Sport Scale (Feltz, Short, & Sullivan, 2008) to assess perceived ability to succeed based on personal feedback; (6) the Winning Profile Athlete Inventory (PsyMetrics Inc, 2006) to assess competitiveness, dependability, commitment, positive attitude, self-confidence, planning, aggressiveness, team orientation, willingness to sacrifice injury, and trust; and (7) the Coping Inventory for Sport (Gaudreau & Blondin, 2002) to assess task-oriented coping, distraction-oriented coping, and disengagement-oriented coping styles in athletes and guide cognitive/behavioral intervention in teaching more adaptive and positive explanatory styles (Peterson & Steen, 2009). Finally, the Performance Failure Appraisal Inventory (Elliot, Conroy, Barron, & Murayama, in press) is a multi-dimensional measure of cognitive, motivational, and relational appraisals that are linked with the sense of fear of failure (FF). This scale provides information that is relevant to five aversive consequences in athletes (i.e., experiencing shame and embarrassment, devaluing one's self-estimate, having an uncertain future, important others losing interest, upsetting important others).

*Behavioral observation.* Once the initial target cognitions are identified, we utilize behavioral observation procedures to more specifically examine how thoughts are related to actions in performance scenarios (Chapter 12, this volume;

Leffingwell, Durand-Bush, Wurzberger, & Cada, 2005). Observations should occur in both competitive and practice settings. In each of these settings, we schedule observations when target behaviors are most and least likely to occur. To decrease the likelihood of response reactivity (an alteration in behavior due to being observed), we initiate our observations in relatively inconspicuous circumstances (e.g., sitting with others watching the event) and maintain neutral affect throughout the process. Observational effects are also minimized by scheduling informal observation prior to recording practices. Schedules of observation are varied to accommodate diversity within settings and circumstances, thus enhancing external validity. We make notes of environmental events that come before, during, and after behaviors that are associated with both failure and success, and subsequently query athletes to explain thoughts they may have experienced at key events or moments during these situations. For instance, a cross-country runner may be observed to run poorly when her competition looks physically intimidating, but may excel when her competition is less daunting. If this finding is reliably observed, it becomes clear that the athlete may experience debilitating cognitions about the competition immediately prior to running, rather than functionally appropriate thoughts about her personal preparation. The latter hypothesis would be substantiated if, upon being queried to report her thoughts immediately before and after the race, it was discovered that she made comments such as "She's too strong for me" before the race and reinforced these cognitive beliefs with confirmatory thoughts after the race (e.g., "I knew she was too much for me"). Comparing cognitions at key behavioral set points during sporting events assists in minimizing inaccuracies associated with self-report methodologies (i.e., faulty memories, biased responses) because the observer is present to substantiate the context in which self-reports are made. Congruence is an excellent method of confirming the accuracy of self-reported information and is demonstrated when self-reported cognitions are consistent with observed behaviors. For example, congruence would be demonstrated if an athlete reported that she evidenced derogatory or self-defeating cognitions before, during, or after crying, pacing, tensing muscles, and rapid breathing.

Interestingly, debilitating thoughts and behaviors are sometimes conditioned to co-occur in ways that can be understood only after formal cognitive assessment. For instance, one elite athlete we treated told jokes and laughed about the competition during warm-ups. Her teammates reported that her comments distracted them from focusing on what they needed to do prior to the race. When queried to report her thoughts before an observed warm-up, it was revealed that she experienced worrisome thoughts about the upcoming race. Therefore, her jokes appeared to be a nonfunctional method of distracting her from the worrisome thoughts. Indeed, the jokes distracted both her teammates and her from thinking about task-important instructions and positive self-statements that have resulted in optimum performance in controlled trials (e.g., Donohue et al., 2001, 2006).

*Self-monitoring.* Encouraging journaling in an open format or use of structured cognitive tracking assignments may provide fruitful information about cognitive functioning. However, these methods are notoriously limited in not providing a representative sample of cognitions, lack reliability and validity, and are dependent on the athletes' self-awareness (see Hackfort & Schwenkmezger, 1989). As an alternative approach, structured self-monitoring exercises may assist in gaining an accurate representation of problems interfering with performance (Gardner & Moore, 2006). Athletes may be instructed to record the frequency of cognitions that occur within a prescribed time frame (e.g., number of positive self-evaluation statements during a 2-h block) and setting (e.g., practice, game, team lunch), or specific thoughts and ratings of intensity can be recorded during critical points of performance. As in behavioral observation, the antecedent stimuli (e.g., being criticized) and consequences (e.g., threw ball away) of monitored thoughts should be recorded to assist in understanding etiological factors maintaining the respective cognitions.

*Functional assessment and analysis.* Although functional analysis has historically been utilized to determine factors maintaining identified problem behaviors, its method is also appropriate in understanding the function of thoughts. In doing so, hypotheses are formulated about the function of operationally defined thoughts in relation to environmental antecedents and consequences. We utilize the ABC model as our method of organization, whereby the "A" stands for antecedents, the "B" refers to beliefs or behaviors, and the "C" refers to consequences (Groden, 1989; Iwata, 1994; Iwata, Kahng, Wallace, & Lindberg, 2000). Of course, in cognitive assessment, the practitioner is primarily interested in gaining an understanding of dysfunctional thoughts that are influenced by antecedents and consequences. We relax the "B" (beliefs or behaviors) part of this model to include dysfunctional thoughts and images. In Table 5.3, we provide two ABC models: one focuses on the "B" as a belief and the second focuses on the "B" as a behavior. To demonstrate these models, in Table 5.3 we create three columns. In the first column, we record stimuli that precede the respective belief or behavior. In the second column, we record the respective belief or behavior, and in the third column, we record consequences of the respective belief or behavior.

The first model at the top of Table 5.3 focuses on a middle-weight boxer's belief that an upcoming bout will result in defeat. This belief is likely influenced

Table 5.3 Examples of two ABC models for use in athletes

| A (antecedents) | B (belief) | C (consequences) |
|---|---|---|
| Missing training days | "I'm going to lose the upcoming match" | Poor effort/motivation |
| Knowledge of competition | | Irritability |
| Lack of sleep | | Withdraw of anxiety |
| Told brother had better attitude | | Quick fuse |
| | | Poor response to feedback |
| A (antecedents) | B (behavior) | C (consequences) |
| "I'm going to lose the fight | Poor effort during practice | Poor timing in skill |
| "I'm not my brother" | | Irritability |
| "They only care if I win" | | Arguments with others |
| Told need to practice harder | | Quick fuse |

by the environmental stimuli and cognitions that are listed in the left and right margins. These stimuli were identified during a behavioral interview. Although other antecedents and consequences influencing this belief may not have been identified, if the assessment was sufficient, then etiological hypotheses for this belief may be drawn. For instance, examining the antecedent factors, it appears missing training days may have influenced low self-efficacy, particularly because the competition is expected to be "tough." Interestingly, lack of sleep is often associated with faulty thinking patterns and irrationality (Durmer & Dinges, 2005), which may lead to poor decision making. Lastly, being told by his father that his brother had a better attitude may be detrimental. That is, this statement suggests he has a bad "attitude." Additionally, being compared with others in a negative light is ill-inspiring. On the consequence side, self-defeating thoughts have been shown to decrease motivation to practice (Elliot & Harackiewicz, 1996) and increase irritability (Cacioppo & Hawkley, 2009), both of which may have resulted in a pattern of negative interactions with others. At first glance it may appear strange to see the boxer's self-defeating thoughts appear to be an influence in reducing his perceptions of anxiety. However, defeat is an easy outcome to predict, and anxiety is centered on the unknown.

The second model in Table 5.3 exemplifies poor effort during practice as a target behavior for this athlete, and the self-defeating thought "I'm going to lose the upcoming match" as an antecedent cognition contributing to his poor effort. Unlike the previous model where the thought "I'm going to lose the upcoming match" was isolated as the target belief, in this model the boxer's thought is put into context with other debilitating thoughts (i.e., "I'm not my brother"). It becomes clear that being told by the boxer's father that the brother had a better attitude was probably upsetting as the boxer spent time away from productive thoughts about practice to instead focus on his brother. It can also be hypothesized that brotherly comparisons contributed to irritability in this boxer. The second model also shows how thoughts are rarely isolated and that being told he had to practice harder by his coach was ineffectual or perhaps deleterious to his efforts. Poor effort appears to be reinforced by poor performance, arguments with others, and potential resentment perhaps due to the belief that others like him only when he wins. The latter hypothesis suggest this boxer may be demonstrating a lack of effort to determine if others continue to support him during defeat because as noted, poor effort is associated with poor performance.

*Testing functional hypotheses.* The next step in functional assessment is to determine which environmental stimuli and thought patterns have greatest influence on sport performance so competing behaviors and cognitions can be emphasized in intervention. From the intervention provided in Table 5.3, it is difficult to determine which factors contribute most to sport performance. However, it may be deduced that self-defeating cognitive sets (e.g., lack of confidence, insecurities, focus on issues relevant to resentment) interact with behavioral problems (e.g., lack of effort during practice, arguments). Therefore, cognitive interventions might incorporate competing positive self-statements, perspective taking skills training, and emphasize the benefits of practice, whereas behavioral interventions might include exercises designed to enhance relationships. It would make sense that the physiological problems (i.e., lack of sleep, irritability, anxiety) would dissipate when the cognitive and behavioral problems are effectively addressed.

Prior to testing these hypotheses, all data and hunches should be revealed to the athlete/performer and relevant significant others to obtain their feedback. First, participants should be queried to explain what they were hoping to gain from the assessment process. Certainly, this permits an informed opportunity to address misconceptions and determine what should be emphasized and avoided while presenting information. We review the implications of each cognitive assessment scale, starting with the results of non-elevated factors and progressing to an interpretation of elevated scales. We frequently ask if the information appears to be accurate, listen to concerns, and make adjustments when discrepancies are reported.

We like to show our clients the completed ABC analysis. We explain the conceptual aspects of the model because understanding it reinforces the intervention process. After the model is understood, competing behaviors and cognitions are generated from the participants. Of course, this helps participants become invested in the intervention plan and often results in useful strategies to complement the previously generated cognitions and behaviors. Competing behaviors and cognitions are prioritized according to the extent to which they are expected to lead to environmental reinforcement, are incompatible with debilitating thoughts and behaviors, can be implemented quickly, are desired by the athlete, have occurred previously or may be acquired without much effort, and have a strong likelihood of generalizability.

Finally, soliciting feedback from athletes and their significant others may be used as a springboard for intervention. Indeed, asking athletes how they would like to think during sport events, asking what they are hoping to get from interventions, and establishing a collaborative approach to intervention are all associated with consumer-driven evidence-based care. Moreover, we have our clients choose which evidence-based cognitive interventions, such as the ones reviewed in this book, they find most appealing and believe will produce the best outcomes.

## References

Abuhamdeh, S., & Csikszentmihalyi, M. (2009). Intrinsic and extrinsic motivational orientations in the competitive context: An examination of person–situation interactions. *Journal of Personality, 77*, 1615–1635.

Anderson, M. (2000). *Doing sport psychology*. Champaign, IL: Human Kinetics.

Baseball Almanac (2010). *Yogi Berra quotes*. Retrieved March 6, 2010, from: http://www.baseball-almanac.com/quotes/quoberra.shtml

Bois, J. E., Sarrazin, P. G., Southon, J., & Boiché, J. C. S. (2009). Psychological characteristics and their relation to performance in professional golfers. *The Sport Psychologist, 23*, 252–270.

Brustad, R. (1993). Who will go out and play? Parental and psychological influences on children's attraction to physical activity. *Pediatric Exercise Science, 5*, 210–223.

Brustad, R. J., & Partridge, J. A. (2002). Parental roles and involvement in youth sport. In F. L. Smoll & R. E. Smith (Eds.), *Children and youth in sport: A biopsychosocial perspective* (2nd ed, pp. 187–210). Dubuque, IA: Kendall/Hunt.

Bunker, L., Williams, J. M., & Zinsser, N. W. (1993). Cognitive techniques for improving performance and building confidence. In J. M. Williams (Ed.), *Applied sport psychology: Personal growth to peak performance* (2nd ed., pp. 225–242). Mountain View, CA: Mayfield.

Cacioppo, J., & Hawkley, L. (2009). Perceived social isolation and cognition. *Trends in Cognitive Sciences, 13*, 447–454.

Callow, N., & Hardy, L. (1997). Kinesthetic imagery and its interaction with visual imagery perspectives during the acquisition and retention of a short gymnastics sequence. *Journal of Sports Sciences, 15*, 75.

Carron, A. V., Colman, M. M., Wheeler, J., & Stevens, D. (2002). Cohesion and performance in sport: A meta analysis. *Journal of Sport & Exercise Psychology, 24*, 168–188.

Cox, R. H., Russell, W. D., & Robb, M. (1998). Development of a CSAI-2 short form for assessing competitive state anxiety during and immediately prior to competition. *Journal of Sport Behavior, 21*, 30–40.

Derogatis, L. R. (1994). *SCL-90-R: Administration, scoring, and procedures manual* (3rd ed.). Minneapolis, MN: Derogatis.

Donohue, B., Barnhart, R., Covassin, T., Carpin, K., & Corb, E. (2001). The development and initial evaluation of two promising mental preparatory methods in a sample of female cross country runners. *Journal of Sport Behavior, 24*, 19–30.

Donohue, B., Covassin, T., Lancer, K., Dickens, Y., Miller, A., Hash, A., et al. (2004). Examination of psychiatric symptoms in student athletes. *Journal of General Psychology, 131*, 29–35.

Donohue, B., Dickens, Y., Lancer, K., Covassin, T., Hash, A., Miller, A., et al. (2004). Improving athletes' perspectives of sport psychology consultation: A controlled evaluation of two interview methods. *Behavior Modification, 28*, 181–193.

Donohue, B., Miller, A., Beisecker, M., Houser, D., Valdez, R., Tiller, S., et al. (2006). Effects of brief yoga exercises and motivational preparatory interventions in distance runners: Results of a controlled trial. *British Journal of Sports Medicine, 40*, 1–4.

Donohue, B., Miller, A., Crammer, L., Cross, C., & Covassin, T. (2007). A standardized method of assessing sport specific problems in the relationships of athletes with their coaches, teammates, family, and peers. *Journal of Sport Behavior, 30*, 375–397.

Donohue, B., Silver, N. C., Dickens, Y., Covassin, T., & Lancer, K. (2007). Development and initial psychometric evaluation of the sport interference checklist. *Behavior Modification, 31*, 937–957.

Durmer, J. S., & Dinges, D. F. (2005). Neurocognitive consequences of sleep deprivation. *Seminars in Neurology, 25*, 117–129.

Elbe, A. M., Wenhold, F., & Muller, D. (2005). The reliability and validity of the achievement motives scale-sport: An instrument for the measurement of sport-specific achievement motivation. *Zeitschrift fur Sportpsychologie, 12*, 57–68.

Elliot, A. J., Conroy, D., Barron, K. E., & Murayama, K. (2010). Achievement motives and goals: A developmental analysis. In M. E. Lamb, & A. M. Freund (Eds.), *Handbook on life-span human development*. John Wiley and Sons Publishers.

Elliot, A. J., & Harackiewicz, J. M. (1996). Approach and avoidance achievement goals and intrinsic motivation: A mediational analysis. *Journal of Personality and Social Psychology, 70*, 461–475.

Ellis, A. (1982). Self-direction in sport and life. *Rational Living, 17*, 26–33.

Feltz, D. L., Short, S., & Sullivan, P. (2008). *Self-efficacy in sport*. Champaign, IL: Human Kinetics.

Gardner, F., & Moore, Z. (2006). Performance impairment-II (PI-II). In F. Gardner & Z. Moore (Eds.), *Clinical sport psychology* (pp. 157–170). Champaign, IL: Human Kinetics.

Gaudreau, P., & Blondin, J. P. (2002). Development of a questionnaire for the assessment of coping strategies employed by athletes in competitive sport settings. *Psychology of Sport and Exercise, 3*, 1–34.

Gordon, R. A. (2008). Attributional style and athletic performance: Strategic optimism and defensive pessimism. *Psychology of Sport and Exercise, 9*, 336–350.

Gould, D., & Udry, E. (1994). Psychological skills for enhancing performance: Arousal regulation strategies. *Medicine and Science in Sports and Exercise, 26*, 478–485.

Gregg, M., Hall, C., & Nederhof, E. (2005). Imagery ability, imagery use, and performance relationship. *The Sport Psychologist, 19*, 93–99.

Grills-Taquechel, A., & Ollendick, T. H. (2008). Diagnostic interviewing. In M. Hersen & A. M. Gross(Eds.), *Handbook of clinical psychology, Volume 2: Children and adolescents* (pp. 458–479). Hoboken, NJ: John Wiley & Sons Inc.

Groden, G. (1989). A guide for conducting a comprehensive behavioral analysis of a target behavior. *Journal of Behavior Therapy and Experimental Psychiatry, 20*, 163–169.

Hackfort, D., & Schwenkmezger, P. (1989). Measuring anxiety in sports: Perspectives and problems. In D. Hackfort & C. D. Spielberger (Eds.), *Anxiety in sports: An international perspective* (pp. 55–74). New York: Hemisphere.

Hardy, L. (1996). A test of catastrophe models of anxiety and sports performance against multidimensional anxiety theory models using the method of dynamic differences. *Anxiety, Stress & Coping: An International Journal, 9*, 69–86.

Hardy, L., Jones, G., & Gould, D. (1996). *Understanding psychological preparation for sport: Theory and practice of elite performers*. New York: John Wiley & Sons.

Hardy, L., Woodman, T., & Carrington, S. (2004). Is self-confidence a bias factor in higher-order catastrophe models? An exploratory analysis. *Journal of Sport & Exercise Psychology, 26*, 359–368.

Hellstedt, J. (1988). Early adolescent perceptions of parental pressure in the sport environment. *Journal of Sport Behavior, 13*, 135–144.

Hewitt, J. P. (2009). The social construction of self-esteem. In S. Lopez & C. R. Snyder (Eds.), *Oxford handbook of positive psychology* (Rev. ed., pp. 217–225). Oxford, NY: Oxford University Press.

Iwata, B. A. (1994). Functional analysis methodology: Some closing comments. *Journal of Applied Behavior Analysis, 27*, 413–418.

Iwata, B. A., Kahng, S., Wallace, M. D., & Lindberg, J. S. (2000). The functional analysis model of behavioral assessment. In J. Austin & J. E. Carr (Eds.), *Handbook of applied behaviour analysis* (pp. 61–90). Reno, NV: Context Press.

Jackson, S. A., & Eklund, R. C. (2002). Assessing flow in physical activity: The flow state scale-2 and dispositional flow scale-2. *Journal of Sport and Exercise Psychology, 24*, 133–150.

Jackson, S. A., & Marsh, H. W. (1996). Development and validation of a scale to measure optimal experience: The flow state scale. *Journal of Sport and Exercise Psychology, 18*, 17–35.

Kirschenbaum, D., & Bale, R. (1980). Cognitive-behavioral skills in golf: Brain power golf. In R. Suinn (Ed.), *Psychology in sports: Methods and applications* (pp. 275–287). Minneapolis, MN: Burgess.

Leffingwell, T. R., Durand-Bush, N., Wurzberger, D., & Cada, P. (2005). Psychological assessment. In J. Taylor & G. Wilson (Eds.), *Applying sport psychology: Four perspectives* (pp. 85–100). Champaign, IL: Human Kinetics.

Louis, M., Guillot, A., Maton, S., Doyon, J., & Collet, C. (2008). Effect of imagined movement speed on subsequent motor performance. *Journal of Motor Behavior, 40*, 117–132.

Maddux, J. E. (2009). Self-efficacy: The power of believing you can. In S. Lopez & C. R. Snyder (Eds.), *Oxford handbook of positive psychology* (Rev. ed., pp. 335–345). Oxford, NY: Oxford University Press.

Martin, S. B. (1998). High school athletes' attitudes toward sport psychology services. *Journal of Applied Sport Psychology, 10*, 151–156.

Martin, E., & Dodder, R. A. (1991). Socialization experiences and level of terminating participation in sports. *Journal of Sport Behavior, 14*, 113–128.

Martin, A., & Jackson, S. (2008). Brief approaches to assessing task absorption and enhanced subjective experience: Examining 'Short' and 'Core' flow in diverse performance domains. *Motivation and Emotion, 32*, 141–157.

Martin, S. B., Wrisberg, C. A., Beitel, P. A., & Lounsbury, J. (1997). NCAA Division I athletes' psychological skills and attitudes toward seeking sport psychology consultation: The development of an objective instrument. *The Sport Psychologist, 11*, 201–218.

Meyers, A. W., Whelan, J. P., & Murphy, S. M. (1996). Cognitive behavioral strategies in athletic performance enhancement. *Progress in Behavioral Modification, 30*, 137–164.

Miller, A., & Donohue, B. (2003). The development and controlled evaluation of athletic mental preparation strategies in high school distance runners. *Journal of Applied Sport Psychology, 15*, 321–334.

Nakamura, J., & Csikszentmihalyi, M. (2009). Flow theory and research. In S. Lopez & C. R. Snyder (Eds.), *Oxford handbook of positive psychology* (Rev. ed., pp. 195–207). Oxford, NY: Oxford University Press.

Orlick, T., & Partington, J. (1988). Mental links to excellence. *The Sport Psychologist, 2*, 105–130.

Parfitt, C. G., & Hardy, L. (1994). The effects of competitive anxiety on memory span and rebound shooting tasks in basketball players. *Journal of Sports Sciences, 11*, 517–525.

Patrick, T. D., & Hrycaiko, D. W. (1998). Effects of a mental training package on an endurance performance. *The Sport Psychologist, 12*, 283–299.

Peterson, C., & Steen, T. (2009). Positive explanatory style. In S. Lopez & C. R. Snyder (Eds.), *Oxford handbook of positive psychology* (Rev. ed., pp. 313–323). Oxford, NY: Oxford University Press.

PsyMetrics (2006). Winning Profile Athlete Inventory (WPAI). Trends Data [E-mailed Data file]. Retrieved June 1, 2010, from http://www.psymetricsinc.com/athlete.htm.

Quested, E., & Duda, J. L. (2010). Exploring the social environmental determinants of well- and ill-being in dancers: A test of basic needs theory. *Journal of Sport & Exercise Psychology, 32*, 39–60.

Raglin, J. S., & Hanin, Y. L. (2000). Competitive anxiety. In Y. L. Hanin (Ed.), *Emotions in sport* (pp. 93–111). Champaign, IL: Human Kinetics.

Robazza, C., Bortoli, L., & Nougier, V. (1998). Physiological arousal and performance in elite archers: A field study. *European Psychologist, 3*, 263–270.

Rushall, B. S. (1975). Psycho-social factors in performance. In J. Taylor (Ed.), *Science and the athlete* (pp. 51–62). Ottawa, ON: Coaching Association of Canada.

Rushall, B. S. (1982). The content of competition thinking strategies. In L. Wankel & R. B. Wilber (Eds.), *Psychology of sport and motor behavior: Research and practice* (pp. 173–184). Edmonton, AB: University of Alberta.

Rushall, B. S. (1984). The content of competition thinking. In W. Straub & J. Williams (Eds.), *Cognitive sport psychology* (pp. 51–62). Lansing, NY: Sport Science Associates.

Sheard, M., Golby, J., & van Wersch, A. (2009). Progress toward construct validation of the Sports Mental Toughness Questionnaire (SMTQ). *European Journal of Psychological Assessment, 25*, 186–193.

Taylor, J., & Wilson, G. S. (2002). Intensity regulation and sport performance. In V. J. L. Raalte & B. W. Brewer (Eds.), *Exploring sport and exercise psychology* (2nd ed, pp. 99–130). Washington, DC: American Psychological Association.

Theodorakis, Y., Weinberg, R., Natsis, P., Douma, I., & Kazakas, P. (2000). The effects of motivational versus instructional self-talk on improving motor performance. *The Sport Psychologist, 14*, 253–272.

Vallejo, M. A., Jordán, C. M., Díaz, M. I., Comeche, M. I., & Ortega, J. (2007). Psychological assessment via the internet: A reliability and validity study of online (vs paper-and-pencil) versions of the general health questionnaire-28 (GHQ-28) and the Symptoms Check-List-90-Revised (SLR-90-R). *Journal of Medical Internet Research, 9*, 1–10.

Van Raalte, J., Brewer, B. W., Lewis, B. P., Linder, D. E., Wildman, G., & Kozimor, J. (1995). Cork! The effects of positive and negative self-talk on dart throwing performance. *Journal of Sport Behavior, 18*, 50–57.

Weinberg, R. S. (1990). Anxiety and motor performance: Where to from here? *Anxiety Research, 2*, 227–242.

Weinberg, R. S., Jackson, A., & Smith, J. (1984). Effects of association, dissociation, and positive self-talk strategies on endurance performance. *Canadian Journal of Applied Sport Science, 9*, 25–32.

Weiss, M. R., & Fretwell, S. D. (2005). The parent-coach/child-athlete relationship in youth sport: Cordial, contentious, or conundrum? *Research Quarterly for Exercise and Sport, 76*, 286–305.

Weiss, M. R., & Friedrichs, W. D. (1986). The influence of leader behaviors, coach attributes, and institutional variables on performance and satisfaction of collegiate basketball teams. *Journal of Sport Psychology, 8*, 332–346.

Williams, J. M., & Krane, V. (2006). Psychological characteristics of peak performance. In J. M. Williams (Ed.), *Applied sport psychology: Personal growth to peak performance* (pp. 204–224). New York: McGraw-Hill.

Woolger, C., & Power, T. (1993). Parent and sport socialization: Views from the achievement literature. *Journal of Sport Behavior, 16*, 171–189.

Wright, C. J., & Smith, D. (2009). The effect of PETTLEP imagery on strength performance. *International Journal of Sport and Exercise Psychology, 7*, 18–31.

Zinnser, N., Bunker, L., & Williams, J. M. (1998). Cognitive techniques for improving performance and building confidence. In J. M. Williams (Ed.), *Applied sport psychology: Personal growth to peak performance* (3rd ed., pp. 225–242). Mountain View, CA: Mayfield.

Zourbanos, N., Theodorakis, Y., & Hatzigeorgiadis, A. (2006). Coaches' behaviour, social support, and athletes' self-talk. *Hellenic Journal of Psychology, 3*, 117–133.

# Part III
# Performance Enhancement

# Chapter 6
# Goal Setting and Performance Feedback

**Phillip Ward**

Goal setting and performance feedback are two of the most used and most studied performance-enhancing strategies in sport. Both strategies have roots outside of sport with the seminal work for goal setting being conducted in organizational management in work settings and for performance feedback in both organizational management and education. Goal setting and performance feedback have been used extensively in sports settings –long before researchers started attending to their effects, and probably as long ago as individuals wanted to improve their performance. Today goal setting and performance feedback are well known to coaches and researchers alike as effective tools for performance improvement.

Goal setting and performance feedback commonly fall under the lay umbrella term of motivation. Motivation is discussed both as a goal of coaches and as a problem with athletes. It is, however, an amorphous term with multiple meanings in both the lay and empirical literature. Brent Rushall, arguably the most influential behavioral sport psychologist in the past 50 years, suggests that athletes are considered motivated if specific behaviors occur at consistently high rates, with seemingly few rewards (Rushall, 1980). The rates of behavior observed are higher than what might be considered "normal" in the setting, and the reinforcers for the behavior may not be obvious to the observers. Sport-specific behaviors can include a variety of behaviors such as attending practices consistently, being punctual to practices and games, completing training tasks and workloads successfully, providing encouragement to peers, engaging in fair play, and organizing team activities. Goal setting and performance feedback are two of the most effective behavioral interventions that can produce the outcomes Rushall described as "motivation."

## Goal Setting

"A goal is a level of performance proficiency that we wish to attain, usually within a specified time period" (Latham & Locke, 2006, p. 332). More specifically, a goal

---

P. Ward (✉)
The Ohio State University, Columbus, OH, USA
e-mail: Ward.116@osu.edu

describes a specific behavior such as the jump shot in basketball or an overhead clear shot in badminton. Goals are typically presented in statements such as the following:

*Soccer player*: "I want to make 2 more shots on goal during this game than I did yesterday."
*Badminton coach*: "I want to see your wrist snap as you contact the shuttle in these next five overhead clears."

From a behavioral perspective, a goal is a rule (Martin, 1997). Rules represent behavior that is initially controlled by its antecedents, but is then maintained by its consequences as the person comes into contact with the consequences of the behavior. Rules alter behavior because they describe the contingency that results from following the rule. Some caveats are warranted here. First, the rule may not describe a contingency (antecedents, the behavior, and its consequences) explicitly, as in the case of a high school basketball coach saying to his team, "Let's make 80% of our free throws tonight during the game." In this example, the consequences for not making the free throws are either implicit or nonexistent. Second, the contingency described in the goal statement may not be the actual contingency that is operating. For example, a coach may say to the team that she is going to recognize players who are performing well using a wall chart to acknowledge their success, but some players may act to avoid getting cut from the team for poor performance.

There is a substantial general sports psychology literature examining goal setting (see Horn, 2009, for a review of this literature). This literature as shown that, in general, goals have been found to be effective at improving performance outcomes for athletes. However, there are studies that have reported equivocal findings (Locke, 1991; Weinberg, 1994). Locke (1991) argued that the equivocal findings have been the result of methodological flaws, many of which concern the internal validity of the studies (e.g., choosing goals that were not actually difficult or relevant). More recently, Mellalieu, Hanton, and O'Brien (2006) were critical of goal-setting studies that (a) too often used a limited number of observations of the dependent variables leading to conclusions based on a non-representative sample of observations; (b) combined skills rather than focusing on specific discrete skills, and thus increasing the task complexity that has been shown to be a strong moderator of goal-setting effects (Latham & Locke, 2006); and (c) too often used dependent variables that were not important variables for athletes and as such there was little commitment from the athletes in achieving the goals.

Within the behavioral sports psychology literature, these issues have not been prevalent because of the nature of single-subject designs that (a) allow participants to serve as their own controls, (b) focus on changing specific behaviors one at a time, and (c) select behaviors as goals that were socially significant for athletes in the context of their sporting lives. There are, however, some limitations in the behavioral literature and these include the following: (a) the packaging of goal-setting interventions with other strategies (e.g., verbal and graphic feedback), making specific interpretations of the effects of goal setting unclear; (b) limitations in the number of studies conducted in different sports settings (college, high school, and clubs represent the majority of research); (c) lack of demonstrated maintenance and generalization effects in many studies; and (d) too few studies that have described completely the behavioral contingencies in place.

## *Evidenced-Based Goal-Setting Principles*

Three primary principles of goal setting can be derived from the behavioral literature. As described below, goals should be specific and difficult, goal statements should define the consequences of meeting or not achieving the goal, and goal setting is more effective when combined with performance feedback.

*Goals should be specific and difficult.* Descriptions of behaviors used to set goals can be defined functionally or topographically (Cooper, Heron, & Heward, 2007). Function-based definitions are used when outcomes of the performance are expected. For example, in a study of collegiate rugby players, Mellalieu et al. (2006) used the following function-based behaviors: number of ball carries, number of tackles, and number of turnovers won. An advantage of function-based behaviors is that they are easy to measure because of their discrete characteristics. To illustrate, a tackle can be defined by its legal definition within the game and if it is effective in stopping the forward motion of the ball carrier.

Topographical-based behaviors are often seen when referring to technique of sports skills. For example, Ward and Carnes (2002) used a topographical description of a performance tactic in collegiate football: "A correct read or drop occurred if the linebacker moved to the correct zone relative to predefined pass coverage described in the coaches' play book" (p. 3). Topographical-based behaviors are more difficult to measure because they involve more complex definitions than function-based behaviors.

Note, however, that there is more to a goal statement than merely describing a specific behavior. The conditions under which a goal is to be performed are either implicitly or explicitly stated. When a goal such as "Successfully increasing the percentage of successful jump shots in basketball" is stated, there should be a description of where the jump is to occur. Will it be measured in the context of free practice, scrimmages, or games as well? Will it be counted from the three-point line, or anywhere on the court? Similarly, performance-orientated goals function best with a criterion tied to the performance, such as making 8 out of 10 jump shots from the free throw line (Martin, 1997). In the vast majority of studies, the coach has set the criterion performance in the goal. Brobst and Ward (2002) in their study of female high school soccer players reported that the coach and the lead researcher set a goal of 90% correct performance for three behaviors, which were movement with the ball, movement during restarts, and movement after the player passed the ball. The three behaviors were selected on the assumptions of the coaches that the skills could be performed by these players at that level.

A typical goal-setting study in a work setting compares the goal-setting condition to a "do your best" encouragement condition. The results of more than a 1,000 studies in organizational management have shown that *difficult*, but *possible to perform* goals produce the most effort and performance compared to being encouraged to "do your best" (Latham & Locke, 2006). These findings have been replicated in sport settings as well. For example, Boyce (1990) showed the effects of instructor-set specific goals versus "do your best" encouragement in rifle shooting in a college physical education class. She later replicated the study in a college tennis setting comparing "do your best" encouragement with self-set goals and instructor-set goals with the same results (Boyce, Wayda, Johnston, Bunker, & Eliot, 2001).

One problem with the recommendation of establishing difficult goals is defining what is meant by the term difficult. To date, no studies have examined the functional definition of "difficult" in sport settings. Latham and Locke (2007) and Locke (1991) argued that findings from the organizational literature show that difficult goals should be defined in terms of a criterion where no more than 10% of participants could reach the criterion without the use of goal setting or some other intervention. Accordingly, two caveats are important in establishing specific and difficult goals that focus on improving performance. First, the behavior should be in the current repertoire of the performer, or if it is a new skill, it must be achievable. Asking for performance improvement of a sports skill when the person cannot perform it is counterproductive and may lead to injury. Thus, determining whether goal is difficult requires some knowledge of the ability of the performer and some knowledge of the difficulty of the behavior to be performed. Second, the goal must be realistically achievable within the time frame targeted for the goal to be achieved. Creating unrealistic performance goals will result in athletes becoming unsuccessful and frustrated.

In single-subject design studies in sports (see Chapter 4, this volume), the baseline phase has typically represented the existing conditions present in the setting. Such conditions might include group expectations, feedback from coaches, and athletes' knowledge of their performance successes. For example, Swain and Jones (1995) examined the effects of goal setting on basketball skills of elite college players over the course of a season. In their study, the existing coaches' practices were treated as a constant and their goal-setting intervention was the primary manipulation. There have been no studies to date that have controlled the baseline conditions to the extent that there was no feedback or instructions from coaches. While this might limit experimental control, it enhances the ecological validity of these studies because goal-setting intervention has been used in the actual context it has been designed for.

Few studies have examined effects of goal setting in sports as a function of skill level. A study by O'Brien, Mellalieu, and Hanton (2009) showed the differential effects of goal setting on the performance of teenage elite and nonelite boxers. Their findings show that elite boxers displayed consistent performance improvement as a result of the goal-setting intervention and the nonelite boxes improved, but did so with less consistency. This finding is important to examine more closely particularly in the context of youth sport settings where athletes are often developing new skills and refining them.

*Goal statements should describe the consequences of meeting or not meeting the goal.* Behavior analysts are well versed in the importance of providing consequences for behavior. It is commonplace that when goals are stated in educational and sports settings, the response consequences either are not stated or if they are stated, the consequences are not applied. Interestingly, most goal-setting studies, behavioral or otherwise, have not described the response consequences as a component of the goal-setting intervention, thus making it difficult to assess the role of variables such as praise, feedback, and the role of social reinforcement.

When studies have described the response consequences, the most common strategy used has been praise and recognition of improved performances. Ward, Smith, and Sharpe (1997) combined goal setting with public posting when assessing the percentage of correct blocks and percentage of correct routes run by wide receivers on a collegiate football team. During the intervention phase of the study, the researchers met with the players following each practice session and congratulated them if they met their goal. Contingent on goal achievement, their names were added to a second poster board called the 90% club. Players who consistently made the 90% club each week were recognized at the end of the season social event.

*Goal setting is more effective when combined with performance feedback.* The majority of studies have combined performance feedback with goal setting to produce significant positive effects in the behaviors of athletes. The performance feedback can be either verbal descriptions or graphic displays (public posting or private) or both. Other interventions have combined goal setting and performance feedback with other components. For example, Wanlin, Hrycaiko, Martin, and Mahon (1997) demonstrated the effects of a package intervention consisting of mission development, athlete-set long- and short-term goals, self-talk, and goal visualization on elite speed skaters practice workloads, off-task behavior, and race times.

Few studies have directly assessed goal setting with and without other interventions. Smith and Ward (2006) used a multiple treatment design to assess the differential and combined effects of goal setting and public posting on the performance of wide receivers in college. While each condition was more effective than baseline, the goal setting and public posting condition was consistently better than public posting or goal setting alone.

## *Goal-Setting Principles Included in Interventions but Not Directly Assessed*

Three additional principles are typically associated with goal setting in sport (Martin, 1997; Rushall, 1980). Although there are no studies in the behavioral sport psychology literature that have directly evaluated these principles, they are often included in sport and in organizational management studies of work settings.

*Public goals may be more effective than private goals.* Despite the fact that when most individuals set goals, they do so privately, there is little research on this topic. In goal-setting studies in sports, someone other than the athlete (i.e., coaches, peer, researchers) has been aware of the goals and the performance objectives, typically on a practice-to-practice and game-to-game schedule. One of the few studies to use private goal setting in sport was conducted by Campbell and Martin (1987), who used private goal setting and private self-monitoring compared to standard coaching conditions in youth tennis players. Campbell and Martin found that private goal setting and private self-monitoring did not improve performance beyond that obtained in the standard coaching conditions. To date, there are no studies that have directly assessed the effects of private versus public goal setting. There are, however, studies that have kept the identities of the athletes and their goals from their coaching staff and other players during the study (e.g., Mellalieu et al., 2006).

There is some evidence that public goals may be better than private goals. Lyman (1984) reported that public goal setting was significantly more effective than private goal setting on the classroom on-task behavior of children with emotional and behavior disorders. Hayes et al. (1985) conducted two experiments examining public versus private goal setting and self-reinforcement of individuals studying for the graduate record examination. In both studies, the public conditions were more effective than the private ones. Hayes et al. (1985, p. 201) concluded, "The two experiments make more plausible the view that self-reinforcement procedures work by setting a socially available standard against which performance can be evaluated. The procedure itself functions as a discriminative stimulus for stringent or lenient social contingencies."

Implicit in the statement that goals should be public is the recommendation that there should be a system for monitoring progress toward goals. This system might include recording of performance by athletes using training logs or by coaching staff. Public posting of daily performance goals also could be included. Ward and Carnes (2002) investigated the effects of publicly posting "Yes" or "No" on a chart to indicate whether collegiate football players had met their daily self-set goals. The actual goals were never made public to the coaching staff. In addition to the intervention being effective, the effects were similar to other studies in which the goals were publicly stated (e.g., Smith & Ward, 2006; Ward et al., 1997).

*Break complex or longer-term or larger goals into smaller subgoals.* To date, there are no studies that have evaluated reducing large goals into smaller sub-goals, although Martin (1997) recommends this approach. However, there is good evidence from the task analysis literature showing that breaking tasks into smaller steps or stages is effective (Cooper et al., 2007). For example, creating smaller steps makes it easier to pinpoint where errors occur and when to provide feedback and consequences (e.g., reinforcement or correction).

*Gain Commitment from Athletes for the Goals.* A recurring finding goal-setting research has been the extent to which the participant is committed to the task. Martin (1997, p. 45) explains:

> Goals are likely to be effective only if there is continuing commitment to them by the individuals involved. From a behavioral perspective, commitment refers to statements or actions by a person setting a goal that imply that the goal is important, that he or she will work towards it, and that he or she recognizes the benefits of doing so.

An efficient approach to commitment is to involve the athlete in the process of setting goals. While there are some studies demonstrating that self-set goals may not work as well as instructor-set goals (Boyce et al., 2001), the difference between these two strategies is not substantial. Yet the majority of studies have shown that self-set goal is an effective goal-setting strategy (e.g., Mellalieu et al., 2006; O'Brien et al., 2009; Ward & Carnes, 2002).

## Performance Feedback

The purpose of performance feedback is to provide information to athletes that allows them to correct or maintain their performance. Similar to the goal-setting literature, the findings for feedback are inconsistent and do not support often-cited assumptions that (a) more feedback is better (Lee, Keh, & Magill, 1993; Magill, 1994), (b) some feedback is better than no feedback (Lee et al., 1993), or (c) positive feedback is better than corrective feedback (Brophy, 1981; Brophy & Good, 1986; Lee et al., 1993; Magill, 1994). Among the reasons for these inconsistent results are that many feedback studies were conducted under laboratory conditions with little ecological validity. Also, feedback studies too often have focused on the topography of the feedback (e.g., positive, corrective, negative) or who provided it (e.g., instructor or peer) without assessing the effects of the feedback. Other limitations are that feedback studies have used pre-post measures of student and athlete learning, have not reported effects of the feedback relative to specific trials, and confused feedback with rienforcement (Ward, 1995). Behavioral studies of performance feedback avoid many of the above limitations.

Note that performance feedback can be provided by coaching staff, peers, self, and even technology. For example,

| | |
|---|---|
| *Basketball coach*: | "I saw that your elbow is moving the side when you make your set shot, this next shot I want you to keep your forearm vertical as you make your shot." |
| *Volleyball teammate*: | "You are standing too high when you bump, bend your knees more!" |
| *Soccer player*: | "I can't believe that I contacted the ball that high, I've got to kick under the ball more." |
| *Technology*: | Heart rate monitors that sound when you are above or below your target heart rate while you are running or electronic beams that make a sound when a body moves between the beams indicating that you had too low a trajectory off the vaulting horse in gymnastics. |

In addition, performance feedback can be presented in graphs or charts that are recorded by coaching staff, peers, self, or researchers. In this overview of performance feedback, I include four strategies that have been studied in the behavioral literature and represent evidence-based methods.

### *Behavioral Coaching*

Studies focusing on behavioral coaching use verbal feedback and instructions as independent variables and compare the package to the baseline or standard coaching occurring in the setting. What distinguishes behavioral coaching using performance feedback from nonbehavioral studies is that the principles of applied behavior analysis are used in the design and application of the intervention (e.g., contingent reinforcement, clearly specified behaviors and contingencies). Behavioral coaching using verbal feedback, instructions, and reinforcement has been effectively demonstrated in many sports settings, improving (a) play execution by youth and high school football athletes (Komaki & Barnett, 1977; Stokes, Luiselli, & Reed, 2010; Stokes, Luiselli, Reed, & Fleming, 2010), (b) stroke performance by youth swimmers (Fitterling & Ayllon, 1983; Koop & Martin, 1983), (c) correct relay tag performance by competitive inline-roller speed skaters (Anderson & Kirkpatrick, 2002), (d) foul shooting performance of a women's collegiate basketball team (Kladopoulos & McComas, 2001), (e) practice and social behaviors by members of a youth swim team (Vogler & Mood, 1986), and (f) the technique of youth tennis players (Buzas & Allyon, 1981).

One very promising strategy, long used by coaches, is the "freeze strategy." In this feedback technique, the coach calls a freeze to the play in a scrimmage or drill and players are questioned about their current physical placements relative to the play. This is followed by modeling and then a replay of the events. The freeze technique has been used successfully to improve performance of technical skills and tactics in gymnastics, tennis, and football (Allison & Ayllon, 1980), youth soccer (Rush & Allyon, 1984), and youth track (Shapiro & Shapiro, 1985).

## *Public Posting of Performance*

Pubic posting is an effective behavioral feedback strategy that has demonstrated utility in a variety of settings (see Brobst & Ward, 2002, for a summary). Van Houten (1980) provided two explanations for the effectiveness of public posting. First, feedback serves to prompt and reinforce athlete performance. Second, public posting provides specific public expectations that become norms for conduct in an instructional environment.

Most public posting studies use goal setting and verbal feedback as components of the intervention because there are advantages to combining them. Goal setting provides an explicit criterion, as opposed to "do your best," while public posting is a technology that makes the performances public and also serves to provide feedback to performers. Verbal feedback is implemented frequently with public posting interventions, though it is often not explicitly described as a component of such interventions. When verbal feedback is used in conjunction with public posting and goal setting, it is typically limited to restating what has been publicly posted (e.g., Swain & Jones, 1995). However, the act of meeting and providing verbal feedback may also function as social reinforcement.

Galvan and Ward (1998) used public posting to effectively reduce unsportsmanlike behavior during tennis matches by male and female collegiate tennis players. In their study they reported that coaches were concerned with inappropriate behaviors such as disrespectful physical gestures, swearing publicly, and throwing and striking objects during tennis matches (e.g., tennis balls and racquets). The intervention consisted of presenting the data to the tennis players individually on the frequency of inappropriate behaviors collected during baseline and establishing an expectation in the form of a goal that these behaviors would be reduced from game to game. The data from games were publically posted in training sessions for all players to see. While the behaviors were not eliminated for any of the players, the overall reductions were from means of 14 per game in baseline to 2–4 occurrences per game during the intervention.

The effects of public posting have also been effectively demonstrated in increasing the success of set plays in scrimmages with measures of generalization to game performances in collegiate football (Smith & Ward, 2006; Ward & Carnes, 2002; Ward et al., 1997) and increasing body checks during collegiate hockey games (Anderson, Crowell, Doman, & Howard, 1988).

## Self-Monitoring

Self-monitoring occurs when individuals notice and record specific behaviors of interest. Several studies have successfully demonstrated the effects of self-monitoring in improving behaviors of athletes. Hume, Martin, Gonzalez, Cracken, and Genthon (1985) used a self-monitoring feedback package to improve the performance of youth figure skaters. Similarly, Wolko, Hrycaiko, and Martin (1993) demonstrated the effectiveness of self-monitoring compared to standard coaching of female youth gymnasts. More recently, Polaha, Allen, and Studley (2004) used a self-monitoring feedback package to decrease stroke counts in college-aged swimmers.

McKenzie and Rushall (1974) conducted one of the earliest studies of self-monitoring in sports. The study took place at a youth swim club where attendance and work rates (i.e., laps swum) were low. The research evaluated a public posting of performance intervention, described as follows:

> A large waterproof display board was constructed, on which each swimmer could indicate his/her cumulative attendance at practice. Spaces were also provided for the recording of each swimmer's present and best attendance records. Prominent spaces were reserved for the posting of the names of those who had the best records. (McKenzie & Rushall, 1974, p. 200)

One of the important characteristics of self-monitoring is the effect on a participant's behavior caused by the act of self-monitoring. This reactivity typically operates in favor of the intervention, but not always. In their study, McKenzie and Rushall (1974) concluded that in addition to the self-monitoring, a part of the effects of their intervention might have been attributable to the coach's verbal feedback. Critchfield and Vargas (1991) replicated the McKenzie and Rushall (1974) study controlling for coach prompting by scripting the amount of verbal instructions provided by the coach. Critchfield and Vargas (1991) reported modest and temporary increases in behavior under their conditions, raising the question about the role of reactivity effects in the self-recording performance. In a follow-up study examining the frequency of self-recording on laps swum (i.e., after 2 laps, after 4 laps, or following completion of all the required laps), Critchfield (1999) showed frequent self-recording was less effective for measuring laps swum than infrequent recording. Collectively, the studies by Critchfield and Vargas (1991) and Critchfield (1999) show that the mechanisms of self-monitoring are unclear and that there are contextual nuances that require elucidation in future studies.

## *Technology*

Technology has become increasingly useful in providing feedback in sporting settings and in fitness and health. Consider a person visiting a fitness center and using exercise cycles, treadmills, and step machines. Once she/he provides information such as body weight, age, and duration of workout, the machines follow a set program regardless of the effect that the activity has on her/his heart rate response to exercise. For some people, their heart rate may be 190 beats per minute (bpm), while for others it may be 114 bpm. If the person was wearing a heart rate monitor or if the machine measured the heart rate using hand sensors, her/his heart rate would be transmitted to a receiver in the machine. For maximum health benefits, exercisers should train within their target heart rate zone (i.e., 60–85% of maximum heart rate). If the machine is tracking the person's heart rate, it will adjust the load it places on the body to maintain a personal target zone. The accuracy and immediacy of technology feedback makes it a useful tool in research and an excellent resource for coaches and athletes.

Several studies have been conducted using technology as a feedback medium. Recently Boyer, Miltenberger, Batche, and Fogel (2009) examined the effects of combining video modeling by experts with video feedback in the performance of gymnastic skills by female youth gymnasts. Following skill performance, the gymnast viewed a video segment showing an expert gymnast performing the same skill and then viewed a video replay of her own performance of the skill. Each gymnast was told to try to match her performance to the expert performance. The gymnast then returned to practice. The intervention was successful for all four gymnasts in the study. A similar study was conducted using youth swimmers by Hazen, Johnston, Martin, and Srikameswaran (1990).

Scott, Scott, and Goldwater (1997) used a shaping procedure with a photoelectric beam to improve the technical skill and performance of a pole vaulter. The task was to help the vaulter extend his arms completely prior to take-off. The intervention involved a verbal prompt of "reach," which was shouted to the vaulter as he ran down the runway. He received immediate feedback in the form of a beep when the photoelectric beam was broken, indicating that he had achieved the desired height set for that vault. The height of the beam was gradually increased until the vaulter reached targeted arm extension at take-off. The increases in arm extension were matched by increases in bar height clearance.

Hume and Crossman (1992) used contingent musical reinforcement to improve swimming behaviors on the dry land portion of swimming practices (e.g., conditioning) and decreased nonproductive behaviors (i.e., eating, taking someone's goggles) of youth swimmers at practices. There were immediate and substantive increases in productive behaviors and decreases in nonproductive behaviors.

Finally, several performance feedback "package" interventions have incorporated combinations of goal setting, relaxation, imagery, self-monitoring, and self-talk with track and field athletes in Special Olympics (Gregg, Hrycaiko, Mactavish, & Martin, 2004; Wanlin et al., 1997), adult tri-athletes and runners (Patrick & Hrycaiko, 1998; Thelwell & Greenlees, 2003), youth figure skaters (Ming & Martin, 1996), youth hockey goaltenders (Rogerson & Hrycaiko, 2002), and collegiate basketball players (Hamilton & Fremouw, 1985; Kendall, Hrycaiko, Martin, & Kendall, 1990).

## Concluding Comments

What is striking about the intervention procedures reviewed in this chapter is the strength of their effects, and the social validity of the goals, procedures, and outcomes that have been used. Additionally, the procedures are low cost, easily implemented, and well accepted in sport settings by coaches and players alike. More research is certainly needed to identify mechanisms at work in these procedures. Furthermore, there should be more practitioner-based articles in coaching journals and more frequent coaching workshops showing how goal setting and performance feedback procedures can be adopted to improve athletic performance.

## References

Allison, M. G., & Ayllon, T. (1980). Behavioral coaching in the development of skills in football, gymnastics, and tennis. *Journal of Applied Behavior Analysis, 13,* 297–314.

Anderson, C. D., Crowell, C. R., Doman, M., & Howard, G. S. (1988). Performance posting, goal setting, and activity-contingent praise as applied to a university hockey team. *Journal of Applied Psychology, 73,* 87–95.

Anderson, G., & Kirkpatrick, M. A. (2002). Variable effects of a behavioral treatment package on the performance of inline roller speed skaters. *Journal of Applied Behavior Analysis, 35,* 195–198.

Boyce, B. A. (1990). The effect of instructor-set goals upon skill acquisition and retention of a selected shooting task. *Journal of Teaching in Physical Education, 9,* 115–122.

Boyce, B. A., Wayda, V. K., Johnston, T., Bunker, L. K., & Eliot, J. (2001). The effects of three types of goal setting conditions on tennis performance: A field based study. *Journal of Teaching in Physical Education, 20,* 188–200.

Boyer, E., Miltenberger, R. G., Batche, C., & Fogel, V. (2009). Video modeling by experts with video feedback to enhance gymnastics skills. *Journal of Applied Behavior Analysis, 42,* 855–860.

Brobst, B., & Ward, P. (2002). Effects of public posting, goal setting, and verbal feedback on the skills of female soccer players. *Journal of Applied Behavior Analysis, 35*(3), 247–257.

Brophy, J. (1981). Teacher praise: A functional Analysis. *Review of Educational Research, 51*(1), 5–32.
Brophy, J., & Good, T. (1986). Teacher behavior and student achievement. In M. C. Wittrock (Ed.), *Handbook of research on teaching* (3rd ed., pp. 328–374). New York: Macmillian.
Buzas, H. P., & Ayllon, T. (1981). Differential reinforcement in coaching tennis skills. *Behavior Modification, 5,* 372–385.
Campbell, R. C., & Martin, G. L. (1987). Private self-management versus a public mastery contingency for improving practice performance of young tennis players. Paper presented at the Annual International Conference of the Association for Behavior Analysis, May.
Cooper, J. O., Heron, T. E., & Heward, W. L. (2007). *Applied Behavior Analysis.* Columbus, OH: Merrill.
Critchfield, T. S. (1999). An unexpected effect of recording frequency in reactive self-monitoring. *Journal of Applied Behavior Analysis, 32,* 389–391.
Critchfield, T. S., & Vargas, E. A. (1991). Self-recording, instructions, and public self-graphing: Effects on swimming in the absence of coach verbal interaction. *Behavior Modification, 15,* 95–112.
Fitterling, J. M., & Ayllon, T. (1983). Behavioral coaching in classical ballet: Enhancing skill development. *Behavior Modification, 7,* 345–368.
Galvan, Z. J., & Ward, P. (1998). Effects of public posting on inappropriate on-court behaviors by collegiate tennis players. *The Sport Psychologist, 12,* 419–426.
Gregg, M. J., Hrycaiko, D., Mactavish, J. B., & Martin, G. L. (2004). A mental skills package for Special Olympics athletes: A preliminary study. *Adapted Physical Activity Quarterly, 21,* 4–18.
Hamilton, S. A., & Fremouw, W. J. (1985). Cognitive behavioral training for college basketball free throw performance. *Cognitive Therapy and Research, 9,* 479–483.
Hayes, S. C., Rosenfarb, I., Wulfert, E., Munt, E. D., Korn, Z., & Zettle, R. D. (1985). Self-reinforcement effects. An artifact of social standard setting. *Journal of Applied Behavior Analysis, 18,* 204–214.
Hazen, A., Johnston, C., Martin, G. L., & Srikameswaran, S. (1990). A videotaping feedback package for improving skills of youth competitive swimmers. *The Sport Psychologist, 4,* 213–227.
Horn, T. S. (2009). *Advances in sport psychology.* Champaign, IL: Human Kinetics.
Hume, K. M., Martin, G. L., Gonzalez, P., Cracklen, C., & Genthon, S. (1985). A self-monitoring feedback package for improving freestyle figure skating practice. *Journal of Sport Psychology, 7,* 333–345.
Hume, K. M., & Crossman, J. (1992). Musical reinforcement of practice behaviors among competitive swimmers. *Journal of Applied Behavior Analysis, 25,* 665–670.
Kendall, G., Hrycaiko, D., Martin, G. L., & Kendall, T. (1990). The effects of an imagery rehearsal, relaxation, and self-talk package on basketball game performance. *Journal of Sport & Exercise Psychology, 12,* 157–166.
Kladopoulos, C. N., & McComas, J. J. (2001). The effects of form training on foul-shooting performance in members of a women's college basketball team. *Journal of Applied Behavior Analysis, 34,* 329–332.
Komaki, J., & Barnett, F. T. (1977). A behavioral approach to coaching football: Improving the play execution of the offensive backfield on a youth football team. *Journal of Applied Behavior Analysis, 7,* 199–206.
Koop, S., & Martin, G. L. (1983). A coaching strategy to reduce swimming stroke errors with beginning age-group swimmers. *Journal of Applied Behavior Analysis, 16,* 447–460.
Latham, G. P., & Locke, E. A. (2007). New developments in and directions for goal-setting research. *European Psychologist, 12,* 290–300.
Lee, A. M., Keh, N. C., & Magill, R. A. (1993). Instructional effects of teacher feedback in physical education. *Journal of Teaching in Physical Education, 12,* 228–243.
Locke, E. A. (1991). Problems with goal setting research in sports-and their solution. *Journal of Sport and Exercise Psychology, 13,* 311–316.

Locke, E. A., & Latham, G. P. (2006). New directions in goal-setting theory. *Current Directions in Psychological Science, 15*, 265–268.

Lyman, R. D. (1984). The effect of private and public goal setting on classroom behavior of emotionally disturbed children. *Behavior Therapy, 15*, 395–402.

Magill, R. A. (1994). The influence of augmented feedback on skill learning depends of characteristics of the skill and the learner. *Quest, 46*, 314–327.

Martin, G. L. (1997). *Sport psychology consulting, practical guidelines from behavior analysis.* Winnipeg, MB: Sport Science Press.

McKenzie, T. L., & Rushall, B. S. (1974). Effects of self-recording on attendance and performance in a competitive swimming training environment. *Journal of Applied Behavior Analysis, 7,* 199–206.

Mellalieu, S., Hanton, S., & O'Brien, M. (2006). The effects of goal setting on rugby performance. *Journal of Applied Behavior Analysis, 39,* 257–261.

Ming, S., & Martin, G. L. (1996). Single-subject evaluation of a self-talk package for improving figure skating performance. *The Sport Psychologist, 10,* 227–238.

O'Brien, M., Mellalieu, S., & Hanton, S. (2009). Goal setting effects in elite and non-elite boxers. *Journal of Applied Sports Psychology, 21,* 293–306.

Patrick, T., & Hrycaiko, D. (1998). Effect of a mental training package on an endurance performance. *Sports Psychologist, 12,* 283–299.

Polaha, J., Allen, K., & Studley, B. (2004). Self-monitoring as an intervention to decrease swimmers stroke counts. *Behavior Modification, 28,* 261–275.

Rogerson, L. J., & Hrycaiko, D. W. (2002). Enhancing competitive performance of ice hockey goaltenders using centering and self-talk. *Journal of Applied Sport Psychology, 14,* 14–26.

Rush, D. B., & Allyon, T. (1984). Peer behavioral coaching: Soccer. *Journal of Sport Psychology, 6,* 325–334.

Rushall, B. S. (1980). Psychological factors in sports performance. In F. S. Pyke (Ed.), *Towards better coaching. The art and science of coaching* (pp. 177–214). Canberra ACT: Australian Government Printing Service.

Scott, D., Scott, L. M., & Goldwater, B. (1997). A performance improvement program for an international-level track and field athlete. *Journal of Applied Behavior Analysis, 30,* 573–575.

Shapiro, E. S., & Shapiro, S. (1985). Behavioral coaching and the development of skills in track. *Behavior Modification, 9,* 211–224.

Smith, S., & Ward, P. (2006). Effects of public posting, goal setting, and public posting with goal setting in collegiate football. *Journal of Applied Behavior Analysis, 39,* 385–391.

Stokes, J. V., Luiselli, J. K., & Reed, D. D. (2010). A behavioral intervention for teaching tackling skills to high school football athletes. *Journal of Applied Behavior Analysis, 43,* 509–512.

Stokes, J. V., Luiselli, J. K., Reed, D. D., & Fleming, R. K. (2010). Behavioral coaching to improve offensive line pass blocking skills of high school football athletes. *Journal of Applied Behavior Analysis, 43,* 463–472.

Swain, A., & Jones, G. (1995). Effects of goal-setting interventions on selected basketball skills: A single-subject design. *Research Quarterly for Exercise and Sport, 66,* 51–63.

Thelwell, R. C., & Greenlees, I. A. (2003). Developing competitive endurance performance using mental skills training. *Sport Psychologist, 17,* 318–337.

Van Houten, R. (1980). *Learning through feedback: A systematic approach for improving academic performance.* New York: Human Sciences Press.

Vogler, W. E., & Mood, D. P. (1986). Management of practice behavior in competitive age group swimming. *Journal of Sport Behavior, 9,* 160–172.

Wanlin, C., Hrycaiko, D., Martin, G. M., & Mahon, M. (1997). The effects of a goal setting package on the performance of young speed skaters. *Journal of Applied Sports Psychology, 9,* 212–228.

Ward, P. (1995). A response to "The negative effects of positive reinforcement in teaching children with developmental delays". *Exceptional Children, 61,* 489–492.

Ward, P., & Carnes, M. (2002). Effects of posting self-set goals on collegiate football players' skill execution during practice and games. *Journal of Applied Behavior Analysis, 35,* 1–12.

Ward, P., Smith, S., & Sharpe, T. (1997). The effects of accountability on task accomplishment in collegiate football. *Journal of Teaching in Physical Education, 17*, 40–51.

Weinberg, R. S. (1994). Goal setting and performance in sport and exercise settings: A synthesis and a critique. *Medicine and Science in Sports and Exercise, 26*, 469–477.

Wolko, K. L., Hrycaiko, D. W., & Martin, G. L. (1993). A comparison of two self-management packages to standard coaching for improving practice performance of gymnasts. *Behavior Modification, 17*, 209–223.

# Chapter 7
# Cognitive–Behavioral Strategies

**Jeffrey L. Brown**

Can you think of any professional baseball player who has brought more attention to the mental aspect of sport than syntactically challenged New York Yankee catcher Yogi Berra? Berra is frequently quoted: "Baseball is 90% mental and the other half is physical." While his quote often prompts a chuckle and a knowing grin, Berra was right about the cognitive aspects of performance. From baseball to swimming, soccer to fencing, and golf to running, the brain is a fascinating ally in performance. Performance *is* mental.

Today, research continues to reveal that the brains of athletes are somewhat different than of non-athletes, due in part to the cognitive–behavioral aspects of deliberate physical and cognitive training (Nakata, Yoshie, Miura, & Kudo, 2010). Cognitive–behavioral interventions can clearly optimize mental performance and, in some cases, even change the landscape of the brain. Today, cognitive–behavioral strategies are fundamental to sport (Williams & Leffingwell, 2002).

When providing psychological services to athletes, it is common for psychologists to help them create an awareness of mental operations and how they are connected to physical aspects of sport. For example, an athlete may concentrate well under pressure or remain motivated even when the score is not in her favor. It is wrong to assume that athletes who do not understand or have never heard of cognitive–behavioral interventions are not using them. Rather, a psychologist should expect that many psychological strategies are at play and that players possess the capacities to hone those cognitive–behavioral skills and learn new ones along the way.

Traditionally, seasoned athletes may already possess mental skills which lead to success. Rather than starting from scratch with the assumption an athlete has no effective psychological skills at all, cognitive–behavioral consultation may be a matter of identifying an athlete's existing mental strengths in order to use them more. Inasmuch, the role of the cognitive–behavioral psychologist is multi-faceted, as is the psychological potential of the athlete. With such a good match between the natural psychological constitution of athletes and the understanding

---

J.L. Brown (✉)
Harvard Medical School, Boston, MA, USA
e-mail: jeffrey_brown@hms.harvard.edu

cognitive–behavioral research and theory can offer them, what could possibly go wrong?

## The Reality

Well-meaning coaches and parents take aim at athletes every season, offering novice psychological advice such as "don't think about it, just shoot the ball," "are you going to let her treat you like that on the field?," or "let your arms and legs do all the work." Such bleacher-coaching can create frustration and reinforce poor cognitive habits, especially for an athlete who has not yet developed a natural ability to utilize mental skills. Further complicating the relationship between athlete and sport psychologist is a cultural expectation that athletes are stalwart, tough, and psychologically invincible.

During the early years of my doctoral training in cognitive–behavioral therapy, a college football player who had been sidelined because of a broken arm was referred to me. A few weeks after his arm was broken, his younger sister was killed in an automobile accident. In the initial session, he appeared kind and reserved. He answered questions with a "yes, sir" and "no, sir" attitude, almost like I was his coach. The player was mildly disinterested and quietly reported that, in spite of the recent events in life, things were going fine.

As the session progressed, the alliance grew only minimally as he talked about what his sister and he used to do for fun. At times, he reported his thoughts and emotions to me almost as if our conversation was a media interview and he needed to stay in the middle of the road. At the time, his response style seemed reasonable given the tremendous trauma and loss he had faced. I concluded his flat affect and his mildly blunted communication was simply the best he could give considering his circumstances.

We finished the session and scheduled a second appointment. Within hours of scheduling the second appointment, the office manager forwarded a message to me. The player had called to cancel the appointment. His message read: "My coach required me to come to one meeting and that's all I'm going to do."

We could have a consultation heyday interpreting and analyzing this first session and resulting phone message, but I can tell you now the most compelling information had to do with what I learned from that athlete. What had been overlooked and could have simply been addressed with an empathic question about it was this athlete's sense of control about being in therapy. He had no control over his arm being broken or his sister's accident. Now, his coach had taken control away once again by requiring him to see a psychologist.

Some of what I had noticed in that first session with the athlete was accurate: the blunted affect, the distance, the lacking energy. But I had forgotten a well-known belief about athletes. Qualitative research and anecdotal accounts consistently reveal athletes avoid the stigma that they believe accompanies mental health treatment. Just like this football player, athletes may routinely struggle with initiating therapy, issues of control, and being vulnerable.

**Table 7.1** Circumstances appropriate for cognitive–behavioral intervention

Learning skill, form, or technique
Developing concentration and focus
Increasing confidence
Increasing leadership abilities
Developing or terminating a career
Managing life stresses and life events
Rehabilitating an injury
Substance use
Aggression or anger management
Perfectionism
Eating disorders
Training compliance
Team cohesion
Communication
Time management

Etzel, Ferrante, and Pinkney (2002) highlight factors such as performance demands and career transitions that can place unique demands on athletes. Athleticism is about strength and formidability. Athletes will have spent hundreds and, in many cases, thousands of hours training their bodies for strength, endurance, agility, and speed. Finding themselves in an unpredictable, vulnerable situation must indeed feel counterintuitive. Therefore, it is critical for the psychologist attempting to work with an athlete to understand how to frame the relationship in a way that it offers strength and avoids the athlete's likely fear of a stereotypical *What About Bob?* or *Good Will Hunting* experience (Glick & Horsfall, 2009). Relative to this topic, see Table 7.1 for typical reasons athletes would actually use cognitive–behavioral therapy in a therapeutic setting. If you do not have an alliance, then cognitive–behavioral work will never happen.

## The Alliance

Because athletes are uncomfortable with the idea of therapy and vulnerability, I have learned to offer psychological services that are characterized by what I have coined as a "personal consultant" model. I ask athletes to think of me as a personal consultant who is an expert in human behavior, rather than thinking of me as a counselor or therapist. To an athlete who is concerned about delving into psychological matters, a personal consultant model seems more acceptable and permits the athlete to seemingly avoid the stigma of "seeing a counselor" or "having a therapist." It is no surprise athletes find it hard to initiate therapy, let alone stay in it. Therapy is both an art and a skill, and cognitive–behavioral theory is a wonderful guide for negotiating and developing the relationship.

This chapter aims at helping readers understand more about how to successfully engage an athlete in cognitive–behavioral therapy, build an alliance, and offer research-based behavioral interventions. I discuss basic tenets of the interventions, how to implement them, and the potential outcomes and pitfalls. My perspective is that a sport psychologist's competence in cognitive–behavioral therapy can be a mitigating factor when engaging an athlete in the process of change and improvement.

## Know Your Clients and the Language They Speak

A lesser known author whose book is wedged on my bookshelf somewhere between Sigmund Freud and B. F. Skinner is George Herman Ruth (1928) – yes, *the* legendary homerun-hitting icon (i.e., "Babe" Ruth), who has been associated with a worn-out cognitive distortion Bostonians called a *curse* until 2004. (After 86 years, Red Sox Nation finally restructured its irrational belief with evidence of a World Series win.) Mr. Ruth was hardly the traditional academic type, but he made a notable assertion in his 1928 book that the baseball players he played with were regular people from different walks of life. Many of them had varied interests ranging from finance and politics to musical skill. Irrespective of a psychologist's theoretical orientation, I suppose most clinicians today would agree with Ruth's revelation from over 80 years ago that athletes are regular people who, by the mere fact of running the human race with everyone else, will likely face psychological adversities. Today, cognitive–behavioral psychology is logically teamed with sport psychology, not just because research has discovered the fit, but because cognitive skills are what athletes use. Thus, working with athletes now requires specialization and expertise, both in understanding the sport culture and in demonstrating competence in cognitive–behavioral psychology.

While I have maintained a traditional cognitive–behavioral practice working with adults and adolescents, I have found that work with athletes and cognitive–behavioral therapy dovetail quite smoothly. My background as a college baseball player no doubt stirred my interest in sport psychology, but it was not until later in graduate school that I was able to develop actual professional competence in sport psychology and cognitive–behavioral therapy.

It is quite compelling and frankly convenient that athletics and a cognitive–behavioral therapy framework share some common terminologies such as goals, practice, evaluation, and feedback. Therefore, a cognitive–behavioral approach is particularly helpful for and interesting to athletes who may need more traditional clinical support from time to time. Additionally, in order to deliver cognitive–behavioral interventions effectively, it is requisite to know its historical and contemporary implications.

## A Very Brief History of Cognitive–Behavioral Psychology and Sport Psychology

Both cognitive–behavioral psychology and sport psychology have been predicated by generations of research and application in various domains of sport. In the 1890s, the study of sport and behavior made its American debut when Norman Triplett researched bicyclists' performances both individually and against each other. Shortly after the turn of the century, Triplett passed the baton to his prodigious student, Coleman Griffith, who is considered the father of American sport psychology (Weinburg & Gould, 1995).

Ghinassi (2010) provides a succinct overview of the development of cognitive–behavioral therapy per se, beginning with the influence of early theorist George Kelly, whose personal construct theory reflected his belief that an individual possesses constructs or representations that are "the way in which an individual understands or construes the world. Constructs help predict what will happen and how to react appropriately" (p. 33). Sport psychologists using cognitive–behavioral approaches in sport settings frequently find Kelly's constructs to be at work (Kelly, 1963). In general, it is commonplace (and frequently preoccupying) for athletes to want to predict outcomes, compare themselves to others, and make decisions about self-confidence in the absence of physical, objective evidence.

While Kelly may have made it to the psychology hall of fame a first, two more inductees who would eventually keep him company are Albert Ellis (2001) and Aaron T. Beck (Beck, 1995). Both men were psychoanalysts-turned-cognitive-behaviorists. Ellis, who died in 2007, developed what is currently known as Rational Emotive Behavior Therapy. I personally saw Ellis in action in his New York City institute on more than one occasion and can attest that his approach was focused more on problem solving through the elimination of cognitive distortions and less on alliance building with the client. Even at the risk of making a client look unintelligent, Ellis would attack illogical and irrational thoughts. Beck, on the other hand, emphasizes a more collaborative approach with a client. The collaboration explores negative beliefs and schemas that lead to negative emotion about the self. A host of other cognitive–behavioral psychologists' influences continue to shape our understanding of therapeutic theory, strategy, and technique in sport psychology.

More than a century after its inception, sport psychology is a clearly defined specialty that is recognized formally by national organizations such as the Association of Applied Sport Psychology and the American Psychological Association's Division 47, Exercise and Sport Psychology. Sport psychology possesses its own ethics code and offers a certification process intended to establish competency through documentation of coursework and supervised training experiences through the Association for Applied Sport Psychology. Sport psychologists who are certified as a consultant in the Association for Applied Sport Psychology may also serve on the United States Olympic Committee (USOC) Registry of Psychologists. Inclusion on the Registry creates an opportunity to work with Olympic athletes and teams who utilize USOC resources throughout the country.

## Myths about Cognitive–Behavioral Therapy: Protecting Theory and the Athlete

The history of cognitive–behavioral psychology and sport psychology was not free of challenges and biases. Today, misunderstandings about cognitive–behavioral therapy exist and directly affect professional practice. Clearly responding to these misunderstandings may help athletes more confidently engage in therapy and have informed expectations. Five myths about cognitive–behavioral therapy and sport seem to exist.

## *Myth 1: Cognitive–Behavioral Therapy Is a Collection of Tricks*

Many prospective clients and some clinicians unfamiliar with cognitive–behavioral therapy erroneously believe it consists of tricks or gimmicks for developing a particular skill. Add to that belief an underlying notion that these alleged tricks require only little effort and what you will quickly have is a recipe for disaster, with the psychologist being blamed for failure. Athletes need to be educated about how cognitive–behavioral therapy is a diverse, research-based approach to healthy thinking, feeling, and behavior. While it should be methodically and characteristically strategic, it is not a secret formula or a series of fancy parlor tricks.

## *Myth 2: Cognitive–Behavioral Therapy Produces Immediate Effects*

In some cases, it is true that clients respond to cognitive–behavioral interventions faster than others. Realistically, cognitive–behavioral therapy is an approach that brings about change over time through cognitive processes such as restructuring, self-monitoring, practice, and experimentation with new thoughts or behaviors. The human physique changes as the result of deliberate, purposeful, and repetitive exercise over time. The same effort is required for the human brain (Brown, Fenske, & Neporent, 2010).

Prospective clients may initiate contact for services because of a performance or critical competition that is to occur in a matter of days or weeks. Not surprising, the telephone call or email has often been prompted by increased anxiety related to the approaching competition. Anxiety in parents or spouses, not just in the athletes, can be a driving force for a referral as well. Psychologists should avoid being driven by the client's anxiety or the unrealistic expectation that any positive outcome will be immediate. Quickly clarify what is to be expected, emphasizing consistent work over time.

## *Myth 3: Once Learned, Cognitive–Behavioral Strategies Should No Longer Be Practiced*

The comparison of cognitive–behavioral training and physical training is a perfect analogy. When helping clients understand how to incorporate and benefit from cognitive–behavioral work on an ongoing basis, it is good to explain it as a developmental process. Be sure to include sport examples. Football players would not start lifting weights a week or two before their first game. Rather, they would be lifting weights months before and throughout the season. Marathon runners do not take a quick jog around the block or make fast friends with a treadmill just days before staring down 26.2 miles. They train months at a time in preparation for a single performance. Mental training, just like physical training, should be strategic and ongoing. Compliance with cognitive–behavioral training can be difficult.

In our win-at-all-cost culture, athletes seem to have an increased interest in psychological aspects of performance. Moreover, research and brain science is progressing at such a rapid pace that the lay public is learning more about the brain's capabilities for success and how they can take an active role in the process. In that same busy culture, however, athletes frequently learn psychological concepts, but fail to practice or apply them. It is much like knowing that the oil in a car needs to be changed regularly, but it does not happen. It is clear the car will run better, be less apt to need repair, and promote overall efficiency. But, nonetheless, it is neglected. Encourage athletes to consistently practice and use cognitive–behavioral strategies as part of ongoing training commitments.

## *Myth 4: Cognitive–Behavioral Therapy Is Used Only for Treating Psychopathology*

A vast collection of research has examined cognitive–behavioral therapy's treatment efficacy across a wide range of psychopathological conditions. Indeed, cognitive–behavioral therapy is the treatment of choice for many conditions, ranging from irritable bowel syndrome and obsessive compulsive disorder to sexual dysfunction and panic disorder (Freeman, 1995). However, it is not limited to just treating uncomfortable or annoying symptoms. Indeed, most people, athletes included, will likely benefit from therapy at some point in life. Even more, athletes and other performers can benefit from cognitive–behavioral interventions prior to experiencing a mental health crisis. It is this differential you will make to your client that can spark interest and build an alliance. Emphasizing the positive health components of cognitive–behavioral psychology will help eliminate the theory's wrong exclusive association with pathology (Brown et al., 2010).

## *Myth 5: Any Clinician Can Provide Cognitive–Behavioral Therapy*

This perception is probably linked to the "bag of tricks mentality" about cognitive–behavioral therapy. Once you know the tricks, you are an expert. Schinke and Watson (2009) draw on the ethics code set forth by the Association of Applied Sport Psychology when directing that "the critical aspect of competence is that it is acquired with time and effort" (p. 17). It is clear that competence as a cognitive–behavioral psychologist does not happen as a matter of chance or by the ability to follow cook-book methodology. Cognitive–behavioral interventions should be uniquely designed and offered to athletes based on their individual strengths and deficits (Hays, Thomas, Maynard, & Bawden, 2009). It is the result of combined formal study, supervision, and practice that develops the competent professional.

Further, sport psychologists are not qualified to practice based on general interest in sports or previous athletic experience. While experience is a good teacher for many aspects of life and drawing on previous athletic experience may be helpful when building an alliance with a client, it is insufficient for meeting professional standards of practice (Brown & Cogan, 2006).

## Behavioral Interventions in Sport

Cognitive–behavioral interventions in sport abound, but I will focus on three necessary strategies that should be in every sport psychologist's toolbox. Each section includes a brief description of the intervention, a vignette, and a discussion. I also point out potential pitfalls when implementing each strategy.

## Goal Setting

As I emphasized previously, cognitive–behavioral therapy and sport psychology complement each other quite naturally. Athletes are goal- and performance-oriented, much like cognitive–behavioral therapy. A foundational element to cognitive–behavioral therapy is to have at least one specific goal. When athletes commit to goals, it is likely they will strive to meet them and, in that pursuit, desire to apply even more psychological strategies (Crust & Azadi, 2010). It is the role of the psychologist to help an athlete define a goal well and offer additional cognitive–behavioral strategies for reaching it.

A well-defined goal not only is a starting point for working together, but also helps the psychologist and athlete immediately share something in common, ultimately strengthening their growing alliance. Goal setting as a cognitive process is valued as an effective cornerstone to all other performance-enhancement strategies (Meyers, Whelan, & Murphy, 1996).

## Goal Setting Vignette: Alexis on the Run

Alexis, a 26-year-old law student, wants "to run better." She runs every day, but thinks she could make her running "more effective." She explained her work in law school is tedious and time consuming. One evening she went running with a friend who was soon moving to a different state. Alexis experienced the run in such a positive way that she was hooked. When asked what she specifically wanted to improve about her running, she said that she did not know, but she just thought something could be different in a better way.

## Goal Setting: Intervention and Discussion

Alexis's intentions are good. She is motivated and wants help. A key piece that is missing for her is a clear goal. In cases of goal setting, it is helpful to explain two types of goals to an athlete. The first type of goal is an *outcome goal*. An outcome goal is exactly what it sounds like. It is the measure of a performance after it is over. Outcome goals come in the form of a final score, a time or some measurement. What an outcome goal ignores, and what is critical to helping an athlete set healthy goals, is the actual behavior during the performance.

The second type of goal that is critical is the *performance goal*. Performance goals are individualized, personal goals that are unique to an individual performer. it is common to have multiple performance goals within one outing or activity where a goal can be reached. Before identifying performance goals for Alexis, I should emphasize that the other critical criteria for goal setting is ensuring that goals are objective and measurable.

Too often an athlete sets vague goals such as "feeling better about how I played" or "making my coach believe in me." While those goals have meaning to the athlete, it may be unclear when the athlete actually meets that goal. Therefore, it is important to make certain a goal is objective and measureable (this is what we call a "behavioral" goal). I use a two-question test for athletes to determine if they have identified a useful goal. First, to test for objectivity, I ask, "If ten people watched you perform, would they all agree that you met your goal?" Next, to test for measurability, I ask, "Did you use some unit of measurement to describe your goal?" For example, did the athlete use minutes, pounds, seconds, or days or, in the case of emotion, rated its strength on a scale of 1–10? If the answer to both of these questions is yes, then the athlete has likely identified a useful, behaviorally focused performance goal. Additional factors that are crucial when setting performance goals include developing an evaluation and feedback system, sharing goals with encouraging support systems, and ensuring that the athlete has the skill necessary to reach the goal.

In Alexis's case, she would fail the test, would not she? It is the psychologist's responsibility to help her clarify those goals. To help Alexis, the two-question test might sound something like this:

| | |
|---|---|
| CBT: | Alexis, when you are running and enjoying it, what would other people who were watching you say you're doing when that happens. |
| Alexis: | They'd see me running through the city in the evening. |
| CBT: | How long would you have been running when they saw you? |
| Alexis: | About 30 minutes into my run. |
| CBT: | If they were watching for you all of the time, how often would they see you running? |
| Alexis: | Twice a week, probably. Law school keeps me busy, you know! |
| CBT: | You said you wanted your running to be better in a different way. What would all of those people see you doing if your running was better? |
| Alexis: | They'd probably see me more often. When I run I enjoy it so much, but it's hard to find the time to do it. They'd probably see me running with friends, too. |

This example of a brief interchange demonstrates a process of converting an athlete's soft goals into objective, measurable goals. There is more work here to do with Alexis, but she and the psychologist are on a better track to understand what she truly desires. Likely her goal will include increased frequency and time, as well as more social contact. As goals solidify for Alexis, it will become more clear what other behavioral strategies might help her in her quest and how her performance goals will become a priority over her outcome goals.

## Evidenced-Based Self-Talk

The positive influence an athlete's thinking can have on emotion and performance can be significant (Tod, Thatcher, McGuigan, & Thatcher, 2009). For example, Medvic, Madey, and Gilovich (1995) described how Olympic athletes who medaled have a range of thought styles about their success, even though they performed expertly. For two reasons, such research is significant to the athlete who is considering cognitive–behavioral therapy. First, it is helpful for athletes to learn from research that focused on successful, not pathological, athletes. Secondly, focusing on how those athletes think normalizes and perhaps even makes the information gleaned from the research desirable to know. As a clinician, you do not have to trick an athlete into utilizing cognitive–behavioral strategies, but it is important to present the most helpful information in a useful manner so the athlete can make an informed decision.

## Evidence-Based Self-Talk Vignette: Theo's Thoughts

Theo is a 17-year-old high school pitcher. His pitching is inconsistent because his confidence wavers. While he denies it to his coach and parents, he revealed in consultation that he is often intimidated by certain teams or strong hitters. He was able to identify an anxious feeling related to lacking confidence, which surfaced a couple of days before a game against strong performers and continued through his pitching outing.

## Evidenced-Based Self-Talk: Discussion and Intervention

Theo was asked to keep a self-talk log. For his convenience and for compliance, he simply kept an index card in his hip pocket and wrote down three pieces of information: (a) the situation, (b) his thoughts, and (c) the resulting emotion or behavior (see Table 7.2 for a sample of Theo's self-talk log).

Fundamental to cognitive–behavioral therapy is making certain that an individual's thoughts are rational and not distorted. I prefer to use the terms "accurate" and "evidence based" when working with athletes, primarily because words like "irrational" and "distorted" can have a negative connotation. Thinking accurately

Table 7.2 A sample self-talk log

| Situation | Thoughts | Resulting emotion or *behavior* |
|---|---|---|
| Reading box scores of opposing team | "They are going to hit me out of the ballpark." | Anxiety, loss of sleep |
| Pre-game team meeting | "My coach doesn't believe I can pitch well." | Anxiety, decreased confidence |
| Listening to teammates talk about how we need to win | "I'm going to let my team down." | Dread, embarrassment |

about oneself and having evidence for those beliefs is essential for a solid performance. Athletes are usually aware of their performance statistics (times, personal records, averages, and so forth); therefore, the evidence-based way of thinking is quite natural and makes sense.

As Theo reviewed his thought log in session, it was easy to take aim at the thoughts section of the log and identify thinking that had no evidence. For example, Theo thought the batters on the opposing team would hit his pitching so well that he would be embarrassed and removed from the game. Helping him identify that he was predicting the future and that any team is expected to hit the opposing team's pitching caused his anxiety to reduce and made him feel better about throwing in the game.

Many different types of cognitive errors can exist, and it is the cognitive–behavioral psychologist's responsibility to understand how inaccurate ways of thinking can be at work both obviously and covertly. The *Feeling Good Handbook* by David Burns (1999) is a classic read and a good starting point for understanding various distortions that can be upheld and can affect emotion and self-perception.

## Imagery

Imagery, sometimes referred to as visualization in sport psychology, is a heavily researched behavioral technique that demonstrates robust efficacy (Gould, Damarjian, & Greenleaf, 2002). Whether it is used for skill acquisition, relaxation in a pre-competition routine, or mastery of emotional balance and control during competition, imagery is a skill that is likely useful to any athlete who integrates it into a training routine on a regular, consistent basis. Two powerful characteristics of imagery that are particularly advantageous to athletes are vividness and controllability.

Vividness refers to the quality of imagery and how detailed it becomes through the use of all the senses. Sight, sound, smell, touch, and taste help enrich the vividness of a rehearsed image. For example, the sounds of the stadium, the taste of salty sweat on one's lips, the pressure of tightly laced cleats, the smell of popcorn, heat rub ointment, or chlorine each adds a dimension to an athlete's imagery. These details probably help the brain rehearse an experience as if it were real and activates similar parts of the brain, whether the activity is imagined or actually motor based

(Guillot et al., 2009). Also, rehearsing and practicing the performance at the speed it naturally occurs are preferable.

The second factor unique to imagery is controllability. Simply, an athlete can control the image to whatever degree she/he prefers. Athletes can create situations utilizing imagery where they may not otherwise experience or experience infrequently. Taking risks, pushing physical limits, or increasing the frequency of repetitions for practice are ways controllability can be used to maximize imagery's benefits.

Two separate but related measures for understanding an athlete's imagery experience is the Sport Imagery Questionnaire (SIQ; Hall, Stevens, & Paivio, 2005) and the Sport Imagery Questionnaire for Children (SIQ-C; Hall, Munroe-Chandler, Fishburne, & Hall, 2009).

## Imagery Vignette: Tristan Sees Himself Improve

Tristan has been a goalie for his local town soccer team for the past 2 years. Even though he started playing soccer later in life than most of his peers, his natural talent quickly catapulted him to being goalie. Knowing that he had started playing soccer several years after his peers did, he often felt behind and still made some rookie mistakes. He wanted to improve his performance and his confidence, but was already maximizing his time with daily practices and college preparatory classes at school.

## Imagery: Intervention and Discussion

While Tristan's schedule was full, he was able to devote 20 min each day to work on imagery in his bedroom. He used his imagery to expose himself to numerous situations where he had to respond as a goalie. Using an assortment of scenarios, Tristan imagined in real-time himself responding positively, effectively, and confidently on the soccer field. When he was ready, he also imagined making typical goalie errors and then successfully and immediately recovering from them. He found he could actually experience more blocks and situations in 20 min of imagery work than he could during 90 min of practice. Additionally, he was able to develop imagery as a skill that he could use for pre-game work or for taking exams in his college preparatory classes.

## Conclusion

Sport is an extraordinary metaphor for life because it aptly teaches social and intrapersonal values such as resilience, motivation, integrity, and cooperation. Historically, sport has been enjoyed as a cultural activity well before any contemporary psychological theory came along to explain what the brain is doing during competition and how to help it do it better. By now, it is clear that cognitive–behavioral psychology has caught up to sport in many aspects. Athletes, coaches, and parents now have volumes of research and interventions about how cognitive—behavioral psychology can improve performance. The professional sport psychologist today has the responsibility and privilege of working with multifaceted players with typically high expectations for performance. Balancing those expectations, reducing stigmas about mental health, developing an working alliance, and delivering interventions in a skillful, ethical manner are all in a day's work.

## References

Beck, J. (1995). *Cognitive therapy: Basics and beyond*. New York: Guilford.
Brown, J., & Cogan, K. (2006). Ethical clinical practice and sport psychology: When two worlds collide. *Ethics and Behavior, 16*, 15–23.
Brown, J., Fenske, M., & Neporent, L. (2010). *The winner's brain: 8 strategies great minds use to achieve success*. Cambridge, MA: Da Capo Life Long Books.
Burns, D. (1999). *The feeling good handbook*. New York: Plume.
Crust, L., & Azadi, K. (2010). Mental toughness and athletes' use of psychological strategies. *European Journal of Sport Sciences, 10*, 43–51.
Ellis, A. (2001). *Overcoming destructive beliefs, feelings, and behaviors*. Amherst, MA: Prometheus.
Etzel, E., Ferrante, A., & Pinkney, J. (2002). *Counseling college student-athletes: Issues and interventions*. Morgantown, WV Fitness Information Technology.
Freeman, A. (Ed.). (1995). *Encyclopedia of cognitive behavior therapy*. New York: Springer.
Ghinassi, C. (2010). *Anxiety*. Santa Barbara, CA: Greenwood.
Glick, I., & Horsfall, J. (2009). Psychiatric conditions in sports: Diagnosis, treatment, and quality of life. *The Physician and Sportsmedicine, 37*, 29–34.
Gould, D., Damarjian, N., & Greenleaf, C. (2002). Imagery training for peak performance. In J. Van Raalte & B. Brewer (Eds.), *Exploring sport and exercise psychology* (pp. 49–74). Washington, DC: American Psychological Association.
Guillot, A., Collet, C., Nguyen, V., Malouin, F., Richards, C., & Doyon, J. (2009). Brain activity during visual versus kinesthetic imagery: An FMRI study. *Human Brain Mapping, 30*, 2157–2172.
Hall, C., Munroe-Chandler, K., Fishburne, G., & Hall, N. (2009). The sport imagery questionnaire for children (siq-c). *Measurement in Physical Education and Exercise Science, 13*, 93–107.
Hall, C., Stevens, D., & Paivio, A. (2005). *The sport imagery questionnaire: Test manual*. Morgantown, WV Fitness Information Technology.
Hays, K., Thomas, O., Maynard, I., & Bawden, M., (2009). The role of confidence in world-class sport performance. *Journal of Sports Sciences, 27*, 1185–1199.
Kelly, G. (1963). *A theory of personality: The psychology of personal constructs*. New York: Norton.
Medvic, V., Madey, S., & Gilovich, T. (1995). Counterfactual thinking and satisfaction among olympic medalists. *Journal of Personality and Social Psychology, 69*, 603–610.
Meyers, A., Whelan, J., & Murphy, S. (1996). Cognitive behavioral strategies in athletic performance enhancement. *Progress in Behavior Modification, 30*, 137–164.
Nakata, H., Yoshie, M., Miura, A., & Kudo, K. (2010). Characteristics of the athletes' brain: Evidence from neurophysiology and neuroimaging. *Brain Research Reviews, 62*, 197–211.
Ruth, G. (1928). *Babe Ruth's own book of baseball*. New York: Putnam.
Schinke, R., & Watson, J. (2009). An invitation to consider general principles through a CSP lens. *Association for Applied Sport Psychology Newsletter, (23)*1, 17–19.

Tod, D., Thatcher, R., McGuigan, M., & Thatcher, J. (2009). Effects of instructional and motivational self-talk on the vertical jump. *Journal of Strength and Conditioning Research, 23*, 196–202.

Weinburg, R., & Gould, D. (1995). *Foundations of sport and exercise psychology.* Champaign, IL: Human Kinetics.

Wiliams, J., & Leffingwell, T. (2002). Cognitive strategies in sport and exercise psychology. In J. Van Raalte & B. Brewer (Eds.), *Exploring sport and exercise psychology* (pp. 75–98). Washington, DC: American Psychological Association.

# Chapter 8
# Establishing and Maintaining Physical Exercise

**Christopher C. Cushing and Ric G. Steele**

Physical exercise can be defined as any goal-directed activity that is intended to improve or maintain physical fitness, and which involves the movement of skeletal muscles resulting in energy expenditure (Caspersen, Powell, & Christenson, 1985). This definition is important because it establishes the goal-directed nature of *physical exercise,* which distinguishes it from *physical activity.* For example, in reading this chapter, a number of physical activity behaviors will be performed (e.g., turning pages, shifting positions, walking to retrieve refreshments). However, these behaviors are not intended to promote or maintain health and therefore do not constitute physical exercise. Despite the importance of this distinction, it is difficult for researchers to objectively measure bouts of physical exercise, and gross measures of physical activity are usually used as a proxy indicator. Because this chapter is focused on physical exercise promotion, we will discuss findings in terms of physical exercise even when the primary studies used physical activity as an outcome variable.

By way of an overview, we begin with a brief review of the physical and psychological benefits of physical exercise to provide the reader with an understanding of the types of outcomes that have been associated with physical exercise. Next, we aim to present two goal-oriented theoretical frameworks that are regularly applied to physical exercise and describe intervention components that map onto these theoretical frameworks. Finally, we conclude with brief recommendations for practice and future research based on theoretical models.

## Benefits of Physical Exercise

Beyond increasing athletic performance, routine physical exercise has a number of benefits for health and well-being across the lifespan. Individuals who are more physically active have a lower risk of cardiovascular and cardiorespiratory disease,

---

R.G. Steele (✉)
Clinical Child Psychology Program, University of Kansas, Lawrence, KS 66045, USA
e-mail: rsteele@ku.edu

cancer, degenerative bone conditions, endocrine system disorders, and the negative physical sequela associated with obesity (Folsom et al., 1997; WHO, 2004). In addition to higher levels of physical health, individuals that are physically active also experience significant psychological benefits (Hamer, Stamatakis, & Mishra, 2009; Ströle, 2009; Walsh, 2011). One area of recent exploration is the impact of physical exercise on hippocampal volume and memory. Animal models have demonstrated significant increases in brain derived neurotrophic factor (BDNF), hippocampal volume, and memory in rats that engage in more physical exercise (van Praag, 2008). Recently, an intervention trial of prescribed moderate physical exercise (40 min per day × 3 days per week) demonstrated significant salutary changes in hippocampal volume among previously sedentary adults, providing preliminary evidence that physical exercise is linked to central nervous system functioning and subsequent psychological ability (Erickson et al., 2011). Similarly, a 13-week after-school exercise intervention study in overweight children demonstrated significant improvements in cognitive ability with a dose–response effect (Davis et al., 2011). Results indicated that children in exercise groups evidence significantly greater changes in executive functioning compared to a control group. In addition, the investigators discovered a dose–response effect for both mathematics achievement scores and executive functioning, indicating that 40 min of exercise produced superior benefits to 20 min of exercise. Taken together, these studies suggest that many biologically mediated psychological benefits of physical activity are available beyond the physical health benefits of exercise.

Physical exercise also impacts a number of subjectively experienced psychological constructs. Routine physical exercise appears to help alleviate depression (possibly through the BDNF pathways described above); in fact, the evidence for the impact of physical exercise on depression is so convincing that some have called for physical exercise interventions as primary or adjunctive treatments for clinical depression (Fox, 1999; Walsh, 2011). Quality of life (QOL) also shows promise as one of the variables that is most sensitive to change in healthy lifestyle interventions. In a recent meta-analysis of physical exercise interventions, Conn, Hafdahl, and Brown (2009) discovered a small but significant effect size in experimental studies that prescribe physical exercise. It is important to note that these interventions were not designed to modulate QOL directly. This means that physical exercise confers a direct benefit on QOL even when interventions hold changes in other variables as their primary focus (e.g., recovery from myocardial infarct). The finding that physical activity interventions produce changes in QOL is consistent with some descriptive work indicating that children who are more active during the school day experience better QOL irrespective of their weight status (Shoup, Gattshall, Dandamudi, & Estabrooks, 2008). An implication of these studies is that engaging in physical activity even when a disease or physical health process is involved can derive important subjective psychological benefits.

## Baseline Levels of Physical Exercise and Recommendations

The Center for Disease Control (CDC) and the Surgeon General recommend that adults participate in a minimum of 150 min of moderate-to-vigorous physical exercise each week, with an ideal target of 300 min, and that children participate in 60 min of moderate-to-vigorous physical exercise every day of the week (Department of Health and Human Services, 2008; CDC, 2011). A recent analysis of objectively reported physical exercise collected as part of the 2003–2004 National Health and Nutritional Examination Survey (NHANES) revealed that 6–11-year-old children are the only group that can be said to meet their broad moderate-to-vigorous physical exercise recommendations, but even this group was not engaged in enough vigorous physical activity (Troiano et al., 2008). Moreover, compliance with physical exercise recommendations is even poorer when considering bouts of physical exercise lasting 10 min or more, which is thought to be a measure of planful sustained exercise (Troiano et al., 2008).

## Theoretical Models of Health Promotion

"There is nothing so practical as a good theory" (Lewin, 1951, p. 169). Lewin's words are not lost on the modern behavioral scientist. In fact, behavioral psychology has seen a large expansion of theoretical work since the time of Lewin's writing, and it can be difficult to find one overarching theory to guide the development and implementation of physical exercise research. Evidence is available to support a number of important and frequently articulated theories governing the promotion of physical exercise, including Social Cognitive Theory (SCT; Bandura, 2004), Control Theory (CT; Carver & Scheier, 1982), the Theory of Reasoned Action (Fishbein & Ajzen, 1975; Fishbein, 1967), and the Theory of Planned Behavior (Ajzen, 1985; see Rapoff, 2010, for a general review of these theories).

In this chapter we focus primarily on two of these (SCT and CT) for a number of reasons. First, both the Theory of Reasoned Action and the Theory of Planned Behavior significantly overlap with each another (Rapoff, 2010) and frequently do not explain variance above what can be explained using SCT (Bandura, 2004; Dzewaltowski, Noble, & Shaw, 1990). Second, CT and SCT are highlighted here because of the clear link to operant psychology and the implications for setting up antecedents and consequences necessary to establish and maintain physical exercise. More specifically, we believe these theories have both heuristic and practical applications, in that they frequently describe contextual preconditions for behavior change. Below we briefly describe the application of SCT and CT to physical exercise promotion. The sections below are brief discussions of complex theories. The interested reader is referred to Bandura's (2004) application of his theory to health behavior change and Carver and Scheier's (1982) seminal article on CT for additional reading. Finally, we conclude with a comment on the importance of determining the effectiveness of individual theoretical/intervention components.

*Social cognitive theory.* As it applies to physical exercise, SCT specifies that five core factors influence an individual's ability to self-regulate their behavior (Bandura, 2004). First, the individual must have sufficient *knowledge* about the risks of sedentary behavior and benefits of engaging in physical exercise. Indeed, many physical exercise interventions attempt to modulate this factor; a recent review article revealed that 55% of physical activity interventions designed for adults include some component of educating participants about the health consequences of their current behavior (Michie, Abraham, Whittington, McAteer, & Gupta, 2009). Further, in a large meta-analysis of clinical trials to promote physical exercise in adults with chronic illness, Conn, Hafdahl, Brown, and Brown (2008) reported that interventions with supervised exercise sessions were no more effective in changing physical activity than those that relied exclusively on educational or motivational sessions. Given the relatively robust overall effect sizes of included studies, these results underscore the importance of educational and/or motivational components of treatments.

The individual's beliefs about the expected costs and benefits for different health habits make up *outcome expectancies,* the second factor in Bandura's (2004) model. This construct is subdivided into physical, social, and self-evaluative areas. Physical outcome expectations are perhaps most obviously related to physical exercise. An individual who believes that physical exercise will make them tired, sweaty, and uncomfortable can be said to have negative physical outcome expectations and will engage in less physical exercise (Nelson, Benson, & Jensen, 2010). For such individuals, the behavior therapist may need to set graded tasks, provide specific encouragement, and model attentional redirection so that the individual can begin to derive pleasure from physical exercise. Social outcome expectancies include the approval or disapproval (i.e., social contingencies) one receives from others for performing a behavior. The behavior therapist should be careful not to overlook this factor when addressing the initiation of a new physical exercise regimen, especially in overweight or obese individuals. Recent research has indicated that overweight young girls who are dissatisfied with their body engage in significantly more physical activity than those who are happy with their body; however, this healthy exercise behavior is negatively moderated by weight-related criticism (Jensen & Steele, 2009). The final outcome expectancy is self-evaluation. This includes the personal standards and positive and negative evaluations used to judge one's health behavior. The role of the behavior therapist is to ensure that the individual is setting concrete and proximal goals (e.g., "walk for 10 min three times this week") rather than distal or abstract goals (e.g., "get healthy"). By setting concrete proximal goals that can be followed by more close approximations of a long-term goal, the behavior therapist can reduce the negative self-evaluations because the individual is more likely to attain their goal and have a positive appraisal of their own ability (i.e., improved self-efficacy).

Understanding and ameliorating *impediments* or *barriers* to goal attainment constitutes a critical component of Bandura's (2004) model of health behavior promotion. Individuals are often able to think of many barriers to physical activity (e.g., low energy, lack of time, etc.). Using SCT, the behavior therapist may be able to help the individual identify and remove barriers to achieving their goals. This is a common component of interventions for physical exercise; Michie and colleagues (2009) discovered that 42% interventions to affect physical exercise in adults use barrier identification and amelioration as an intervention component. However, Conn et al. (2008) reported that interventions that included barriers management (among adults with chronic illness) were no more effective than interventions that did not include such strategies. Clearly, more work in this area is needed to resolve the unique contribution of barriers management to exercise promotion.

Bandura (2004) has argued that *perceived self-efficacy* is the most central tenet of his theory to explain behavior. Self-efficacy is the belief in one's ability to accomplish a goal. Individuals with higher self-efficacy set loftier goals and remain more firmly committed to them (Bandura, 2004). Bandura posits that self-efficacy has a direct impact on individual behaviors as well as indirect effects, through the four processes detailed above. For example, a person may know that exercise is important to attain cardiovascular health and set a goal to adhere to the Surgeon General's recommendations for physical activity. However, if the individual does not believe that they can engage in aerobic exercise or if they believe that exercise will not lead to their end goal of cardiovascular health, then motivation to engage in the behavior will remain low. They may also believe that their efforts generally do not produce the outcomes that they desire (low self-evaluative outcome expectations). Because self-efficacy is so central to Bandura's (2004) theory, there is not a single intervention component that is thought to modulate self-efficacy; rather, all intervention components of social cognitive interventions affect self-efficacy in each of the four domains identified above.

Two large tests of SCT variables have demonstrated indirect effects of self-efficacy on physical exercise. The largest study to date was conducted by Anderson, Wojcik, Winett, and Williams (2006) in the context of a church-based health-promotion intervention. The investigators used structural equation modeling (SEM) to test the impact of social support, self-efficacy, physical outcome expectations, and self-regulation on physical activity in a group of 999 primarily overweight and obese churchgoers in southwest Virginia. The results of the SEM analysis explained 46% of the variance in objectively measured physical activity. SCT variables that impacted physical exercise were social support mediated by self-efficacy, and self-regulation, underscoring the importance of self-regulation and social support to a healthy lifestyle. In their discussion of the findings, the authors suggested that self-efficacy may be an important intermediate step to physical exercise adoption; however, self-regulation conferred the largest independent effect.

Similarly, Rovniak, Anderson, Winett, and Stephens (2002) examined SCT variables as a predictor of physical exercise in a structural equation model of data from a large sample of undergraduate students. Specifically, the model (which explained 55% of the variance in the data) suggested that social support significantly influenced self-efficacy for exercise and that this relationship was mediated by self-regulation. That is, participants who experienced higher self-efficacy also engaged in more self-regulatory behaviors leading to greater physical exercise adoption. Taken together, the results of Rovniak et al. (2002) and Anderson et al. (2006) indicate that self-efficacy may be the cognitive set that increases the probability of physical exercise occurring, but self-regulation is the observable behavioral support that facilitates an individual's engagement in physical exercise. These are particularly important to the behavioral therapist in that they highlight the importance of assessing social support and self-efficacy for exercise followed by coaching in adoption of self-regulatory behaviors.

*Control theory.* In their seminal article, Carver and Scheier (1982) described interdisciplinary cybernetic control theory and how it can be applied to goal-oriented cognitive–behavioral psychology. CT posits that behavior is a part of a negative feedback loop. The loop is negative because it serves always to reduce the discrepancy between a current state and a reference value (e.g., a goal). The loop functions such that information from the environment (e.g., self-monitoring) is perceived by an individual and compared against a reference value (e.g., goal). According to CT, if the individual perceives a discrepancy between the current state and the reference value, the individual performs a behavior to decrease the discrepancy. Once goals are formulated, individual behaviors are simply an effort to correct the discrepancy between the ideal goal and the current state.

Within CT, all behavior is hierarchically organized. Therefore, an individual can engage in multiple goal-oriented behaviors simultaneously, and each of these behaviors can serve to move the individual closer to multiple hierarchically organized goals at one given time point. Due to this hierarchical organization, CT can be used to explain thoroughly expansive concepts such as engaging in a level of exercise consistent with the sociocultural ideal (e.g., achieving health through exercise, adhering to exercise recommendations, becoming a fit person) as well as lower-order goals such as the contraction of individual muscle groups that produce voluntary running. Therefore, CT is simultaneously more expansive and reductionistic than social learning theory.

Practically, CT requires that an individual sets a goal for physical exercise. For example, an individual may set a goal to walk for 40 min per day 3 days per week. The next step is to monitor one's compliance with the goal. If a self-monitoring record shows that exercise was performed on 2 of 3 days, then the individual uses this feedback to resolve the discrepancy between the goal and the performance. In this system, if the superordinate goal (see above) is "overall health," then the individual will produce a behavioral change to increase physical exercise. By this point, the experienced behaviorist can probably predict that the key intervention components in CT are goal setting (including frequency, intensity, and duration), self-monitoring, feedback, and review of goals. It is important to note, however, that CT would suggest that these processes have a synergistic effect on each other. This does not necessarily require that intervention components always be used in conjunction with one another. For example, modulating self-monitoring may change the feedback available to an individual without requiring that the interventionist actively participate in providing feedback. Nonetheless, interventions that attempt to modulate more than one component of a synergistic system ought to have a larger impact on behavior than those that affect only one component.

A major piece of supporting evidence for the use of CT in physical exercise promotion comes from a meta-regression conducted by Michie and colleagues (2009). The investigators were not able to identify a large number of intervention studies that employed all components of CT (See Table 8.1); however, when CT components were used in combination, they produced larger effect sizes than the largest effect size produced by any one technique alone. This finding argues for the synergistic effect of the theoretically derived intervention components reviewed above. In contrast (and perhaps surprisingly), Conn et al. (2008) reported that though the use of any one CT component (i.e., behavioral strategy) was associated with larger effect sizes than interventions that included none, the inclusion of multiple CT components (e.g., contracting, feedback, goal setting, and self-monitoring) provided no net increase in effect size.

*Importance of self-monitoring.* As we noted previously, it is important to consider individual intervention strategies that appear to affect engagement in physical exercise. Table 8.1 provides a list of Michie and colleagues' (i.e., Abraham & Michie, 2008; Michie et al., 2009) taxonomy of intervention components from the two theoretical frameworks reviewed above.

When considering the importance of individual program components, behavioral interventionists should understand the importance of self-monitoring in physical exercise interventions. Most interventions reviewed by Abraham and Michie (2008) employed self-monitoring of physical exercise as a method of gathering assessment data and providing feedback about goal attainment. Indeed, Michie and colleagues' (2009) meta-analysis revealed self-monitoring to be the most important component of behavioral interventions designed to produce changes in physical exercise.

**Table 8.1** Taxonomy of behavior change techniques from Abraham and Michie (2008) and Michie et al. (2009)

| Theoretical framework | |
| --- | --- |
| Social cognitive theory | Control theory |
| Provide information on consequences | Prompt specific goal setting |
| Prompt intention formation | Prompt review of behavioral goals |
| Prompt barrier identification | Prompt self-monitoring of behavior |
| Provide general encouragement | Provide feedback on performance |
| Set graded tasks | Prompt intention formation |
| Provide instruction | |
| Model or demonstrate the behavior | |

Note: For a review of health behavior change studies using each of the intervention components listed above, see Michie et al. (2009).

Further, in their meta-analysis of exercise promotion programs for adults with chronic illness, Conn et al. (2008) reported that interventions that included self-monitoring produced significantly greater effect sizes than interventions that did not include self-monitoring.

Self-monitoring can include objective data such as a pedometer, which gathers step counts to be recorded in a log and returned to an interventionist. These protocols are remarkably effective at increasing physical exercise. A recent systematic review by Bravata et al. (2007) revealed that participants in randomized controlled trials who used a pedometer significantly increased their physical exercise by 2,491 steps more than control participants; participants in single-group observational studies increased their step count by 2,183 steps per day. An important consideration is that the inclusion of a step goal (e.g., 10,000 steps per day) was a significant predictor of step count, which is also consistent with CT. The evidence is clear, when attempting to modulate physical exercise, there are remarkably sound theoretical and empirical grounds for the inclusion of self-monitoring as an intervention component.

## Typical Intervention Delivery Mechanisms

*Primary care.* Visits to primary care physicians are obvious opportunities to address physical exercise with individuals in need of lifestyle change. Physicians themselves have demonstrated that they are willing and able to participate in brief (<10 min) consultations to promote physical exercise in their patients (Pinto, Goldstein, DePue, & Milan, 1998). However, time constraints in primary care offices leave physicians with barely enough time to make brief verbal and written recommendations, which are largely ineffective at changing physical exercise behaviors (e.g., Hillsdon, Foster, & Thorogood, 2005; Lawlor & Hanratty, 2001).

Nevertheless, some examples do exist that show an additive effect of physician advice, behavioral counseling, and self-monitoring for improving adherence to physical exercise recommendations. For example, Armit and colleagues (2009) recruited a sedentary sample of 50–70-year-old patients presenting to a primary care physician's office. Participants were assigned to receive a brief recommendation from a physician, a brief physician consultation plus a behavioral counseling session with an exercise physiologist, or a brief consultation plus behavioral counseling session and a pedometer for self-monitoring. All participants demonstrated improvements in physical exercise, but the group receiving all three intervention components demonstrated better physical fitness and greater adherence to physical activity recommendations. Therefore, direct recommendations from a physician may be part of helping individuals increase physical exercise, while the ideal primary care intervention will include additional behavioral counseling components.

Future work is needed to help ensure appropriate allocation of resources to individual patients. Baseline patient characteristics such as social support, self-efficacy, and barriers to physical activity mediate the effectiveness of brief behavioral counseling sessions targeting physical exercise (Steptoe, Rink, & Kerry, 2000). Therefore, it is possible that relatively low-effort inexpensive interventions may work for a large portion of the population with good social support, high self-efficacy, and low barriers to physical activity. In these cases, physicians may be able to provide a recommendation for exercise, a low-cost pedometer, and materials for self-management. Before such a program can be effective, however, more emphasis will need to be placed on the assessment of psychosocial variables during primary care visits.

*Community-based programs.* Compared to primary care interventions, community-based physical activity interventions are more well established and better researched. In fact, the evidence base for such programs is so large that a recent cost-effectiveness computer simulation study concluded that seven types of community-based interventions are appropriate for broad dissemination to promote physical activity (Roux et al., 2008). Of the programs that intervened at the individual level (Kriska et al., 1986; Lombard, Lombard, & Winett, 1995), both programs used components of SCT and CT to produce behavior change: program activities were tailored to individual's preferences, interests, or readiness to change; participants were taught specific skills to help improve self-efficacy for exercise activities; and assistance was provided to help participants build social support for healthy behaviors. These characteristics are noteworthy in their similarity to the model evaluated by Anderson and colleagues (2006) above. In addition to the SCT components, individuals were assisted in setting behavioral goals for physical exercise and taught to self-monitor their goal attainment. Beyond SCT and CT, participants were also taught specific operant conditioning skills for self-reward and reinforcement of positive health behaviors.

*School-based interventions.* Not surprisingly, theories of physical activity promotion that are effective in adults are also useful in school-age children and adolescents. Principles of SCT and CT are observed in interventions for school-age children; however, less time is spent identifying barriers to physical exercise, and more structure is placed around opportunities for exercise. For example, in a 2-year trial of the Sports, Play, and Active Recreation for Kids (SPARK) program, Sallis et al. (1997) delivered health-related curriculum combined with self-management strategies such as self-monitoring, goal setting, stimulus control, and self-reinforcement to fourth- and fifth-grade students. Ultimately, the intervention was successful in increasing physical exercise during school, but not during leisure time. This finding is consistent with the larger literature on school physical exercise promotion programs (Dobbins, De Corby, Robeson, Husson, & Tirilis, 2009). The SPARK program was limited to the school setting; however, programs that have included a community-based component in addition to the school curriculum have also demonstrated poor adoption of physical exercise outside the classroom (Nader et al., 1996).

Future work to increase the impact of school-based interventions should consider a socioecological model that includes family involvement. Within the pediatric overweight literature, a consistent predictor of child and adolescent weight loss is parental weight loss (Hunter, Steele, & Steele, 2008; Sato et al., 2011). Such findings indicate that the environmental contingencies at work in children's homes are as important as those in their schools when helping children adopt healthy behaviors.

Dramatic improvements in physical exercise are possible using CT interventions when parents are put in control of making television watching contingent on the performance of physical activity (Roemmich, Gurgol, & Epstein, 2004). In addition, recent work has demonstrated that the natural decline in physical activity observed in adolescence is accelerated in eighth grade when family support for physical activity is low (Dowda, Dishman, Pfeiffer, & Pate, 2007). Taken together, these findings indicate that parents should be targeted for direct intervention regarding their own health behavior as well as their management of their child's behavior.

*Innovative delivery mechanisms.* With the success of fact-to-face interventions for physical exercise, behavior change researchers have begun to look to technology as the next wave of intervention delivery for physical exercise interventions. Within the broad health behavior change literature, it is known that technologically driven interventions are best when they are modeled after what works in face-to-face interventions, are more interactive, and use theoretically meaningful behavior change principles such as goal setting, immediate feedback, self-monitoring, and barriers identification (Cushing & Steele, 2010; Hurling, Fairley, & Dias, 2006; Ritterband et al., 2003). Specific work in the area of physical exercise is relatively limited but appears to hold promise for technologically delivered interventions (e.g., van den Berg, Schoones, & Vilet Vieland, 2007). A recent review of technologically based interventions for general health behavior revealed that theoretically based interventions produce larger effects than atheoretical interventions (Webb, Joseph, Yardley, & Michie, 2010). The results of the review also indicate that many of the theoretically consistent strategies identified above are effective in modifying behavior such as modeling, goal setting, prompt feedback, barrier identification and amelioration, plan for developing social support, self-monitoring, feedback on performance, and education about consequences of behavior.

One successful technologically delivered intervention utilized a totally automated Internet, email, and mobile phone system to increase physical exercise (Hurling et al., 2008). In this study, Hurling and colleagues collected baseline information using a Web-based system to conduct an assessment of barriers to physical exercise and make a plan for participating in physical exercise. The 9-week program was designed to provide both normative and ipsative feedback on physical exercise behavior and employed some cognitive strategies for modifying beliefs about barriers to physical activity. At the end of the trial, participants receiving the intervention demonstrated a significantly greater increase in physical exercise than the control group, and consequently lost more body fat.

## Conclusions and Future Directions

Drawing from the above review of the literature on SCT and CT as it relates to the promotion and maintenance of physical exercise, the following conclusions and recommendations appear warranted. When working with typical individuals (i.e., individuals not engaged in elite athletic competition), the interventionist is encouraged to consider family or peer support for exercise behaviors. Consistent with SCT, the best practice is to create an expectation that support is available to help the individual attain reasonable goals. Consistent with Anderson et al.'s (2006) findings, a "team" approach may facilitate self-efficacy and self-regulation. Further, inclusion of family and/or peers may increase opportunities for modeling of healthy behaviors and social reinforcement of approximations to health-related goals.

Relatedly, the literature suggests that the successful behavior therapist will assess an individual's self-efficacy for exercise and the appropriateness of her/his exercise goals. In individuals with particularly low self-efficacy for physical exercise, the behavior therapist should pay particular attention to ensure that the client has set easily reached proximal goals. This will serve to build self-efficacy and set the stage for self-regulatory interventions, both of which have been shown to be related to successful outcomes in terms of exercise promotion.

As detailed above, both SCT and CT underscore the importance of self-monitoring. Depending on the individual goals, self-monitoring can involve the use of a pedometer, heart-rate monitor, or exercise log. The individual should be instructed to review self-monitoring promptly and to either seek corrective feedback from the behavior therapist in session or to use the self-monitoring record to adjust behavior themselves. The behavior therapist should help the individual identify and remove barriers to exercise. Depending on the individual's level of preparedness for exercise, it may be necessary to provide education, encouragement, and modeling of basic exercise behaviors.

With regard to the adoption of technologically based interventions, we encourage the behavior therapist to hone their skill in applying Abraham and Michie (2008) behavior change taxonomy to commercially available products. For example, sites such as www.livestrong.com help individuals set goals, self-monitor, receive social support, and provide feedback on performance. A recent multiple-baseline study examining the utility of self-monitoring on an iPod Touch$^{TM}$ demonstrated marked and sustained improvement in self-monitoring compliance among three overweight adolescent girls, providing evidence that commercially available products can serve as a helpful adjunct to treatment (Cushing, Jensen, & Steele, 2011).

With regard to the research literature, we argue that research on exercise promotion has reached a point that developing new theories for behavior change has relatively limited utility. As suggested by the similarities in the two theoretical models presented here (as well as the similarity of these models to others not reviewed), there appear to be a set of core principles that can be successfully applied to exercise promotion. In fact, most intervention programs appear to integrate effective aspects of several theories (see Conn et al., 2008; Michie et al., 2009).

Rather, instead of generating new theories to explain the promotion and maintenance of physical exercise, we argue for further elaboration of the conditions and contexts under which known efficacious principles can be effectively implemented (see Glasgow, Lichtenstein, & Marcus, 2003; Steele, Mize-Nelson, & Nelson, 2008). As eloquently explained by Glasgow and colleagues, *efficacy* studies provide evidence that an intervention can be beneficial under "ideal" circumstances, whereas *effectiveness* studies provide evidence that the intervention is beneficial when implemented under "real world" (and usually considerably more difficult) conditions. Our read of the literature suggests that the field has much to offer in terms of *efficacy* (i.e., "what can work"), but somewhat less depth in terms of what "does work" when scaled at the community level.

To this end, Abraham and Michie's (2008) taxonomy for categorizing intervention components may provide a conceptual framework for further studies aimed at "scaling the science up" to programs that can impact larger numbers of individuals. In addition to this conceptual framework, Glasgow, Vogt, and Boles's (1999) RE-AIM dimensions for program evaluation provide a structural framework for understanding the reach, adoption, implementation, and maintenance of health promotion interventions and programs in terms of both efficacy and effectiveness. A great deal of the retrospective work in the area of exercise promotion is reviewed in this chapter. However, prospective component analyses of behavior change components will be necessary to help streamline interventions, and methodologically complex studies may be necessary to fully explore "What components work, for whom, and under what circumstances?" (Elkin, Roberts, & Steele, 2008).

## References

Abraham, C., & Michie, S. (2008). A taxonomy of behavior change techniques used in interventions. *Health Psychology, 27*, 379–387.

Ajzen, I. (1985). From intentions to actions: A theory of planned behavior. In J. Kuhl & J. Beckmann (Eds.), *Action control: From cognition to behavior* (pp. 11–39). Berlin, Heidelberg, New York: Springer.

Anderson, E. S., Wojcik, J. R., Winett, R. A., & Williams, D. M. (2006). Social-cognitive determinants of physical activity: The influence of social support, self-efficacy, outcome expectations, and self-regulation among participants in a church-based health promotion study. *Health Psychology, 25*, 510–520.

Armit, C. M., Brown, W. J., Marshall, A. L., Ritchie, C. B., Trost, S. G., Green, A., et al. (2009). Randomized trial of three strategies to promote physical activity in general practice. *Preventive Medicine, 48*, 156–163.

Bandura, A. (2004). Health promotion by social cognitive means. *Health Education and Behavior, 31*, 143–164.

Bravata, D. M., Smith-Spangler, C., Sundaram, V., Gienger, A. L., Lin, N., Lewis, R., et al. (2007). Using pedometers to increase physical activity and improve health: A systematic review. *JAMA, 298*, 2296–2304.

Carver, C. S., & Scheier, M. F. (1982). Control theory: A useful conceptual framework for personality-social, clinical, and health psychology. *Psychological Bulletin, 92*, 111–135.

Caspersen, C. J., Powell, K. E., & Christenson, G. M. (1985). Physical activity, exercise, and physical fitness: Definitions and distinctions for health-related research. *Public Health Reports, 100*, 126–131.

Centers for Disease Control and Prevention (2011). How much physical activity do children need? Retrieved from http://www.cdc.gov/physicalactivity/everyone/guidelines/children.html.

Conn, V. S., Hafdahl, A. R., & Brown, L. M. (2009). Meta-analysis of quality-of-life outcomes from physical activity interventions. *Journal of Nursing Research, 58*, 175–183.

Conn, V. S., Hafdahl, A. R., Brown, S. A., & Brown, L. M. (2008). Meta-analysis of patient education interventions to increase physical activity among chronically ill adults. *Patient Education and Counseling, 70*, 157–172.

Cushing, C. C., Jensen, C. D., & Steele, R. G. (2011). An evaluation of a personal electronic device to enhance self-monitoring adherence in a pediatric weight management program using a multiple baseline design. *Journal of Pediatric Psychology, 36*, 301–307.

Cushing, C. C., & Steele, R. G. (2010). A meta-analytic review of eHealth interventions for pediatric health promoting and maintaining behaviors. *Journal of Pediatric Psychology, 35*, 937–949.

Davis, C. L., Tomporowski, P. A., McDowell, J. E., Austin, B. P., Miller, P. H., Yanasak, N. E., et al. (2011). Exercise improves executive function and achievement and alters brain activation in overweight children: A randomized controlled trial. *Health Psychology, 30*, 91–98.

Dobbins, M., De Corby, K., Robeson, P., Husson, H., & Tirilis, D. (2009). School-based physical activity programs for promoting physical activity and fitness in children and adolescents aged 6–18. *Cochrane Database Systematic Reviews, 1*, CD007651.

Dowda, M., Dishman, R. K., Pfeiffer, K. A., & Pate, R. R. (2007). Family support for physical activity in girls from 8th to 12th grade in South Carolina. *American Journal of Preventive Medicine, 44*, 153–159.

Dzewaltowski, D. A., Noble, J. M., & Shaw, J. M. (1990). Physical activity participation: Social cognitive theory versus the theories of reasoned action and planned behavior. *Journal of Sport & Exercise Psychology, 12*, 388–405.

Elkin, T. D., Roberts, M. C., & Steele, R. G. (2008). Emerging issues in the continuing evolution of evidence-based practice. In R. G. Steele, T. D. Elkin, & M. C. Roberts (Eds.), *Handbook of evidence-based therapies for children and adolescents: Bridging science and practice* (pp. 569–574). New York: Springer.

Erickson, K. I., Voss, M. W., Prakash, R. S., Basak, C., Szabo, A., Chaddock, L., et al. (2011). Exercise training increases size of hippocampus and improves memory. *Proceedings of the National Academy of Science U S A, 108*, 3017–3022.

Fishbein, M. (1967). *Readings in attitude theory and measurement*. New York: Wiley.

Fishbein, M., & Ajzen, I. (1975). *Belief, attitude, intention, and behavior: An introduction to theory and research*. Reading, MA: Addison-Wesley.

Folsom, A. R., Arnett, D. K., Hutchinson, R. G., Liao, F., Clegg, L. X., & Cooper, L. S. (1997). Physical activity and incidence of coronary heart disease in middle-aged women and men. *Medicine and Science in Sports and Exercise, 29*, 901–909.

Fox, K. R. (1999). The influence of physical activity on mental well-being. *Public Health and Nutrition, 2*(3A), 411–418.

Glasgow, R. E., Lichtenstein, E., & Marcus, A. C. (2003). Why don't we see more translation of health promotion research to practice? Rethinking the efficacy to effectiveness transition. *American Journal of Public Health, 93*, 1261–1267.

Glasgow, R. E., Vogt, T. M., & Boles, S. M. (1999). Evaluating the public health impact of health promotion interventions: The RE-AIM framework. *American Journal of Public Health, 89*, 1322–1327.

Hamer, M., Stamatakis, E., & Mishra, G. (2009). Psychological distress, television viewing, and physical activity in children aged 4 to 12 years. *Pediatrics, 123*, 1263–1268.

Hillsdon, M., Foster, C., & Thorogood, M. (2005). Interventions for promoting physical activity. *Cochrane Database Systematic Reviews, 1*, CD003180.

Hunter, H. L., Steele, R. G., & Steele, M. M. (2008). Family based treatment for pediatric overweight: Parental weight loss as a predictor of children's treatment success. *Children's Health Care, 37*, 112–125.

Hurling, R., Catt, M., De Boni, M., Fairley, B. W., Hurst, T., Murray, P., et al. (2008). Using internet and mobile phone technology to deliver an automated physical activity program: Randomized controlled trial. *Journal of Medical Internet Research, 9*, 1–12.

Hurling, R., Fairley, B. W., & Dias, M. B. (2006). Internet-based exercise intervention systems: Are more interactive designs better? *Psychology and Health, 21*, 757–772.

Jensen, C. D., & Steele, R. G. (2009). Body dissatisfaction, weight criticism, and self-reported physical activity in preadolescent children. *Journal of Pediatric Psychology, 34*, 822–826.

Kriska, A. M., Bayles, C., Cauley, J. A., LaPorte, R. E., Sandler, R. B., & Pambianco, G. (1986). A randomized exercise trial in older women: Increased activity over two years and the factors associated with compliance. *Medicine and Science in Sports and Exercise, 18*, 557–562.

Lawlor, D. A., & Hanratty, B. (2001). The effect of physical activity advice given in routine primary care consultations: A systematic review. *Journal of Public Health Medicine, 23*, 219–226.

Lewin, K. (1951). *Field theory in social science: Selected theoretical papers*. New York: Harper & Row.

Lombard, D. N., Lombard, T. N., & Winett, R. A. (1995). Walking to meet health guidelines: The effect of prompting frequency and prompt structure. *Health Psychology, 14*, 164–170.

Michie, S., Abraham, C., Whittington, C., McAteer, J., & Gupta, S. (2009). Effective techniques in healthy eating and physical activity interventions: A meta-regression. *Health Psychology, 28*, 690–701.

Nader, P. R., Sellers, D. E., Johnson, C. C., Perry, C. L., Stone, E. J., Cook, K. C., et al. (1996). The effect of adult participation in a school-based family intervention to improve children's diet and physical activity: The child and adolescent trial for cardiovascular health. *American Journal of Preventive Medicine, 25*, 455–464.

Nelson, T. D., Benson, E. R., & Jensen, C. D. (2010). Negative attitudes toward physical activity: Measurement and role in predicting physical activity among preadolescents. *Journal of Pediatric Psychology, 35*, 89–98.

Pinto, B. M., Goldstein, M. G., DePue, J. D., & Milan, F. B. (1998). Acceptability and feasibility of physician-based activity counseling. The PAL project. *American Journal of Preventive Medicine, 15*, 95–102.

Rapoff, M. A. (2010). *Adherence to pediatric medical regimens* (2nd Ed.). New York: Springer.

Ritterband, L. M., Gonder-Frederick, L. A., Cox, D. J., Clifton, A. D., West, R. W., & Borowitz, S. M. (2003). Internet interventions: In review, in use, and into the future. *Professional Psychology Research and Practice, 34*, 527–534.

Roemmich, J. N., Gurgol, C. M., & Epstein, L. H. (2004). Open-loop feedback increases physical activity of youth. *Medicine and Science in Sports and Exercise, 36*, 668–673.

Roux, L., Pratt, M., Tengs, T. O., Yore, M. M., Yanagawa, T. L., Van Den Bos, J., et al. (2008). Cost effectiveness of community-based physical activity interventions. *American Journal of Preventive Medicine, 35*, 578–588.

Rovniak, L. S., Anderson, E. S., Winett, R. A., & Stephens, R. S. (2002). Social cognitive determinants of physical activity in young adults: A prospective structural equation analysis. *Annals of Behavioral Medicine, 24*, 149–156.

Sallis, J. F., McKenzie, T. L., Alcaraz, J. E., Kolody, B., Faucette, N., & Hovell, M. F. (1997). The effects of a 2-year physical education program (SPARK) on physical activity and fitness in elementary school students. Sports, play and active recreation for kids. *American Journal of Public Health, 87*, 1328–1334.

Sato, A. F., Jelalian, E., Hart, C. N., Lloyd-Richardson, E. E., Mehlenbeck, R. S., Neill, M., et al. (2011). Associations between parent behavior and adolescent weight control. *Journal of Pediatric Psychology, 36*, 451–460.

Shoup, J. A., Gattshall, M., Dandamudi, P., & Estabrooks, P. (2008). Physical activity, quality of life, and weight status in overweight children. *Quality of Life Research, 17*, 407–412.

Steele, R. G., Mize-Nelson, J. A., & Nelson, T. D. (2008). Methodological issues in the evaluation of therapies. In R. G. Steele, T. D. Elkin, & M. C. Roberts (Eds.), *Handbook of evidence-based therapies for children and adolescents: Bridging science and practice* (pp. 25–43). New York: Springer.

Steptoe, A., Rink, E., & Kerry, S. (2000). Psychosocial predictors of changes in physical activity in overweight sedentary adults following counseling in primary care. *American Journal of Preventive Medicine, 31*(2 Pt 1), 183–194, doi: 10.1006/pmed.2000.0688.

Ströle, A. (2009). Physical activity, exercise, depression and anxiety disorders. *Journal of Neural Transmission, 116*, 777–784.

Troiano, R. P., Berrigan, D., Dodd, K. W., Masse, L. C., Tilert, T., & McDowell, M. (2008). Physical activity in the United States measured by accelerometer. *Medicine and Science in Sports and Exercise, 40*, 181–188.

U.S. Department of Health and Human Services (2008). Physical activity guidelines for Americans. Retrieved from http://www.health.gov/paguidelines/factsheetprof.aspx.

van den Berg, M. H., Schoones, J. W., & Vilet Vieland, T. P. M. (2007). Internet-based physical activity interventions: A systematic review of the literature. *Journal of Medical Internet Research, 9*, 71–86.

van Praag, H. (2008). Neurogenesis and exercise: Past and future directions. *Neuromolecular Medicine, 10*, 128–140.

Walsh, R. (2011). Lifestyle and mental health. *American Psychologist*, Advance online publication. www.apa.org/pubs/journals/releases/amp-ofp-walsh.pdf.

Webb, T. L., Joseph, J., Yardley, L., & Michie, S. (2010). Using the internet to promote health behavior change: A systematic review and meta-analysis of the impact of theoretical basis, use of behavior change techniques, and mode of delivery on efficacy. *Journal of Medical Internet Research, 12*(1), e4.

World Health Organization (2004). *Global strategy on diet, nutrition, and physical activity*. Geneva: World Health Organization.

# Chapter 9
# Behavioral Momentum in Sports

Henry S. Roane

## Introduction

The property of momentum is one of the most fundamental principles of physics. The basis of physical momentum is Newton's second law of motion, which states that the change in the movement of an object is inversely related to its mass. Thus, momentum describes the relationship between the velocity of an object and the mass of that object. This relationship is expressed as $p = mv$, where momentum ($p$) is a product of the mass ($m$) and velocity ($v$) of an object. Thus, the greater physical mass or velocity an object has, the greater is its momentum. Conversely, the greater an object's momentum, the more opposing force required to alter the object's momentum.

The property of momentum applies to multiple dimensions of the physical world, including sports performance. It is common for athletic competition to involve physical momentum that is altered by some alternative physical event. To illustrate, a running back weighing 93 kg running at a speed of 8 m/s would have momentum of 744 kg m/s. If the running back's forward progress is disrupted by an external event (e.g., a linebacker), his velocity would decrease, thus decreasing his momentum. Likewise, the amount of force applied by the opposing player (e.g., a 143-kg defensive lineman or an 86-kg cornerback) to the running back will affect the degree to which the running back's momentum is disrupted. Alternatively, a player who is smaller than the running back (e.g., a wide receiver) might have less momentum and, consequently, might be differentially affected when hit by a defensive lineman or cornerback.

All sports, whether they are considered "contact" sports (e.g., hockey, rugby) or "non-contact" sports (e.g., tennis, baseball), involve manipulations of physical momentum in some form. For example, in American football, a particularly hard tackle might be affected by momentum (e.g., a fast-moving linebacker hits a

---

H.S. Roane (✉)
Department of Pediatrics and Psychiatry, SUNY Upstate Medical University, Syracuse, NY 13210, USA
e-mail: roaneh@upstate.edu

quarterback who is slowing down while running out of bounds). Likewise, in racing, the momentum of one car coming out of a turn might be greater than that of a competitor, thus allowing the first car to overtake the second one (e.g., "Schumacher had the momentum going into Turn 1, which allowed him to get by Button," *SpeedTV* coverage of the Spanish Grand Prix, May 9, 2010). In both cases, the term momentum is correctly applied in that the objects in question (a car or the linebacker) have physical attributes that are measurable. Understanding the impact of physical momentum might affect the development and enforcement of rules regarding safety in sports. For example, in baseball a metal bat is usually lighter than a wooden bat. Consequently, a swing with a metal bat is likely to generate more velocity than one with a wooden bat, resulting in the batter hitting the ball harder, which might be beneficial in gameplay (e.g., more likely to hit a homerun). However, harder hit balls might also increase the likelihood of more severe injuries, which has led to some bans on the use of metal bats in baseball (Rivera, 2007).

Although the term momentum can be technically applied to some physical aspects of sporting behavior, this is not the most common manner in which momentum is discussed in sports. Rather, momentum is a term commonly used to describe some aspect of psychological behavior in sports. Any sports fan is familiar hearing about a player having momentum in a sporting contest (e.g., a shooter with a "hot hand") or a team gaining/losing momentum over the course of a season (Bresnahan, 2010). In addition, the term "momentum" is frequently applied to describe the behavior of an individual or a team in sports. It is not uncommon to hear commentary on a team carrying momentum into a coming season, an individual building on the momentum established from a previous game, or, within the context of a game, a team gaining or losing momentum (Deford, 1999). Even some popular sports video games have a measure of momentum to indicate which team is more likely to play better throughout a contest. As noted by Mace, Lalli, Shea, and Nevin (1992), this form of momentum is based on the notion that "success breeds success." Conversely, there is the implication that playing poorly will lead to additional poor play (i.e., the wheels coming off), which might be interpreted as "losing" momentum. In these descriptions, the term momentum is applied as a metaphor. That is, the behavior described (e.g., winning several games at the end of the season) has no true mass or velocity per se; rather the term is used to describe what might be considered a psychological form of momentum.

## Psychological Momentum in Sports

The term momentum is frequently applied to describe individual or team sports performance. And, unsurprisingly, there is literature in the field of sports psychology that discusses this type of momentum. Within athletic competition, psychological momentum has been described in the simplest form as winning the first match or scoring first (e.g., Weinberg, Richardson, & Jackson, 1981). More complex definitions of psychological momentum are multidimensional and incorporate a variety of psychological constructs. For example, Iso-Ahola and Mobily (1980) described momentum as changes in the perceptions of events that occurred early in a given competition and the impact of those events on subsequent gameplay (defined as cognitive and physiological changes in behavior that are associated with better or worse success later in the game). Taylor and Demick (1994) described a model of psychological momentum in sports in which momentum is accounted for by changes in precipitating events (i.e., events in the course of a game that might be deemed positive or negative by the players), cognition/affect (e.g., reports of how likely a player/team was to make another goal, shot, etc.), and changes in behavioral persistence and performance (e.g., altering shot selection), which result in changes in the behavior of the target individual or team and the opponent.

As might be expected from the varying ways in which momentum has been conceptualized and quantified, research in sports psychology has demonstrated wide-ranging results about the extent to which certain variables affect momentum. Gayton, Very, and Hearns (1993) examined momentum (defined as scoring first or "winning" the first period of play) within professional hockey. These results found that scoring first or winning the first period was associated with winning the game in 66.5% and 72.5% of cases, respectively. These results are, of course, correlational, as many other variables can affect the outcome of a game; yet the results of Gayton et al. are similar to other results involving individual sports performance (e.g., scoring first in a tennis match increases the probability of winning that match; Silva, Hardy, & Grace, 1988).

Regarding more complex models of psychological momentum, Taylor and Demick (1994) found that individuals who won a tennis match were more likely to have experienced a preponderance of positive precipitating events than negative precipitating events (with the inverse being true for losers of the match). In a follow-up investigation, Mack and Stephens (2000) used a basketball shooting task to evaluate psychological momentum. These results showed that poorer momentum (defined as making or missing one of three shots) was associated with changes in cognition (i.e., lower self-efficacy and affect ratings). However, poorer momentum was not clearly correlated with response persistence, a finding that was somewhat contradictory with previous research.

In sum, the field of sports psychology has presented a range of conceptual models for approaching an analysis of momentum in sports. Collectively, the results of previous investigations afford the following conclusions: (a) scoring first is better in terms of an increased likelihood of winning a game, (b) experiencing events that are more favorable is associated with a greater probability of winning, and (c) good performance is associated with reports of better psychological function regarding gameplay. Although this research may offer insights into sports performance, methods of consultation, and coaching strategies, the types of procedures used in the studies noted above are uncommon within the context of behavior analysis. Two of the defining characteristics of behavior analysis are a focus on observable events (rather than self-report of psychological constructs) and a link between the behavior being observed and some well-researched conceptual model of behavior (Baer, Wolf, & Risley, 1968). Consequently, behavior analytic examinations of momentum in sports have involved direct observation and quantification of sports-related behavior and linking this behavior to a broader conceptualization of response persistence. Prior to discussing previous behavior analytic research on momentum in sports, it is important to introduce the theoretical underpinning of that research.

## Momentum and Behavior Analysis

Within the field of behavior analysis, the property of momentum has been applied metaphorically to describe the behavior of various organisms under differing conditions. Although this description of momentum is not technically accurate (e.g., behavior has no specific mass), the metaphor of "behavioral momentum" is used to describe the relationship between response rate and resistance to behavior change when certain "disrupter" events occur (Nevin, 1996). Within the framework of behavioral momentum, the velocity of a response is analogous to the rate of reinforcement. Mass is conceptualized as the persistence of behavior over time following at least one event change (e.g., no longer providing reinforcement for responding). Thus, behavioral momentum is a two-component variable that includes the ongoing rate of the response and the resistance of change in response rate when responding is disrupted by programmed (or unprogrammed) variables (Nevin, Mandell, & Atak, 1983). Though an in-depth discussion of behavioral momentum is beyond the scope of this chapter, a brief overview of the procedures and general findings of this conceptualization of behavior is necessary to understand the role of behavioral momentum in sports performance.

In basic laboratory research, behavioral momentum is commonly evaluated in a multiple-schedule paradigm. In a multiple schedule, there are at least two distinct behavioral contingencies presented, each of which is associated with a unique discriminative stimulus. The combination of the contingency and its respective discriminative stimulus is referred to as a component. To evaluate behavioral momentum, the researcher first establishes stabile patterns of responding in one component. Next, that component is removed and the second component (different contingency and different discriminative stimulus) is introduced. The second component might involve reinforcing the behavior less frequently or not at all (i.e., extinction). The variable of interest is how long responding persists when the contingencies change from the first component to the second (e.g., responses that persist longer in the second component are deemed to have greater momentum).

Using an approach similar to that described above, Nevin, Tota, Torquato, and Shull (1990) evaluated resistance to change in a laboratory environment using pigeons as subjects. The birds were trained to peck colored light panels, each of which was associated with a different rate of reinforcement (e.g., 15 reinforcers per hour). In one condition, responding on the left panel produced reinforcement at a rate of 45 per hour and responding on the right panel resulted in 15 reinforcers per hour. In two other conditions, responding on the left panel resulted in no reinforcement, whereas responding on the right panel resulted in relatively low (15 reinforcers per hour) or relatively high (60 reinforcers per hour) rates of reinforcement. Once stabile responding was achieved in these conditions, this responding was disrupted either by giving the pigeons extra food (satiation) or by presenting a situation in which responding on the panels no longer produced reinforcement (extinction). Resistance to behavioral change was assessed by comparing responding under each of these conditions to behavior under the disrupter context for extended period of time (e.g., 4 h). Each condition produced a different slope of responding in relation to how much behavior persisted after exposure to the disruptor. Responding under some conditions (left panel responding for 15 reinforcers per hour) decreased more quickly than under other contexts (e.g., when left panel responding resulted in 15 reinforcers per hour and right panel responding resulted in 45 reinforcers per hour). These results showed that resistance to change varied as a function of the context in which initial responding was trained (i.e., responding in the different contexts varied in terms of behavioral momentum).

The roots of behavioral momentum lie within the experimental analysis of behavior. However, this general principle has been applied frequently to issues of clinical concern. Initially, this application consisted of procedures designed to increase client compliance with difficult-to-complete instructions. For example, Mace et al. (1988) applied Nevin's model of behavioral momentum to decrease noncompliance with instructions for four individuals with developmental disabilities. Participants were identified to be noncompliant with specific tasks (e.g., cleaning the bathroom). These tasks were deemed low-probability tasks in reference to the participants' uncommon rate of completion. By contrast, a series a "high probability" tasks were identified for each participant (e.g., prompting the participants to give a high five). In general, noncompliance with low-probability requests was high when these tasks were presented sequentially. However, when these same tasks were embedded within a sequence of high-probability tasks (e.g., four high-probability instructions preceded a low-probability instruction), noncompliance with the low-probability tasks decreased significantly. From the perspective of behavioral momentum, the higher rate of reinforcement obtained with the high-probability instructions produced a response sequence that was more resistant to change when a disrupter event (i.e., a low-probability instruction) was presented. Said another way, the momentum of compliance with the high-probability requests led to greater compliance with low-probability requests. Since Mace's initial application of the behavioral momentum metaphor to the treatment of problematic behavior, the efficacy of the high-probability instructional sequence has been replicated repeatedly in various response-acquisition programs (e.g., Belfiore, Lee, Vargas, & Skinner, 1997) and in the treatment of problematic behavior disorders (e.g., Dawson et al., 2003; Zarcone, Iwata, Mazaleski, & Smith, 1994). In addition, the effects of response persistence have recently been evaluated within the context of treatments for problematic behavior displayed by individuals with developmental disabilities (Mace et al., 2010).

## Previous Research on Behavioral Momentum and Sports

Although there are likely sport-specific variables that affect an individual's or a team's momentum, some researchers have catalogued events that seem to influence an observer's interpretation of momentum. Burke, Burke, and Joyner (1999) had a seasoned (former player and coach) basketball observer watch 14 basketball games (11 college and 3 high school) and report when a team started to show "momentum." The observer then indicated the events that preceded the team's momentum (e.g., a dunk, causing a turnover, a string of unanswered points, crowd noise), events that occurred during momentum (e.g., steals, blocked shots, dunks, 3-point goals), and events that ended the momentum (e.g., time-out, steal, turnover). The latter category was scored for both the team that possessed momentum and their opponent. Across 50 observed momentum events, the most common momentum started was good play by one team and poor play by the other. Specific to events that started momentum, 3-point shots, defensive stops, and steals were the most often cited events. Within a momentum run, the primary observed events were turnovers (favoring the momentum team), increased crowd noise, defensive stops, and steals. Finally, the events that were most often associated with the end of momentum were a turnover by the momentum team, missed shots by the momentum team, and time-outs called by the opponent. As might be expected, the momentum team was found to outscore the opponent by a margin of 7.58 to 2.62 during the momentum interval.

The descriptive results of Burke et al. (1999) are interesting because they contribute to a number of events that could be categorized as potential reinforcers or, in the case of momentum-ending events, disruptors. As noted in the previous section, responses that result in a high rate of reinforcement are more likely to be resistant to a disruptor event. That is, those responses may be said to have greater behavioral momentum. In other words, as an individual's behavior results in more and more reinforcer delivery, the responding of that behavior should be more likely to persist (i.e., greater momentum) than the behavior of a responder who contacts less reinforcement. As noted previously, this procedure has been the focus of a number of investigations in both experimental and applied research (see Nevin, 1996, for a review). In addition, the generality of the behavioral momentum metaphor has also been examined within the context of sport performance (albeit in a relatively small set of investigations).

Mace et al. (1992) applied the concept of behavioral momentum to men's college basketball. The premise of their research was similar to that of others who have examined the notion of momentum in sports. However, rather than evaluating psychological interpretations of momentum, Mace et al. conceptualized momentum in relation to the property of momentum in physics. Specifically, good gameplay was conceptualized as "velocity" (i.e., response rate), and continued good game performance when faced with some adverse event (e.g., a turnover favoring the opponent) was equated with "mass." Using a sample of college basketball games, Mace et al. sought to address the performance within the framework of behavioral momentum along two dimensions: (a) whether a team would perform better after an adverse event if their pre-event scoring rate was relatively high or low and (b) whether a team's scoring rate would persist following a period of time-out.

Mace et al. (1992) examined the responding of 14 teams across seven college tournament basketball games (although two teams were dropped from data analysis given atypical distributions of local reinforcement rates; described below). Data were collected on three classes of events: (a) reinforcers obtained by the target team (i.e., 3-point goals, 2-point goals, 1-point foul shots, steals/turnovers favoring the target team), (b) adversities encountered by the target team (i.e., turnovers favoring the opponent team, missed field goals or free throws, committing a shooting foul), and (c) responses to those adversities (i.e., a reinforcer or adversity that occurred during the first possession following an adversity). Responses to adversities were categorized as favorable or unfavorable depending on the nature of the target team's first response following an adversity (i.e., whether they encountered a reinforcer or another adversity).

Using these data, Mace et al. (1992) calculated an overall rate of reinforcement for the entire sample. These results indicated that, on average, reinforcers occurred once per minute. Next, the data collected by Mace et al. were examined to address the two principal research questions. To determine if a team's response to an adversity was associated with their rate of reinforcement before that adversity, the authors calculated the number of reinforcers that occurred during each 3-min interval that preceded an adversity (i.e., a local rate of reinforcement). These local reinforcement rates were then grouped into three categories: relatively low (0 or 0.33), medium (0.67 or 1.0), and high (1.33 or better). Following computation of the local reinforcement rates, the data on each team's response to a given adversity was assessed by examining the percentage of those adversities that were responded to favorably relative to the local rate of reinforcement. Mace et al. noted a positive correlation between a team's local rate of reinforcement and their having a positive response to an adversity. To illustrate, teams with a low local rate of reinforcement (0 or 0.33) responded favorably to an adversity 44.1% of the time, whereas teams with high local rates of reinforcement (1.33 or more) responded favorably 68% of the time. Overall, the likelihood of a favorable response to an adversity increased as the local rate of reinforcement increased for 67% of the teams in the analysis.

To address the second research question, how a team's performance would be affected by an opponent calling a time-out, Mace et al. (1992) calculated a ratio of the target team's and their opponent's local rates of reinforcement. The presentation of these ratios permitted a comparison of the two team's reinforcement rates at any given point in the game. The authors then evaluated these ratios for each 3-min interval that preceded a time-out, each 3-min interval that followed a time-out, and the overall course of the game (independent of 3-min intervals before time-outs). In general, teams were more likely to call a time-out when their opponent's rate of reinforcement was 2.63 times greater than their own. Interestingly, the results showed that the average reinforcement ratio dropped from 2.63 before the time-out to 1.11 following the time-out. This outcome clearly suggests that calling a time-out was an effective method of disrupting a team's rate of reinforcement. Said another way, calling a time-out was an effective method of altering a team's momentum.

In a follow-up investigation, Roane, Kelley, Trosclair, and Hauer (2004) examined the generality of the Mace et al. (1992) findings by examining the influence of behavioral momentum with women's college basketball. The rationale for the Roane et al. investigation was that women's college basketball was associated with unique differences relative to men's basketball. These variables could have affected gameplay and, correspondingly, relative rate of reinforcement. To illustrate, Roane et al. noted that women's basketball was associated with different rules regarding ball advancement and the shot clock (5 s shorter in women's basketball at the time of the investigation). In effect, these variables could alter the "pace" of a game. Likewise, women's basketball often differs from men's basketball in terms of the style of play (e.g., more perimeter play in women's basketball) and gender differences for certain basketball-related abilities (Smith, 2002). Again, these variables could have resulted in alterations in reinforcement obtainment (e.g., outside shots are generally less accurate than shots made in the post). The authors postulated that these two variables, differences in rules and style of play, could have altered obtained rates of reinforcement, which might have made women's basketball less resistant to the influence of disruptor events.

Roane et al. (2004) used data collection procedures and operational definitions that were similar to those developed by Mace et al. (1992). Specifically, data were collected on three class of events for each of the 12 teams (i.e., each game was watched twice, and each team was recorded as the target team in the separate viewings). The events included reinforcers obtained by the target team (i.e., 3-point goals, 2-point goals, 1-point foul shots, steals/turnovers favoring the target team), adversities encountered by the target team (i.e., turnovers favoring the opponent team, missed field goals or free throws, committing a shooting foul), and responses to those adversities (i.e., a reinforcer or adversity that occurred during the first possession following an adversity). Data were collected across a series of six college basketball games during a national women's championship tournament.

Results of the Roane et al. (2004) analysis were examined using the same data analysis procedures described by Mace et al. (1992). First, an overall rate of reinforcement was calculated for each team by dividing the number of reinforcers obtained by the length of the game (i.e., total game time consisted of all play time and time-out periods but did not include the halftime duration). As expected, Roane et al. observed a lower overall rate of reinforcement for women's basketball (0.67 reinforcers per min) than that observed by Mace et al. for men's basketball (1.0 reinforcers per min). Next, local rates of reinforcement were examined to evaluate the extent to which a team's local rate of reinforcement would affect that team's response to an adversity. This measure was calculated by counting the number of reinforcers that occurred in a 4.5-min period prior to an adversity (Note: Roane et al. used a 4.5-min interval, rather than a 3-min interval used by Mace et al., to hold constant an average of three reinforcers before an adversity; recall that the average rate of reinforcement was lower in the Roane et al. sample than in the Mace et al. sample). The local rates of reinforcement were then grouped into categories that characterized generally poor performance (reinforcement rate of 0–0.44), better performance (reinforcement rate of 0.67–1.11), and good performance (reinforcement rate of 1.33 or greater). These rates were then examined as to each team's responses to adversities given their local reinforcement rate. Across teams, Roane et al. found a general relation between local rate of reinforcement and favorable responses to adversities. For example, at a low level of performance (0 or 0.44 reinforcers per min), 37% of adversities were responded to favorably; this increased to 49% for good levels of performance (1.33 or greater). This outcome was similar to the positive correlation observed by Mace et al., though Roane et al. found no such differences in response to adversities when unweighted means were used to analyze the results. On a team-by-team basis, the results of Roane et al. also differed slightly from those of Mace et al. Specifically, Roane et al. found that responses to adversities increased as a function of rate of reinforcement for the minority of teams (4 of 12) in their sample, whereas this effect was noted for more teams (8 of 12) in the Mace et al. investigation.

By contrast, the results of the Mace et al. (1992) and Roane et al. (2004) investigations yielded similar outcomes regarding the extent to which a time-out called by the opponent effectively functioned as a disruptor event. Both studies found that a target team calling a time-out was an effective disruptor event in terms of decreasing the opponent's reinforcement ratio. Specifically, Roane et al. found that calling a time-out decreased average reinforcement ratios from 2.35 before the time-out to 0.64 after the time-out (similar to the respective 2.63 and 1.11 reinforcement ratios noted by Mace et al. under the same contexts).

Although somewhat disparate results were found in aspects of the Mace et al. (1992) and Roane et al. (2004) investigations, the general conclusion suggests that sports behavior is amenable to the application of the behavioral momentum metaphor. In light of the differences found regarding individual team's responses to adversities, one might argue that the Roane et al. results actually strengthen the conclusions drawn by Mace et al. That is, Roane et al. noted lower overall reinforcement rates (0.67 reinforcers per min) than Mace et al. (1.0 reinforcers per min) and also found less favorable responses to adversities for the women's sample relative to the men's sample. These data support the use of the behavioral momentum metaphor in that resistance to change is dependent upon the rate of reinforcement. Thus, it is consistent with the findings of previous research on behavioral momentum that the overall lower rate of reinforcement in women's basketball would be associated with a general less favorable response to adversities.

## Extension of the Behavioral Momentum Metaphor to Other Sports

The combined results of Mace et al. (1992) and Roane et al. (2004) suggest that the behavioral momentum metaphor can be applied to the sports performance. The impact of behavioral momentum can be felt upon the performance of a team and (perhaps) that of individual athletes. Also, there are two potential avenues of ongoing research regarding the application of behavioral momentum to sports performance. The first involves examining the generality of the Mace et al. and Roane et al. results to sports other than college basketball. The second involves extending the momentum metaphor as an intervention to improve sports performance. This section will briefly discuss the potential use of data derived from momentum analysis and sports and potential areas of future investigation.

The results of Mace et al. (1992) and Roane et al. (2004) suggest that calling a time-out is an effective strategy for decreasing an opponent's rate of reinforcement.

Having said that, both studies found that certain teams were more effective at being able to determine when it was best to call a time-out. Mace et al. noted that one team in their sample (Illinois) called a time-out at a much less disparate reinforcement ratio than did another team (Michigan). Similar individual team differences were noted in the sample obtained by Roane et al. This could be because coaches tend to base their decisions for calling a time-out on factors other than relative reinforcement rates (Duke & Corlett, 1992). However, these combined results suggest that coaches should pay greater attention to ongoing reinforcement ratios for their team and for individual players such that coaches can make empirically based decisions about when it is best to call a time-out. It is not uncommon for a college basketball team to have approximately five assistants on a bench during a given game. One of these assistants could be charged with calculating ongoing rates for this purpose such that coaches make decisions regarding the use of time-out on more quantitative data.

Rates of reinforcement during basketball games could also be assessed on an individual-player basis. Such information might be useful for determining offensive strategy (i.e., increasing the probability of getting the ball to a player with a higher rate of reinforcement in a given timeframe) or defensive strategy (e.g., double-teaming such a player). Anecdotally, many sports observers would likely agree that teams try to give the ball to a player who is having a "hot streak," though the notion of getting "hot" in basketball has been challenged (Gilovich, Valone, & Tversky, 1985). However, it appears that such decisions are primarily made on a player's scoring performance as opposed to his or her obtainment of other reinforcers (e.g., taking a charge, generating a steal). Mace et al. (1992) noted that identifying "hot" players and targeting them accordingly might be an effective way of affecting overall team performance. For example, if the "hot" player scores when the ball is passed to him/her, this would also reinforce the player who passed the ball or another player who set up a screen that would, in turn, affect the class of responses that are generally thought of as good team play.

Basketball is unique among team sports. For example, in basketball there is a fairly high rate of possession changes. Other sports such as hockey and soccer also have a high rate of possession change; however, these sports are associated with less obtainment of points (a reinforcer) than basketball. Such differences obviously affect the overall rate of reinforcement that occurs in a game. When attempting to apply the behavioral momentum metaphor to other sports, one must consider the types of reinforcers and adversities encountered in those sports. For example, soccer is associated with adversities (e.g., offsides) and reinforcers (e.g., corner kicks) that are unique to that sport. A relative abundance of either event could affect overall team performance even though the number of points obtained in a match is relatively low. Managers already make attempts to address such events by "slowing down the game" through shorter passes, more controlled ball handling, etc. However, it would be of interest to see how such events affect team performance in soccer and other sports.

A second line of investigation with regard to individual and team sports performance would be to apply the methods used in behavioral momentum analyses to tactics already employed by coaches and players. For example, a common strategy in American football is to call a time-out just before an attempted field goal at the close of a half (i.e., "icing" the kicker). In baseball, batters have a tendency to call for a brief time-out or step out of the batter's box as a pitcher nears his windup in an apparent attempt to disrupt the pitcher's performance. The effects of these events as disruptors are unknown. Although these tactics seem to be work infrequently, their persistence of use seems to suggest it might be effective intermittently. An analysis of momentum in such a situation might be assessed by comparing a kicker's rate of reinforcement in the presence or absence of such a disruptor (though this analysis would be quite limited given the limited number of potential reinforcers a kicker might obtain) or the degree to which the frequency of batter time-outs affects a pitchers rate of reinforcement (e.g., throwing strikes, forcing a putout).

Coaching tactics to affect the isolated performance of a single player could also impact the performance of a team. Using the tactic of icing a kicker as an example, the impact of this tactic could have widespread effects beyond the accuracy of the kick. For example, a missed kick could be considered a defensive reinforcer (for the non-kicking team), which could reinforce other behavior in that same class of responses. Alternatively, a successful kick could influence a class of offensive reinforcers. The relation between coaching tactics to isolate individual performance and the impact of this on overall team obtained reinforcement (beyond points generated or missed from the kick attempt) would be an interesting line of future investigation.

Many sports have designed defensive strategies specifically to combat an opponent's offensive capabilities. Examples include penalty kill substitutions in hockey, a defensive player "spying" on a specific offensive player in American football, or substituting in a defensive specialist in basketball. Again, the effects of such procedures seem to justify the continued use of such procedure. However, these changes could each be examined as disrupter events and their effects quantified within the context of the behavioral momentum metaphor (i.e., an examination of how such events affect an opponent's ongoing rate of reinforcement).

Finally, there are specific terms used to describe a player's performance over a period of time. It is not uncommon to hear a soccer player described as being "in form" or a baseball player being described as "in the zone." Both terms imply that the player in question has a recent history of obtaining a relatively high rate of reinforcement (e.g., more base hits, higher on-base percentage), and such behavior seems similar to that of a player who is having a streak (e.g., goals scored, homeruns hit). However, such descriptive labels have not been quantified. Examining various rates of reinforcement for players would enable coaching staff to select advantageous substitutions, team rosters, batting orders, etc. Alternatively, examining these data might indicate to an opponent how best to counter players whose rate of reinforcement is relatively high.

Sports performance and coaching are behaviors that appear to be based less on objective data and more on subjective notions of a specific strategy given the occurrence of certain events. Previous research (e.g., Mace et al., 1992; Roane et al., 2004) suggests that examining within-game performance can lead to optimal play calling (e.g., calling a time-out before two team's reinforcement ratios become too disparate). The quantification of sports performance via the conceptualization of behavioral momentum holds promise for enhancing the performance of sports teams and individuals competitors.

## References

Baer, D. M., Wolf, M. M., & Risley, T. R. (1968). Some current dimensions of applied behavior analysis. *Journal of Applied Behavior Analysis, 1*, 91–97.
Belfiore, P. J., Lee, D. L., Vargas, A. U., & Skinner, C. H. (1997). Effects of high-preference single-digit mathematics problem completion on multiple-digit mathematics problem performance. *Journal of Applied Behavior Analysis, 30*, 327–330.
Bresnahan, M. (2010, April 14). Lakers have no playoff momentum. *Los Angeles Times*.
Burke, K. L., Burke, M. M., & Joyner, A. B. (1999). Perceptions of momentum in college and high school basketball: An exploratory, case study investigation. *Journal of Sport Behavior, 22*, 303–309.
Dawson, J. E., Piazza, C. C., Sevin, B. M., Gulotta, C. S., Lerman, D., & Kelley, M. L. (2003). Use of the high-probability instructional sequence and escape extinction in a child with food refusal. *Journal of Applied Behavior Analysis, 36*, 105–108.
Deford, F. (1999, February 3). Momentum gains momentum. Retrieved from http://sportsillustrated.cnn.com/inside_game/deford/990127/
Duke, A., & Corlett, J. (1992). Factors affecting university women's basketball coaches' timeout decisions. *Canadian Journal of Sports Sciences, 17*, 333–337.
Gayton, W. F., Very, M., & Hearns, J. (1993). Psychological momentum in team sports. *Journal of Sport Behavior, 16*, 121–123.
Gilovich, T., Valone, R., & Tversky, A. (1985). The hot hand in basketball: On the misperception of random sequences. *Cognitive Psychology, 17*, 295–314.
Iso-Ahola, S. E., & Mobily, K. (1980). "Psychological momentum": A phenomenon and an empirical (unobtrusive) validation of its influence in a competitive sport tournament. *Psychological Reports, 46*, 391–401.
Mace, F. C., Hock, M. L., Lalli, J. S., West, B. J., Belfiore, P., Pinter, E., et al. (1988). Behavioral momentum in the treatment of noncompliance. *Journal of Applied Behavior Analysis, 21*, 123–141.
Mace, F. C., Lalli, J. S., Shea, M. C., & Nevin, J. A. (1992). Behavioral momentum in college basketball. *Journal of Applied Behavior Analysis, 25*, 657–663.
Mace, F. C., McComas, J. J., Mauro, B. C., Progar, P. R., Taylor, B., Ervin, R., et al. (2010). Differential reinforcement of alternative behavior increases resistance to extinction: Clinical demonstration, animal modeling, and clinical test of one solution. *Journal of the Experimental Analysis of Behavior, 93*, 349–367.
Mack, M. G., & Stephens, D. E. (2000). An empirical test of Taylor and Demick's multidimensional model of momentum in sport. *Journal of Sport Behavior, 23*, 349–363.
Nevin, J. A. (1996). The momentum of compliance. *Journal of Applied Behavior Analysis, 29*, 535–547.
Nevin, J. A., Mandell, C., & Atak, J. R. (1983). The analysis of behavioral momentum. *Journal of the Experimental Analysis of Behavior, 39*, 49–59.
Nevin, J. A., Tota, M. E., Torquato, R. D., & Shull, R. L. (1990). Alternative reinforcement increases resistance to change: Pavlovian or operant contingencies? *Journal of the Experimental Analysis of Behavior, 53*, 359–379.
Rivera, R. (2007, March 14). New York City Council approves ban on metal bats. *The New York Times*.
Roane, H. S., Kelley, M. E., Trosclair, N. M., & Hauer, L. S. (2004). Behavioral momentum in sports: A partial replication with women's basketball. *Journal of Applied Behavior Analysis, 37*, 385–390.

Silva, J. M., Hardy, C. J., & Grace, R. K. (1988). Analysis of psychological momentum in intercollegiate tennis. *Journal of Sport and Exercise Psychology, 10,* 346–354.

Smith, M. C. (2002, February 6). Ability, not gender, is shaping women's sports identity. *The Orange County Register.*

Taylor, J., & Demick, A. (1994). A multidimensional model of momentum in sports. *Journal of Applied Sports Psychology, 6,* 51–70.

Weinberg, R. S., Richardson, P. A., & Jackson, A. (1981). Effects of situation criticality on tennis performance of males and females. *International Journal of Sport Psychology, 12,* 253–259.

Zarcone, J. R., Iwata, B. A., Mazaleski, J. L., & Smith, R. G. (1994). Momentum and extinction effects on self-injurious escape behavior and noncompliance. *Journal of Applied Behavior Analysis, 27,* 649–658.

# Part IV
# Special Topics

# Chapter 10
# Developing Fluent, Efficient, and Automatic Repertoires of Athletic Performance

**Brian K. Martens and Scott R. Collier**

*To master a form, it must be practiced 10,000 times.*
*– Unknown martial arts master*

Some years back, the first author was conversing with a catcher for a minor league baseball team and asked the naïve question, "So what do you think about when deciding where to throw the ball to make a play?" The catcher immediately replied, "There's no time to think, I just react automatically. If you have to think, then it's already too late." This statement captures the essence of much of the research reviewed in this chapter. Namely, accomplished athletes in a variety of domains (e.g., fast ball sports, team sports, martial arts) are able to execute complex chains of behavior so accurately and quickly in response to changing situations that their performance appears both effortless and automatic. In interactive sports, master athletes seem at times to move in unison with their opponents as if in a coordinated dance, rather than in response to the other's actions (Ueshiba, 1987). In individual sports such as golf, elite players are known for their ability to consistently execute difficult shots under seemingly impossible conditions (e.g., Phil Mickelson's 200+ yard shot from behind a tree on pine straw during the 2010 Masters Tournament that landed only feet away from the 13th pin).

Despite domain-specific differences in skills, it is widely believed that a lengthy period of *deliberate practice* is essential for developing expert performance (Ericsson, Krampe, & Tesch-Romer, 1993; Ward, Hodges, Williams, & Starkes, 2004). Estimates of how long a period of time is required to reach elite or master status in sports have been compared to the 10 year/10,000 h rule required for expertise in other domains (e.g., chess and music; Ericsson et al., 1993; Simon & Chase, 1973). Although a good rule of thumb, the number of years required to reach elite status in sports is generally more than 10 years, and accumulated practice hours are usually less than 10,000 due to resource, motivational, and effort constraints inherent in participating in sports over a long period of time (Baker, Cote, & Abernethy, 2003; Ericsson et al., 1993). For example, Baker et al. asked a sample of Australian

B.K. Martens (✉)
Department of Psychology, Syracuse University, Syracuse, NY, USA
e-mail: bkmarten@syr.edu

national team players from three sports (netball, basketball, and field hockey) to report on when they began participating in sports, how many hours per week they practiced, and how long it took to reach the elite level (i.e., selection to the national team). On average, the athletes reported 12.9 years of participation and 3,939 h of accumulated practice prior to team selection. Using similar retrospective recall methods, Helsen, Starkes, and Hodges (1998) examined the amount of time spent in practice by Belgian international-, national-, and provincial-level soccer and field hockey players. Both international- and national-level soccer players peaked in their reported number of weekly practice hours (an indication of maturity in the sport) 15 years into their careers. By 18 years into their careers, international players had accumulated an average of 9,332 practice hours. International field hockey players reached their peak of weekly practice 18 years into their careers, accumulating a total of 10,237 h of practice time. At 12 years into their careers, international-level wrestlers reported accumulating an average of 5,882 h of practice time (Ward et al., 2004).

According to Ericsson et al. (1993), deliberate practice is not simply drill or repetition but is a "highly structured activity, the explicit goal of which is to improve performance" (p. 368). As such, deliberate practice is typically individualized and involves periodic instruction by a coach; increasingly more difficult, domain-relevant training tasks; close monitoring of performance (by both the athlete and the coach); feedback and reinforcement; and re-teaching of poorly executed skills. Another defining feature of deliberate practice is that it requires sustained effort and attention and therefore can be engaged in only for relatively brief intervals (i.e., 1–2 h at a time). In sports, the duration of practice sessions is constrained even further by muscle fatigue and the risk of injury. Therefore, athletes who are committed to achieving expert levels of performance typically adhere to a practice schedule involving one or two sessions a day, every day, for 10+ years (Ericsson & Charness, 1994).

The astute reader will no doubt notice that many of the strategies involved in deliberate practice (i.e., a well-sequenced curriculum, direct instruction of component skills, brief repeated opportunities to respond with feedback and reinforcement) are consistent with other domains of behavioral skill training such as adaptive behavior, communication, and basic academic competency (Martens, Daly, Begeny, & VanDerHeyden, in press; Martens & Witt, 2004). A considerable amount of research exists concerning the use of these strategies to improve athletic performance, particularly goal setting, feedback, and public posting (e.g., Brobst & Ward, 2002; Koop & Martin, 1983; Mellalieu, Hanton, & O'Brien, 2006; Smith & Ward, 2006; Ward & Carnes, 2002). This research is discussed at length in Chapters 6 and 7 of this volume. In contrast, monotonic increases in proficiency that result from deliberate practice over a long period of time (Ericsson et al., 1993) exhibit unique features and benefits (e.g., efficiency, automaticity, resistance to distraction), which, in turn, alter both goals and strategies of practice itself. Surprisingly, these goals and strategies are consistent with ancient wisdom concerning the development of complex performance repertoires (e.g., martial arts training), and it is these unique features that we focus on in the present chapter.

The first half of the chapter describes how behavioral principles (e.g., stimulus control, chaining of component skills) are involved in the development of fluent, efficient, and automatic performance. Specifically, we describe the goals of long-term deliberate practice and how performance changes as a result, and review research concerning how practice should be structured to maximize performance gains and maintain motivation for more accomplished athletes. The second half of the chapter describes neuromuscular adaptations that result from prolonged practice and that underlie efficient and automatic performance. Here we describe both neuromuscular (e.g., neuromuscular facilitation and recruitment efficiency) and physiological (e.g., mechanistic and muscle plasticity) changes produced by prolonged engagement at high levels in athletic activities.

## Behavioral Principles Underlying Automaticity

### Goals of Prolonged Deliberate Practice

> *If your opponent does not move, you remain still. If there is even the slightest movement, you have already moved accordingly.*
> *– Tai chi master, Wu Yu-hsiang (1812–1880)*

A useful model for summarizing research into the development of proficient performance is known as the *Instructional Hierarchy* (IH; Daly, Martens, Barnett, Witt, & Olson, 2007; Haring, Lovitt, Eaton, & Hansen, 1978; Martens et al., in press; Martens & Witt, 2004). According to the IH, learning any new skill involves progression through a series of stages that correspond to increasingly higher levels of proficiency. First, one must learn to perform the skill or its component behaviors correctly in the absence of assistance and in response to key discriminative stimuli (*acquisition*). Discriminative stimuli signal *when* to execute a skill and *whether* it is likely to be reinforced (i.e., produce the desired outcome). In the context of sports training, discriminative stimuli might involve short directives from a coach ("Pass!), the coach's whistle, the location of the ball, or a certain configuration of players on the field. Once a skill has been acquired, focus shifts to performing it both accurately and quickly, or at rates approximating those of competent performers (*fluency*; Binder, 1996). Because emphasis is placed on the speed of responding during fluency building, skills are often practiced in isolation and at levels of difficulty commensurate with the learner's ability (i.e., drill with instructionally matched materials; Martens et al., 2007). Practice under more demanding, difficult, and varied conditions strengthens control over responding by more naturalistic, game-like discriminative stimuli (*maintenance*), and eventually produces the ability to perform behaviors under novel conditions and as part of more complex, composite skills (*generalization*). After a variety of composite skills have been mastered, the learner becomes capable of reorganizing and reconstituting these skills to meet the demands of changing situations (*adaptation*) (Binder, 1996; Johnson & Layng, 1996).

With respect to athletic performance, component behaviors are typically comprised of short motor segments that constitute the basics or fundamentals of a particular sport (e.g., hitting a forehand in tennis, trapping and passing a ball in soccer). From the perspective of the IH, the first goal of prolonged deliberate practice is to build fluency (i.e., accuracy and speed) in these component motor skills so they can be combined into composite motor chains (Mechner, 1995). *Chaining* refers to the procedure by which one learns to perform a series of behaviors in sequence following presentation of a discriminative stimulus and ending with reinforcement (Alberto & Troutman, 2003). Completion of each behavior in the sequence (i.e., link in the chain) serves two functions: (a) as a discriminative stimulus for executing the next behavior in the chain and (b) as a conditioned reinforcer for executing the previous behavior in the chain.

When teaching chains of responses that do not already exist in a learner's repertoire, each component behavior must be taught directly. Depending on the number of behaviors involved, the initial acquisition of these response chains can be a time-consuming process requiring tens and even hundreds of prompted trials (e.g., Luyben, Funk, Morgan, Clark, & Delulio, 1986). Several methods for teaching chained responses have been reported in the literature and include backward chaining (teach behaviors in reverse order from the terminal response), forward chaining (teach behaviors in sequence starting with the initial response), and total task presentation (teach all behaviors each trial; Test, Spooner, Keul, & Grossi, 1990). For example, Luyben et al. used the forward chaining method to teach three adults with mental retardation a nine-step sequence for executing a soccer pass. Five levels of most-to-least prompting (i.e., full physical guidance, partial physical guidance, modeling, gestural prompt, verbal prompt) were used to produce a correct response at each step, and all correct responses were reinforced with verbal praise. Although all three participants reached criterion performance for passing a ball within 29 training sessions, the number of prompted trials (approximately 20 per session) ranged from 440 to 580.

For learners who are already fluent in component skills, composite motor chains can be trained relatively rapidly (Hodge & Deakin, 1998). It is not uncommon for accomplished athletes to periodically reorganize their skill sets (e.g., "make over" their swing), adopt more effective game strategies, and/or alter their attentional focus (Bell & Hardy, 2009). Changes such as these constitute refinements in skill execution and are reinforced when they lead to better outcomes in competition. For more proficient players, novel chains of composite skills can be shaped through instruction and reinforcement (Scott, Scott, & Goldwater, 1997) and may even emerge spontaneously with continued, attentive practice. For example, Kladopoulos and McComas (2001) used the total task presentation method to teach correct foul-shooting form to three NCAA Division II women's basketball players. The study began with a component analysis of techniques reported in instructional manuals, resulting in a chain of five target behaviors. Dependent variables included the percentage of shots made without touching the backboard and the percentage of shots executed with correct form. During the training condition, proper form requirements were reviewed prior to each block of 10 trials, and descriptive praise was provided for their use. Results showed that the percentage of shots taken with correct form increased immediately (i.e., from 1 to 3 sessions or 10–30 trials) to 100%. The percentage of shots made also increased for all three participants.

Harding, Wacker, Berg, Rick, and Lee (2004) attempted to shape novel sequences of techniques in martial arts students by directly reinforcing variability in responding. In this study, two adult Kenpo karate students participated in both drill and sparring sessions with their instructor. During baseline, the students were instructed to use any of 54 different hand-and-foot techniques in any combination in response to the instructor's punches. Students were also told to use the techniques in different combinations, and the number of different techniques executed by the students was recorded each session. In the differential reinforcement condition, the instructor provided brief verbal feedback and praise during training drills when the students executed a different technique or combination of techniques. Repeated techniques were ignored. Results showed an increase in the variability of techniques performed by both students during drills, and these increases in variability generalized to sparring sessions.

Once a number of composite motor chains have been acquired, the second goal of deliberate practice is to develop increasingly more ballistic execution of these chains so they can be performed repeatedly in the same way under different conditions (Mechner, 2009). A well-known finding of basic operant research is that reinforcement makes behavior more frequent, stereotyped, and efficient (Daly, Martens, Skinner, & Noell, 2009; Reynolds, 1975). Moreover, decreases in variability that result from the practice and reinforcement of motor skills appear to be accompanied by a shift in neural activation from widely distributed cortical regions (e.g., sensorimotor, temporal, and occipital cortexes) to subcortical regions (e.g., basal ganglia) (Floyer-Lea & Matthews, 2004; MacPherson, Collins, & Obhi, 2009). This suggests that with practice, the execution of composite motor chains gradually shifts from conscious to unconscious (i.e., automatic) control (MacPherson et al.). In the context of deliberate practice, expert athletes are likely to experience repeated cycles of effortful and attentive learning, a gradual reduction in effort following practice, and a shift to unconscious control as they master subsequent skill sets. Over time, this cycle is likely to be well discriminated and perhaps even anticipated, leading to the negative reinforcement of practice behavior by a reduction in effort. Once a skill set has been practiced to automaticity, it is essentially forgotten (i.e., no longer requires conscious control) and the learner can concentrate on other or more advanced skills.

Practicing a skill to high levels of fluency or automaticity carries additional benefits for the performer that have been summarized by fluency researchers with the acronym RESAA (Johnson & Layng, 1996). These benefits have been used as markers in other domains (e.g., training academic skills) to determine how much practice is necessary for a skill to be functional, and as such represent functional fluency criteria. These benefits would seem particularly applicable to sports and suggest that athletic skills practiced to functional fluency aims are more likely to exhibit *(R)etention* in the absence of practice, *(E)ndurance* over longer practice intervals, *(S)tability* in the face of anxiety or distraction, *(A)pplication* to composite skills and untrained conditions, and *(A)dduction* (spontaneous modification) to meet novel demands (Martens et al., in press). In support of this position, Driskell, Willis, and Copper (1992) conducted a meta-analysis of research concerning the effects of overlearning (i.e., practicing skills beyond an initial accuracy criterion) on retention. They found a mean effect size of 0.44 for physical tasks and a mean effect size of 0.75 for cognitive tasks. In addition, the effect size for retention was significantly correlated ($r = 0.48$) with the degree of overlearning (e.g., 50% vs. 200%) but not the retention interval ($r = -0.0021$). The authors concluded that overlearning produces moderate and significant increases in retention, and this benefit "may be particularly important for team training, in that integrated team performance requires that each team member retain a high level of proficiency to support overall team performance" (p. 620).

A third goal of deliberate practice is to bring the automatic execution of complex skills under control of key discriminative stimuli in the competitive environment. In sports, athletes are required to respond quickly and accurately to changing arrays of complex stimuli (Ericsson & Charness, 1994). As an example, a player receiving service in tennis may have only 500–600 ms in which to organize and execute a return (Abernethy, 1991). Doing so requires attention to relevant features of the stimulus complex (e.g., the location and speed of the approaching ball), movement to a favorable position on the court, execution of the return in a fashion similar to how it was practiced, evaluation of the outcomes of the action, preparation for the next response, and so on. Research in this area falls under the general rubric of decision making and has compared decision accuracy, reaction times, response uncertainty, and anticipatory strategies of athletes at different levels of expertise (Abernethy, 1991; Ericsson & Charness, 1994). Findings have suggested that (a) reaction time increases with increases in stimulus-response uncertainty, (b) reaction time is affected less when the task is highly practiced, and (c) reaction times for skilled athletes are actually similar to those of novice performers on laboratory tasks (Abernethy, 1991).

Findings such as these led Abernethy and his colleagues to examine why highly skilled fast ball and racquet sport athletes appeared to be unhurried when returning a shot even though they were subject to the same uncertainty and reaction time constraints as novices. Through a series of investigations, these researchers examined expert–novice differences in the use of visual cues (i.e., discriminative stimuli) that provide "reliable anticipatory information" (Abernethy, 1991, p. 203) about the flight of the approaching shot. The hypothesis was that elite athletes move into position and begin executing a return much sooner than novices and in response to visual cues (e.g., arm position) from their opponents that occur well before the shot is actually struck. By selectively masking different portions of an opponent's body in video presentations, they found that international-level badminton players did indeed make use of earlier cues in the motor behavior of the other player to predict the landing position of the shuttle. Put another way, expert athletes essentially circumvented reaction time constraints in deciding where the shuttle would land by attending to visual cues more proximal to the opponent's movement. This suggests that one reason why elite athletes appear unhurried and to move almost in unison with their opponents is that prolonged practice under varying conditions allows them to develop increasingly more accurate anticipation or "looking ahead" capacity by attending to much earlier visual cues (see also Mechner, 2009). Athletes who have truly mastered a sport respond automatically to stimuli, of which novices may not even be aware.

## *Practice Techniques for More Proficient Athletes*

> *If you pay attention to your spirit and ignore your breathing, your striking force will be as strong as steel. If you pay attention to your breathing, your force will be inactive and ineffective.*
> – *Tai chi master Wu Yu-hsiang (1812–1880)*

As noted previously, achieving high levels of proficiency in a sport generally requires a well-sequenced set of skill-building activities, direct instruction and feedback by a coach, and a long period of effortful, attentive practice aimed at improving performance. Although these strategies can be used with athletes of all skill levels, several training methods have been shown to be differentially effective for more proficient performers. In general, these strategies are designed to help athletes make more subtle refinements in the execution of complex skills and to reduce the disruptive effects of anxiety on performance.

*Modeling by experts.* One training strategy for helping athletes at more advanced levels refine their skills is simply exposure to expert models. Weissensteiner, Abernethy, and Farrow (2009) conducted an interview-based qualitative study of the developmental histories of 14 elite male cricket players, administrators, and coaches. Several key developmental factors were found to support the progression to elite status (e.g., strong parental support, access to resources) including an extensive history of observational learning in the sport. Specifically, expert batters reported spending hours carefully observing cricket games as well as the techniques of their favorite sports heroes. Apparently, by observing more accomplished players, the developing athletes were able to learn nuances in performance that could not be adequately described in words. Along these lines, Hodge and Deakin (1998) examined the effects of modeling with and without accompanying verbal descriptions (what the investigators termed "context") on the ability of expert and novice Canadian martial artists to replicate novel *kata* (i.e., sequenced patterns of already acquired offensive and defensive techniques). Expert practitioners (first-degree black belts) exhibited higher percentages of serial accuracy than novices (green and orange belts) across all conditions, presumably due to "their extensive experience in the martial arts domain" (p. 268). In addition, the results indicated that the increased recall demands of the running verbal context actually hindered the performance of the novice group, particularly on initial trials.

*Use of metaphors.* Another potentially useful strategy for promoting more nuanced performance of skills is to make use of metaphors during training. As noted by Mechner (1995), metaphors are commonly used by coaches to elicit associations regarding the features of movement that are relevant to a particular skill. For example, by invoking the image of being "like the eagle which glides serenely on the wind, but which can swoop instantly to pluck a rabbit from the ground" (Liao, 1990, p. 115), a martial artist may be encouraged to evade attacks by calmly moving in circles, each one connected to the next and then abruptly exiting or closing these circles when the time comes to attack.

Due to the large number of character ideograms in the Chinese language, the Chinese continued to rely on block printing well after the invention of movable-type presses. As a result, early efforts to document key training principles in the martial arts were necessarily terse in an attempt to capture the essence of a movement as efficiently as possible. In tai chi chuan, for example, this explains the often poetic names of postures (e.g., high pat horse, snake creeps down) as well as the frequent use of metaphors (e.g., "When in stillness you should be as the mountain"; Liao, 1990, p. 115) in classic writings.

*Attentional focus prompts.* As skills become increasingly well practiced, a performer's attention gradually shifts from the conscious and deliberate execution of component behaviors to execution of the entire chain. Through repetition, chained sequences of behavior become more stereotypical and automatic, allowing the focus of attention to shift to intended performance outcomes (e.g., positioning of the ball in an opponent's court, moving an opponent into position for a strike). Even after extensive practice, the latter stages of this progression can be disrupted when athletes experience anxiety, or what is commonly referred to as "choking" in high-stakes competition. One hypothesis for why this occurs is that under anxiety-provoking conditions, athletes redirect their attention internally (e.g., to the execution of component behaviors), which interferes with the automatic control of highly practiced skills (Bell & Hardy, 2009). This suggests also that providing prompts to help an athlete reestablish an external focus might facilitate performance under such conditions. Bell and Hardy tested this hypothesis by assigning 33 skilled male golfers (mean handicap of 5.5) to one of three conditions: an internal focus group (position of the wrist), a proximal external focus group (position of the club face), and a distal external focus group (flight of the ball). After warming up, each participant was required to hit three blocks of 10 chip shots from approximately 22 yards (20 m) while the distance from the pin of each ball was scored. The attentional focus manipulation was conducted by having each player repeat a brief phrase that corresponded to their assigned condition prior to each shot (e.g., "wrist hinge"). Blocks of trials were repeated under a neutral condition and an anxiety-provoking condition in which participants were told that their performance would be evaluated by a PGA professional, publicly posted, and monetarily rewarded if they showed improvement.

Manipulation checks revealed significant differences in self-reported attentional focus as well as state anxiety levels across the relevant conditions. In terms of performance, significant differences were found among all three groups under both neutral and anxiety conditions, with shot accuracy being the highest for the distal external focus group followed by the proximal external focus group and then the internal focus group. Although mean performance for both the internal focus group and the proximal external focus group was slightly less accurate under the anxiety condition, the distal external focus group was slightly more accurate. The authors concluded that it is preferable for highly skilled performers to adopt a distal external focus under varying performance conditions, the exception being if they are attempting to consciously remake aspects of a skill (Bell & Hardy, 2009).

*Rhythmic priming cues.* An interesting but sometimes overlooked component of highly trained motor sequences is their rhythm or temporal phasing (MacPherson et al., 2009). For example, research has suggested that skilled competitive cyclists ($M = 11$ years in competition) have a preferred rhythm or cadence that is less variable than that of unskilled cyclists and is associated with lower heart rate and oxygen uptake (i.e., requires less effort and is more efficient; MacPherson, Turner, & Collins, 2007). Moreover, the more experienced the athlete, the more rapidly they are able to return to their optimal cadence following disruption (e.g., matching pedal strokes to a metronome), suggesting that domain-specific practice and experience are "important factors in establishing stable movement parameters" (MacPherson et al., 2007, p. 52).

Just as anxiety can disrupt performance by interfering with the automatic regulation of well-practiced movement sequences, MacPherson et al. (2007) have suggested that it may also interfere with a movement's temporal phasing. That is, negative emotional states may hinder performance of complex skills by destabilizing previously established rhythms. This being the case, MacPherson et al. have suggested that one possible training technique for more proficient athletes is to provide external cues that help reestablish these optimal rhythms. As an example of the potential effects of this technique, Southard and Miracle (1993) had eight female college varsity basketball players alter the relative timing and duration of their pre-shot rituals for foul shooting. Each participant completed 15 foul shots under standard-time ritual, halftime ritual, double-time ritual, and variable-time ritual conditions. The relative timing of behaviors was preserved under the first three conditions but not the last (i.e., variable time condition). Results showed that participants made significantly more foul shots under the standard-, halftime, and double-time conditions in comparison to the variable-time condition, suggesting that maintaining the relative timing of their eight-step, pre-shot rituals was an important determinant of shot success.

*Reinforcing deliberate practice.* A final consideration concerning training techniques for elite athletes is the problem of how to maintain the motivation to practice over a 10+-year period. In their seminal paper on deliberate practice, Ericsson et al. (1993) characterized effortful practice as lacking inherent enjoyment but rather being engaged in as a means of improving performance. In contrast to this assertion, several studies in which athletes were asked to rate their enjoyment of various practice activities (e.g., team practice, watching games, weight training) have suggested that many of these activities were moderately to highly enjoyable (Helsen et al., 1998; Hodge & Deakin, 1998). Using an 11-point scale with $0 =$ low enjoyment and $10 =$ high enjoyment, Belgian soccer players in the Helsen et al. study gave mean ratings above 5 on 13 of 19 items. Items rated the highest included watching soccer and analyzing game videos individually, working one on one with a coach, and practicing technical and tactical skills in team. Similar results were reported for a sample of Canadian martial artists who gave mean ratings above 5 on 21 of

26 different activities (Hodge & Deakin, 1998). For this sample, the highest rated items included training with others in kata or sparring, training one on one with the instructor, and practicing kata individually.

These data as well as research into developmental factors contributing to the achievement of elite status suggest that reinforcement for deliberate practice comes from multiple sources. These sources are likely to include social-positive reinforcers from a parent, coach, or other players (e.g., praise, corrective feedback, shared experiences of hardship), social-negative reinforcers in the context of competition (e.g., avoiding being benched, losing the game, or having a losing season), and automatic or self-mediated reinforcers that arise from closely monitoring one's own performance (e.g., the experience of being "in the zone," a reduction in effort that comes from achieving automaticity, matching of performance to a valued model, improvement over time). Given that deliberate practice is geared toward the attainment of a goal (i.e., improving performance) and requires a considerable amount of time practicing alone, this latter category of reinforcers would seem particularly important for maintaining motivation.

## Neuromuscular Correlates of Automatic Performance

> *Xian Tian means inborn, congenital, or first nature. Hou Tian refers to those qualities that arise after birth. To reach the highest level, you must turn Hou Tian abilities into Xian Tian abilities.*
> *– Tai chi master, Tung Ying Chieh (1897–1961)*

Deliberate practice produces movements that become "second nature" to individuals who spend years perfecting these movements. Early in the 1900s, Sherrington's work revealed that movement is controlled in the central nervous system by central pattern generators (CPGs), which are specialized neural networks that, when provoked, provide oscillatory motor output without oscillatory input (Sherrington, 1910). Subsequent work in this area has shown that these centers control tasks such as respiration and locomotion. It would appear that repeated activity provides localization in specific centers of the brain, which help develop spinal cord–mediated responses that are crucial for fluid and efficient movements. For example, consider learning to walk or acquiring gait pattern as part of a maturational process that begins in the toddler stage. This is a task we rarely think about, yet we come to exhibit smooth fluid movements during locomotion as a result of practice over an extended period of time. Locomotion is the most extensively studied of the CPGs within the central nervous system, although more recent studies have examined other CPG-controlled movements (Guertin & Steuer, 2009). This section provides an overview of the physiological concepts for spinal cord–mediated responses and rate coding of motorneurons to facilitate "deliberate practice" so performance can become consistent and automatic. Second, in this section we discuss neuromuscular adaptations that arise from prolonged engagement in a domain-specific training regimen.

## *Repeated Practice and Muscle Fiber Recruitment*

Force output during a voluntary contraction can be increased by two methods: either by increasing the number of active motor units or by increasing the firing frequency of the active motor units. The Henneman size principle of motor unit recruitment demonstrates that the smallest units are recruited first, and thereafter, other motor units are recruited in a sequential order based on physical size (Henneman, 1957). This lends to orderly recruitment of muscle fiber, which has specific energy relationships between muscle fiber recruitment to task. For example, one would not want to maximally recruit their forearm muscles to pick up a pencil, as the force required for the task is low. However, if one needed to pick up a much heavier object, the muscle recruitment would demand the involvement of more powerful muscle fiber. The motor unit recruitment progression would typically go through type I → type IIa → type IIx, so activities requiring low force would typically need to recruit only type I muscle fiber to complete the required task. This lends to energy conservation since activities requiring low force need to recruit only muscle fiber that will be most efficient at completing the desired task. Incremental force increases will lead to greater recruitment of muscle fiber involving the larger, yet more fatiguing motor units to meet the demands necessary to complete the task (Henneman, Somjen, & Carpenter, 1965). This orderly recruitment also minimizes the development of fatigue by allowing the most fatigue resistant fibers to be used most of the time, holding the more fatigable fibers in reserve until needed for higher forces, thus allowing for greater fine motor control.

The precise mechanisms of fatigue vary depending on the specifics of the task. Fatigue ultimately depends on the intensity of the activity, the type of contraction, and the muscle group utilized. Deliberate practice increases time to fatigue by adapting muscles to the style of training; hence, if power training is undertaken, the muscles become faster and stronger, yet endurance training (long duration) will result in less readily fatigued muscles.

Skeletal muscle shows great plasticity in adapting to the type of training environment in which it is placed. Mechanisms responsible for muscular adaptation for power (force) or endurance are various and include increased skeletal muscle blood flow and mitochondrial adaptation, increases in muscle growth factors, increases in neural adaptation, increases in muscle cross-sectional area, and enzymatic changes in fiber-type specificity. Training for muscle power relies on a strength regimen that is best explained by the SAID principle where we realize a Specific Adaptation to an Increased Demand on the muscle. When a training load becomes easier to lift, the demand on the muscle becomes less; therefore, one must increase the demand on the muscle and the resistance to facilitate improvements in strength. Without an overload on the muscles, there will be no improvement in strength. When training in this fashion, one realizes that improvements in strength are specific to the movement that is being repeated, which can be explained by neural adaptation. Over time, there is a marked improvement in muscle strength due to increases in muscle growth factors that increase the cross-sectional area of the muscle fiber. It is important to note that humans do not add more fiber, but increase the size of existing fibers. This increase in size will increase the velocity of muscle shortening, which will increase speed, leading to enhanced peak rate of force generation and also a higher frequency of excitation, which will permit a higher rate of force development. We know that type II muscle fiber shows the greatest propensity for hypertrophy, yet fatigue quicker than type I muscle fiber (greater endurance). Since we cannot change the type of muscle fiber from type I to type II and vice versa, we change the enzyme characteristics enabling each type to behave more like the type characteristic of the training we are performing. Typically, resistance training for power results in the use of type II fiber and Staron et al. (1990) have shown an increase in type IIa with a concomitant decrease in type IIb fibers over 20 weeks of progressive resistance training. Power lifters make poor marathoners and vice versa, which is the premise behind fiber-type specificity.

Marathon training is considered a form of endurance training where the muscles undergoing frequent repetition become more fatigue resistant. This decrease in fatigability is in part due to an increase in the sheer numbers of mitochondria (Hoppeler et al., 1985) and an increase in types I and IIa enzyme expression (Friden, Sjostrom, & Ekblom, 1984). While an individual is exercising, the more mitochondria results in a superior supply of energy (ATP) for aerobic activities resulting in longer performance times with less fatigue. Aerobic training also increases the blood supply to the active muscle by creating larger capillary networks or beds that improves oxygen and nutrient delivery to the exercising fibers and a more efficacious removal of metabolic wastes ($K^+$, $H^+$) (Collier et al., 2008; Hudlicka, 1990). The smaller circumference of these muscle fibers may possess an advantage over their power training counterparts as the adaptation may allow for greater diffusion of metabolites and nutrients allowing the body to continue with exercise further over time without the build-up of exercise-limiting factors.

## *Training for Muscle Strength and Efficiency*

As one continues with their training regimen, the frequency and type of training can contribute to more effective gains in their respective competition and/or fitness. The question of single vs. multiple sets has been an issue for decades in the exercise science literature. It has been shown that single sets are as effective as multiple sets on variables such as strength (Starkey et al., 1996), yet multiple progressively heavier sets show greater increases in muscle hypertrophy (Kraemer et al., 2002). It is necessary to keep in mind that as one continues with their training regimen, recent data show that highly trained athletes require multiple sets of resistance exercises per muscle group to elicit maximal strength gains (Peterson, Rhea, & Alvar, 2005), whereas untrained individuals seem to benefit most from programs using fewer sets per muscle group (Galvao & Taaffe, 2004; Peterson et al., 2005). Much like the SAID principle, any individual undertaking a weight-training regimen should increase the intensity of their program by adding sets as time progresses or their program will not keep progressing with increases in strength.

Perhaps not fully understood is the combination of strength and endurance-training programs, which are expected to yield the best of both training regimens in less combined time. Termed "cross-fit" programs, athletes and fitness gurus alike purport gains in overall aerobic fitness while maintaining or improving overall strength. As mentioned previously, it may be best to separate training by the specific outcome desired, such as dedicating strength training to one day and cardiovascular training to a separate day. It has been shown that both untrained and trained participants who undertake combined endurance and strength training during the same workout show attenuated strength gains in comparison to individuals who undertook separate training days for strength and cardiovascular fitness (Dudley & Djamil, 1985; McCarthy, Pozniak, & Agre, 2002; Sale, Jacobs, MacDougall, & Garner, 1990).

It is well known that men are generally stronger than women when total force is compared, and the upper body shows the greatest sex differences as men have been shown to be 50% stronger than their female counterparts (Morrow & Hosler, 1981). These sex differences are attributed to the larger muscle mass with which men are genetically predisposed, due to 20–30 times higher concentrations of testosterone than in women. Yet women show greater gains in strength after a weight-training regimen. However, in terms of fatigue, women show less fatigue during acute endurance bouts than age-matched men (Clark, Collier, Manini, & Ploutz-Snyder, 2005). This could be due to less active hyperemia, where women can keep the muscle perfused with blood due to less occlusive force when compared to the greater contraction force of men, which cuts off blood supply to the active muscle. Further, women may show a greater propensity to utilize accessory muscles to keep the fatiguing contraction to produce measurable force over longer periods of time.

When an individual undertakes a resistance or endurance training activity, one common result is the onset of muscle soreness. For novice athletes, the greatest degree of muscle soreness usually results in 48 h after the completion of their training session. Delayed onset muscle soreness (DOMS) is still not fully explained; however, it is commonly thought of as a muscle tissue injury resulting from the excessive force on the connective and muscle tissue that causes an inflammatory response resulting in edema. The edema is what causes pain until the swelling subsides and movement becomes pain free. In athletes and individuals with years of fitness training, one experiences soreness when they change exercises, intensity, or duration of their current regimen. This changes the angle of pull on the muscle and connective tissue, causing inflammation and pain even in the well trained. However, the pain and edema will be much less after repeated bouts as training results in adaptation of the neural system, metabolites, and active tissues.

Previously it was thought that strength training would lead to a decrease in flexibility, and the myth of becoming "muscle bound" was propagated. This is counterintuitive since an increase in muscle around the joint actually leads to an increase in flexibility (Kraemer, Ratamess, & French, 2002). Stretching or flexibility training may increase flexibility, but it has recently been shown that improved flexibility may not decrease the incidence of sports or exercise-induced injuries (Hart, 2005). Yet it is well known that stretching exercises lead to gains in flexibility, which is needed to optimize the efficiency of movements used in many martial arts, gymnastics, and other sports where flexibility is of great importance.

## *Summary*

In 2004, Timothy Noakes and colleagues hypothesized that physical activity was controlled by a central governor in higher centers of the brain and that the human body synergistically functioned as an extremely complex system during exercise. They proposed a continuously altering pacing strategy, a "black box theory," which theorized that exercising skeletal muscle responded to afferent feedback from different physiological systems and the sensation of fatigue was the conscious interpretation of these homoeostatic, central governor control mechanisms (Noakes, St Clair Gibson, & Lambert, 2005).

With repeated bouts of exercise, an exercise training effect is shown where the body responds almost with previous knowledge of the task. Physiological responses are closely tied with psychological responses to produce a calculated amount of effort. If we increase the intensity or demand on the physiological system, we will realize a physiological adaptation resulting in a greater tolerance (i.e., training effect) that enables the physiological system to work at the heightened level. After several years of this training routine, the central movements will seem effortless and even automatic.

The keys to training for automaticity, then, are to understand the component behaviors that relate to the task, repeatedly practice these behaviors, and add training conditions that will aid one's ultimate training goal. If one requires speed, then the addition of resistance training will help lengthen the muscle, which in turn makes it faster and stronger. If endurance is the desired outcome, the application of aerobic training will increase the time one will be able to endure the higher metabolic cost of endurance events. It is important to remember that fatigue during any form of exercise occurs without evidence of related failure of physiological homoeostasis. This means that the body may still be able to perform, but attention and concentration may be compromised by fatigue. This clearly suggests that psychological training is an integral part of the training regimen and should occur at the same intensity as one's physical preparation.

## Conclusion

A basic tenet of this chapter is that for any voluntary activity, reaching the level of automaticity requires a large number of opportunities to respond. Developing automaticity in the complex repertoires of skilled athletic performance requires a complete commitment to one's sport followed by a long period of deliberate practice (Weissensteiner et al., 2009). What does an athlete gain in return for this investment? The answer to this question requires an appreciation for human beings as highly adaptive organisms. One mechanism by which we adapt to our environment is what Skinner (1987) termed *operant selection,* or when certain behaviors in a person's repertoire come to predominate because they are functional (i.e., repeatedly reinforced) by that environment. From this perspective, automaticity can be viewed as both a behavioral and a physiological adaptation to participating in sports. Behaviorally, deliberate practice produces a large repertoire of skilled performance, the components of which can be executed with high levels of fluency, can be instantly reorganized to meet changing demands, and are under strong stimulus control of subtle cues in the competitive environment. Physiologically, deliberate practice produces a shift from conscious to automatic control over behavior, increasing optimization of muscle recruitment strategies, and changes in muscle physiology to support more efficient movement. In short, in return for a long period of deliberate practice, research suggests that an athlete literally becomes a different person – one uniquely suited both behaviorally and physiologically to meet the unique demands of their sport.

## References

Abernethy, B. (1991). Visual search strategies and decision-making in sport. *International Journal of Sport Psychology, 22,* 189–210.

Alberto, P. A., & Troutman, A. C. (2003). *Applied behavior analysis for teachers* (6th ed.). Upper Saddle River, NJ: Prentice Hall.

Baker, J., Cote, J., & Abernethy, B. (2003). Sport-specific practice and the development of expert decision making in team ball sports. *Journal of Applied Sport Psychology, 15,* 12–25.

Bell, J. J., & Hardy, J. (2009). Effects of attentional focus on skilled performance in golf. *Journal of Applied Sport Psychology, 21,* 163–177.

Binder, C. (1996). Behavioral fluency: Evolution of a new paradigm. *The Behavior Analyst, 19,* 163–197.

Brobst, B., & Ward, P. (2002). Effects of posting, goal setting, and oral feedback on the skills of female soccer players. *Journal of Applied Behavior Analysis, 35,* 247–257.

Clark, B. C., Collier, S. R., Manini, T. M., & Ploutz-Snyder, L. L. (2005). Sex differences in muscle fatigability and activation patterns of the human quadriceps femoris. *European Journal of Applied Physiology, 94*(1–2), 196–206.

Collier, S. R., Kanaley, J. A., Carhart, R., Jr., Frechette, V., Tobin, M. M., Hall, A. K., et al. (2008). Effect of 4 weeks of aerobic or resistance exercise training on arterial stiffness, blood flow and blood pressure in pre- and stage-1 hypertensives. *Journal of Human Hypertension, 22*(10), 678–686.

Daly, E. J., Martens, B. K., Barnett, D., Witt, J. D., & Olson, S. C. (2007). Varying intervention delivery in response to intervention: Confronting and resolving challenges with measurement, instruction, and intensity. *School Psychology Review, 36,* 562–581.

Daly, E. J., III, Martens, B. K., Skinner, C. H., & Noell, G. H. (2009). Contributions of applied behavior analysis. In T. B. Gutkin & C. R. Reynolds (Eds.), *The handbook of school psychology* (4th ed., pp. 84–106). New York: Wiley.

Driskell, J. E., Willis, R. P., & Copper, C. (1992). Effect of overlearning on retention. *Journal of Applied Psychology, 77,* 615–622.

Dudley, G. A., & Djamil, R. (1985). Incompatibility of endurance- and strength-training modes of exercise. *Journal of Applied Physiology, 59*(5), 1446–1451.

Ericsson, K. A., & Charness, N. (1994). Expert performance: Its structure and acquisition. *American Psychologist, 49,* 725–747.

Ericsson, K. A., Krampe, R. Th., & Tesch-Romer, C. (1993). The role of deliberate practice in the acquisition of expert performance. *Psychological Review, 100*, 363–406.
Floyer-Lea, A., & Matthews, P. M. (2004). Changing brain networks for visuomotor control with increased movement automaticity. *Journal of Neurophysiology, 92*, 2405–2412.
Friden, J., Sjostrom, M., & Ekblom, B. (1984). Muscle fibre type characteristics in endurance trained and untrained individuals. *European Journal of Applied Physiology and Occupational Physiology, 52*(3), 266–271.
Galvao, D. A., & Taaffe, D. R. (2004). Single- vs. multiple-set resistance training: Recent developments in the controversy. *Journal of Strength and Conditioning Research, 18*(3), 660–667.
Guertin, P. A., & Steuer, I. (2009). Key central pattern generators of the spinal cord. *Journal of Neuroscience Research, 87*(11), 2399–2405.
Harding, J. W., Wacker, D. P., Berg, W., Rick, G., & Lee, J. F. (2004). Promoting response variability and stimulus generalization in martial arts training. *Journal of Applied Behavior Analysis, 37*, 185–195.
Haring, N. G., Lovitt, T. C., Eaton, M. D., & Hansen, C. L. (1978). *The fourth R: Research in the classroom*. Columbus, OH: Merrill.
Hart, L. (2005). Effect of stretching on sport injury risk: A review. *Clinical Journal of Sports Medicine, 15*(2), 113.
Helsen, W. F., Starkes, J. L., & Hodges, N. J. (1998). Team sports and the theory of deliberate practice. *Journal of Sport and Exercise Psychology, 20*, 12–34.
Henneman, E. (1957). Relation between size of neurons and their susceptibility to discharge. *Science, 126*(3287), 1345–1347.
Henneman, E., Somjen, G., & Carpenter, D. O. (1965). Functional significance of cell size in spinal motoneurons. *Journal of Neurophysiology, 28*, 560–580.
Hodge, T., & Deakin, J. M. (1998). Deliberate practice and expertise in the martial arts: The role of context in motor recall. *Journal of Sport and Exercise Psychology, 20*, 260–279.
Hoppeler, H., Howald, H., Conley, K., Lindstedt, S. L., Claassen, H., Vock, P., et al. (1985). Endurance training in humans: Aerobic capacity and structure of skeletal muscle. *Journal of Applied Physiology, 59*(2), 320–327.
Hudlicka, O. (1990). The response of muscle to enhanced and reduced activity. *Baillieres Clinical Endocrinology and Metabolism, 4*(3), 417–439.
Johnson, K. R., & Layng, T. V. J. (1996). On terms and procedures: Fluency. *The Behavior Analyst, 19*, 281–288.
Kladopoulos, C. N., & McComas, J. J. (2001). The effects of form training on foul-shooting performance in members of a women's college basketball team. *Journal of Applied Behavior Analysis, 34*, 329–332.
Koop, S., & Martin, H. L. (1983). Evaluation of a coaching strategy to reduce swimming stroke errors with beginning age-group swimmers. *Journal of Applied Behavior Analysis, 16*, 447–460.
Kraemer, W. J., Adams, K., Cafarelli, E., Dudley, G. A., Dooly, C., Feigenbaum, M. S., et al. (2002). American college of sports medicine position stand. Progression models in resistance training for healthy adults. *Medicine and Science in Sports and Exercise, 34*(2), 364–380.
Kraemer, W. J., Ratamess, N. A., & French, D. N. (2002). Resistance training for health and performance. *Current Sports Medicine Report, 1*(3), 165–171.
Liao, W. (1990). *Tai chi classics*. Boston: Shambhala.
Luyben, P. D., Funk, D. M., Morgan, J. K., Clark, K. A., & Delulio, D. W. (1986). Team sports for the severely retarded: Training a side-of-the-foot soccer pass using a maximum-to- minimum prompt reduction strategy. *Journal of Applied Behavior Analysis, 19*, 431–436.
MacPherson, A. C., Collins, D., & Obhi, S. S. (2009). The importance of temporal structure and rhythm for the optimum performance of motor skills: A new focus for practitioners of sport psychology. *Journal of Applied Sport Psychology, 21*(Suppl. 1), S48–S61.

MacPherson, A. C., Turner, A. P., & Collins, D. (2007). An investigation of the natural cadence between cyclists and non-cyclists. *Research Quarterly for Exercise and Sport, 78*, 396–400.

Martens, B. K., Daly, E. J., Begeny, J. C., & VanDerHeyden, A. (in press). Behavioral approaches to education. In W. Fisher, C. Piazza, & H. S. Roane (Eds.), *Handbook of applied behavior analysis*. New York: Guilford.

Martens, B. K., Eckert, T. L., Begeny, J. C., Lewandowski, L. J., DiGennaro, F., Montarello, S., et al. (2007). Effects of a fluency-building program on the reading performance of low-achieving second and third grade students. *Journal of Behavioral Education, 16*, 39–54.

Martens, B. K., & Witt, J. C. (2004). Competence, persistence, and success: The positive psychology of behavioral skill instruction. *Psychology in the Schools, 41*, 19–30.

McCarthy, J. P., Pozniak, M. A., & Agre, J. C. (2002). Neuromuscular adaptations to concurrent strength and endurance training. *Medicine and Science in Sports and Exercise, 34*(3), 511–519.

Mechner, F. (1995). *Learning and practicing skilled performance*. Retrieved January 11, 2010, from http://mechnerfoundation.org/newsite/downloads.html

Mechner, F. (2009). Analyzing variable behavioral contingencies: Are certain complex skills homologous with locomotion? *Behavioural Processes, 81*, 316–321.

Mellalieu, S. D., Hanton, S., & O'Brien, M. (2006). The effects of goal setting on rugby performance. *Journal of Applied Behavior Analysis, 39*, 257–261.

Morrow, J. R., Jr., & Hosler, W. W. (1981). Strength comparisons in untrained men and trained women athletes. *Medicine and Science in Sports and Exercise, 13*(3), 194–197.

Noakes, T. D., St Clair Gibson, A., & Lambert, E. V. (2005). From catastrophe to complexity: A novel model of integrative central neural regulation of effort and fatigue during exercise in humans: Summary and conclusions. *British Journal of Sports Medicine, 39*(2), 120–124.

Peterson, M. D., Rhea, M. R., & Alvar, B. A. (2005). Applications of the dose-response for muscular strength development: A review of meta-analytic efficacy and reliability for designing training prescription. *Journal of Strength and Conditioning Research, 19*(4), 950–958.

Reynolds, G. S. (1975). *A primer of operant conditioning*. Glenview, IL: Scott, Foresman, and Company.

Sale, D. G., Jacobs, I., MacDougall, J. D., & Garner, S. (1990). Comparison of two regimens of concurrent strength and endurance training. *Medicine and Science in Sports and Exercise, 22*(3), 348–356.

Scott, D., Scott, L. M., & Goldwater, B. (1997). A performance improvement program for an international-level track and field athlete. *Journal of Applied Behavior Analysis, 30*, 573–575.

Sherrington, C. (1910). Flexion Reflex of the limb, crossed extension reflex, and reflex stepping and standing. *Journal of Physiology, 40*, 28–121.

Simon, H. A., & Chase, W. (1973). Skill in chess. *American Scientist, 61*, 394–403.

Skinner, B. F. (1987). Whatever happened to psychology as the science of behavior? *American Psychologist, 42*, 780–786.

Smith, S. L., & Ward, P. (2006). Behavioral interventions to improve performance in collegiate football. *Journal of Applied Behavior Analysis, 39*, 385–391.

Southard, D., & Miracle, A. (1993). Rhythmicity, ritual, and motor performance: A study of free throw shooting in basketball. *Research Quarterly for Exercise and Sport, 64*, 284–290.

Starkey, D. B., Pollock, M. L., Ishida, Y., Welsch, M. A., Brechue, W. F., Graves, J. E., et al. (1996). Effect of resistance training volume on strength and muscle thickness. *Medicine and Science in Sports and Exercise, 28*(10), 1311–1320.

Staron, R. S., Malicky, E. S., Leonardi, M. J., Falkel, J. E., Hagerman, F. C., & Dudley, G. A. (1990). Muscle hypertrophy and fast fiber type conversions in heavy resistance-trained women. *European Journal of Applied Physiology and Occupational Physiology, 60*(1), 71–79.

Test, D. W., Spooner, F., Keul, P. K., & Grossi, T. (1990). Teaching adolescents with severe disabilities to use the public telephone. *Behavior Modification, 14*, 157–171.

Ueshiba, K. (1987). *The spirit of aikido*. Tokyo, Japan: Kodansha International.

Ward, P., & Carnes, M. (2002). Effects of posting self-set goals on collegiate football players' skill execution during practice and games. *Journal of Applied Behavior Analysis, 35*, 1–12.

Ward, P., Hodges, N. J., Williams, A. M., & Starkes, J. L. (2004). Deliberate practice and expert performance: Defining the path to excellence. In A. M. Williams & N. J. Hodges (Eds.), *Skill acquisition in sport: Research, theory and practice* (pp. 232–258). London: Routledge.

Weissensteiner, J., Abernethy, B., & Farrow, D. (2009). Towards the development of a conceptual model of expertise in cricket batting: A grounded theory approach. *Journal of Applied Sport Psychology, 21*, 276–292.

# Chapter 11
# Sport Neuropsychology and Cerebral Concussion

Frank M. Webbe

Sport neuropsychology defines a discipline of recent origin that combines the two stand-alone disciplines of sport psychology and neuropsychology. Sport psychology can be defined as "the scientific study of people and their behaviors in sport and exercise activities and the practical application of that knowledge" (Weinberg & Gould, 2007, p. 4). Neuropsychology studies the relationship between the functioning brain and behavior, with behavior often broken down into intellectual, emotional, and control components (Lezak, 1983). Both parent fields exhibit several similarities, and each has its scientific and applied sides. Experimental neuropsychology uses methods from experimental psychology to uncover the relationship between the nervous system and behavior, where behavior includes overt as well as within-brain cognitions. Both human and animal experimentation are common in experimental neuropsychology for the same methodological and ethical reasons that both exist in more standard behavior analytic approaches. Clinical neuropsychology applies neuropsychological knowledge to the assessment, management, and rehabilitation of people with neurobehavioral problems due to illness or brain injury. It brings a psychological viewpoint to treatment, to understand how such illness and injury may affect, and be affected by, psychological factors.

In sport psychology, the split is more complex. Exercise science is the predominant scientific side, but the psychology half also is divided into clinical versus scientific aspects. Obvious areas of overlapping interest exist between sport psychology and neuropsychology. For example, exercise science studies motor control and motor learning in sport. Brain injuries might obviously impact such learning and performance, and the rehabilitative effects of relearning motor behavior might in turn affect recovery processes in the brain. A sport neuropsychological approach would map such relationships. Sport science also includes exercise physiology, which details how the demands of exercise alter homeostatic levels and contribute to phenomena such as fatigue, motor errors, and disoriented thinking. For example, marathon runners and other endurance athletes ultimately endure compromise of normal metabolic functioning. Exercise physiologists might be interested

---

F.M. Webbe (✉)
Florida Institute of Technology, Melbourne, FL, USA
e-mail: webbe@fit.edu

**Table 11.1** Comparison of sport psychology vs. sport science disciplines

| Sport science – exercise | Sport psychology |
| --- | --- |
| Biomechanics | Abnormal psychology |
| Exercise physiology | Clinical/counseling psychology |
| Motor development | Developmental psychology |
| Motor learning and control | Learning/behavior analysis |
| Sport pedagogy | Personality psychology |
| Sport sociology | Physiological psychology |

in knowing when such compromise occurs, what the biomarkers are, whether it can be prevented or delayed, and how the altered physiology will impact performance. Table 11.1, adapted from Weinberg and Gould (2007), indicates the various subareas within the sport science-exercise versus psychology domains.

The areas of research and practice that define modern sport neuropsychology include (1) sport-related concussion, (2) role of exercise in enhancing neurocognitive functioning, (3) neurodevelopmental contributions of sport participation, (4) exercise and sport in the rehabilitation of persons with brain damage, and (5) psychoeducational interventions with athletes playing contact sports.

One of the more exciting aspects of this discipline is the heterogeneity of topics that are studied. However, one topic that actually originated the discipline and that has assumed its greatest prominence in the past year is the study of concussions in sport.

## Sport-Related Concussion

### What Is a Concussion?

The most elaborated area of interest in sport neuropsychology is the study of sport-related concussion. There have been many definitions of concussion over the years, with no single one achieving unanimous acceptance. However, at the 3rd International Conference on Concussion in Sport held in Zurich in November 2008, the A-list of attendees arrived at the following consensus definition (McCrory et al., 2009, p. 186):

Concussion is defined as a complex pathophysiological process affecting the brain, induced by traumatic biomechanical forces. Several common features that incorporate clinical, pathologic and biomechanical injury constructs that may be utilized in defining the nature of a concussive head injury include:

1. Concussion may be caused either by a direct blow to the head, face, neck or elsewhere on the body with an impulsive force transmitted to the head.
2. Concussion typically results in the rapid onset of short-lived impairment of neurologic function that resolves spontaneously.
3. Concussion may result in neuropathological changes, but the acute clinical symptoms largely reflect a functional disturbance rather than a structural injury.

Table 11.2 Concussion severity grading guidelines

|  | AAN | Cantu |
|---|---|---|
| Grade I | Symptoms < 15 min *and* No LOC | All symptoms < 30 min *and* No LOC |
| Grade II | Symptoms > 15 min *and* No LOC | Symptoms > 30 min but < 7 days *and/or* PTA > 30 min but < 24 h *and/or* LOC < 1 min |
| Grade III | Any LOC | Symptoms > 7 days *and/or* PTA >24 h *and/or* LOC > 1 min |

4. Concussion results in a graded set of clinical symptoms that may or may not involve loss of consciousness. Resolution of the clinical and cognitive symptoms typically follows a sequential course; however, it is important to note that, in a small percentage of cases, post-concussive symptoms may be prolonged.
5. No abnormality on standard structural neuroimaging studies is seen in concussion.

In order to create standardized approaches for discussing concussion severity that can be of functional use to health-care personnel, systems for grading concussions have been developed that concentrate primarily on loss of consciousness (LOC) and posttraumatic amnesia (PTA), two common symptoms of the many that may occur following concussion. Although many such systems have been developed over the years, two predominate and are summarized in Table 11.2.

The guidelines of the American Academy of Neurology (AAN; Kelly & Rosenberg, 1997) emphasize the qualitative importance of LOC, whereas the guidelines developed by neurosurgeon Robert Cantu (Cantu, 1986, 2001) distinguish between brief and extended LOC, and also emphasize the duration of PTA. Injuries are classified as Grade I (mild), Grade II (moderate), or Grade III (severe).

As was strongly emphasized in the Zurich Conference and is hinted at in the Cantu grading guidelines, duration of recovery is a key element in determining the severity of concussion. This often not only puts diagnosticians in a quandary, but also provides a challenge to sufferers, their families, and their teams, not to know fully the severity until recovery actually occurs.

## *Sport-Related Concussion*

Sport-related concussion defines the phenomenon of concussion as occurring within a sport context. For example, when two soccer players leap into the air, each attempting to head the ball but instead crashing their heads into each other with a resulting impairment in brain functioning, the mechanics of a sport-related concussion have occurred. As one or both players slowly rise to their feet and receive assistance in leaving the field, a trainer may already be asking them questions to determine the extent of amnesia, confusion, and disorientation that is present. They also will have noted whether any loss of consciousness has occurred. The presence of such symptoms affirms functionally that a concussion has taken place. Such an incident represents a sport-related concussion. In subsequent hours and days, issues of symptom severity and duration will be assessed with an eye toward subsequent return to play.

## Concussion Pathophysiology

As the definition given above indicates, cerebral concussion is a closed head injury that follows either impact blows to the skull and/or abrupt acceleration of the brain within the skull. Examples of such trauma are a punch to the face or the rapid deceleration that occurs when a body in motion suddenly is blocked or thrown to the ground. When the concussive event causes a rotational acceleration such that the brain tissue moves against itself inside the skull, the risk for significant functional impairment increases (Barth, Freeman, Broshek, & Varney, 2001). Once such physical forces have been applied to the brain, a succession of morbid outcomes ensue, including rapid increase followed by massive decrease in intracranial pressure (Hovda et al., 1999) and decrease in cerebral blood flow even as metabolic demands for oxygen and glucose increase drastically (Giza & Hovda, 2001). Shortly after the concussive event, electrical activity of the brain is depressed (West, Parkinson, & Havlicek, 1982). The metabolic conversion of glucose and oxygen to cellular energy first increases tremendously, consuming all available energy stores, and then stays in decline for at least several days (Giza & Hovda, 2001). (See Webbe, 2006, for a more detailed summary of the pathophysiology of sports-related concussion). The pressure wave induced by accelerative forces acting on the brain within the skull may produce differential accelerations of tissues (e.g., gray vs. white) that can result in stretching or even shearing. Stretching of neural tissue, especially the axons, causes cytoarchitectural changes that can include the unregulated opening of ion channels followed by a flux of ions that produce massive cellular excitation, and consequent depletion of cellular metabolic resources. The brain remains in a very unstable state of metabolic demands uncoupled from cerebral blood flow for several days to several weeks on the average (Giza & Hovda, 2001).

Traditional neuroradiological tools used in clinical practice such as computed tomography (CT) and magnetic resonance imaging (MRI) are of little value in determining the severity of concussive injury (Johnston, Ptito, Chankowsky, & Chen, 2001) or in predicting recovery for two reasons. First, the structural damage caused by concussion most likely happens at a level far more microscopic than can be detected by any but the most sophisticated research scanners. Second, the extent of structural injury even when detected appears to be a poor predictor of functional deficit (Bigler & Orrison, 2004). Functional MRI (fMRI) and positron emission tomography (PET) are much more likely to detect post-concussion anomalies since the primary abnormalities are physiological/metabolic in nature (Chen, Johnston, Collie, McCrory, & Ptito, 2007). We do know from research studies of concussed patients that cortical brain activity declines following the trauma. Electrophysiological techniques also show promise for detecting the presence of and severity of brain trauma, although such measures as event-related potential and evoked potential measurement rarely stray from the research laboratory. Neuropsychological testing not only represents a functional assessment, but also is objective (compared with simple symptom surveys), relatively inexpensive, and widely available.

## Concussion Epidemiology

Participation in sports is at an all-time high. In 2003, at the high school and college levels where the sanctioning organizations carefully track participation, student-athletes numbered 6,844,572 and 377,641 participants, respectively – an increase of nearly 6% over the 5-year period beginning 1998 (NFHS, 2005; NCAA, 2004). Although participation trends in youth sports are maintained less rigorously, the National Council of Youth Sports estimated recently that 38,259,845 children (63% boys) were engaged in some type of formal participation with teams or leagues (NCYS, 2001).

Athletes of any age are at risk for concussion, the most common form of neurologic head injury. Generally speaking, concussion risk increases as a function of the speed of movement in the sport coupled with the intensity of physical contact. The resultant collision frequency is one accepted measure of risk (Powell, 2001). Thus, sports with the highest concussion risk include American football, soccer, ice hockey, rugby, and lacrosse. However, there are some sleepers that might not be considered at first because participation rates are much lower. These include equestrian sports, rodeo, and wrestling. Boxing, mixed martial arts, and other ring and cage fighting events award a victory to a contestant who causes a brain injury to the opponent. It is not surprising that concussion risk in these events is exceptionally high (Powell, 2001). Both adults and children are subject to injury in any sport, whether it is organized or informal. The United States Consumer Product Safety Commission (CPSC) has listed the top 10 sports and activities in the United States that result in the most head injuries for children under 14. The sport/activity and the number of admissions reported in hospital emergency departments in 2007 are shown in Table 11.3 (CPSC, 2007).

Particularly with the publicity generated by the forced retirements of high-profile professional athletes and recent discoveries of chronic effects of repetitive head trauma (to be discussed later), sports-related concussion has become a very visible public health issue. According to the Centers for Disease Control and Prevention, more than 300,000 athletes per year suffer sport-related head injuries in the United States (Centers for Disease Control and Prevention, 2010; Sosin, Sniezek, & Thurman, 1996). Since this estimate is based only on athletes who lost consciousness – a phenomenon that occurs in only about 10% of diagnosed concussions – the likely incidence of these injuries is much higher. Furthermore, many concussions go unrecognized. In a recent study that examined reporting of concussions, 620 Canadian collegiate athletes were asked to complete symptom checklists based upon their experiences of the previous year. Seventy percent of

**Table 11.3** Emergency room admissions for head injury 2007

| | |
|---|---|
| Cycling | 32,899 |
| Football | 17,441 |
| Baseball and softball | 13,508 |
| Skateboards/scooters (powered) | 11,848 |
| Basketball | 10,844 |
| Skateboards/scooters | 10,256 |
| Winter sports (skiing, sledding, snowboarding, snowmobiling) | 7,546 |
| Powered recreational vehicles | 7,460 |
| Water sports (diving, scuba diving, surfing, swimming, water polo, water skiing) | 6,498 |
| Trampolines | 6,360 |

football players and 63% of soccer players reported that they had experienced symptoms during the prior season that were consistent with concussion. Of these, only 23% of the football players and 20% of the soccer players actually recognized that they had likely suffered a concussion or had been treated for a concussion (Delaney, Lacroix, Leclerc, & Johnston, 2002). Even taking into account the weak reliability of self-report data, these findings of underreporting are fully supported by additional outcome reports from other studies using both self-report and documentary data (Goodman, Gaetz, & Meichenbaum, 2001; McCrea, Hammeke, Olsen, Leo, & Guskiewicz, 2004; Williamson & Goodman, 2006). Moreover, athletes are notorious for hiding concussion symptoms when they do occur, often in attempts to prevent removal from an athletic contest and/or hasten return to play (Echemendia & Julian, 2001; Gerberich, Priest, Boen, Straub, & Maxwell, 1983).

## *Gender*

Concussion in sport is not an equal-opportunity injury in incidence, severity, or symptom duration. Most recent studies have indicated that women and girls tend to fare worse with these injuries than do men and boys. Regarding incidence, Dick (2009) has reviewed key studies reported in PubMed going back to at least 10 years. These included studies of concussion in all major contact sports played by both men and women. He reported that in 9 of the 10 incidence studies covering football, soccer, basketball, and ice hockey, women suffered a higher frequency of concussions than did men, with outcomes reaching statistical significance in four of the nine comparisons. Regarding symptoms, Broshek et al. (2005) and Lovell et al. (2006) found that women reported more symptoms and greater severity of those symptoms than did men. Regarding severity, Broshek et al. (2005) found that across several sports, women's baseline scores on key neurocognitive measures declined significantly more following concussion than did those of men injured in the same sports. Colvin et al. (2009) reported similar outcomses for soccer-specific concussions.

It appears clear that gender represents a risk factor in sport-related concussion and posttrauma symptom and cognitive status. This conclusion naturally stimulates the question *why*. We could theorize that women may be at greater risk for more severe injury and post-concussion effects due to lower body mass and smaller neck size and supporting musculature. Conversely, it could be argued that concussion-inducing collisions in women's sports may be less severe because of overall lower body mass entering into the force–mass relationship. Either way, studies have not yet supported these kinds of theories. Indeed, Colvin et al. (2009) report that it is gender and not mass that appears to be most critical.

Some studies have reported that women appear to be more forthcoming in their symptom reports than men (Broshek et al., 2005; Lovell et al., 2006), so the possibility exists that some differences may be due to gender-discrepant incidence and symptom reports. However, the authors of both these studies argue against such an interpretation since the neurocognitive testing outcomes also supported gender differences.

From a physiological standpoint, gender differences in hormonal systems, cerebral organization, and musculature may partially explain the differential findings. Results of studies with animals have implicated the sex steroid hormone, estrogen, as important in gendered differences in outcome from experimentally induced brain injury. However, some studies support a protective effect of estrogen; some demonstrate an exacerbation of injury (Roof & Hall, 2000). These discrepant findings may be due to major differences in methodology including the mechanism for producing traumatic brain injury (TBI), pretreatment regimen, and even inherent differences in effects of exogenous versus endogenous estrogen. Progesterone appears to reduce post-TBI neural impairment in humans, most likely by inhibiting destructive membrane changes and the resulting vasogenic edema (Roof & Hall, 2000; Roof, Duvdevani, & Stein, 1993). In summary, despite some conflicting studies regarding estrogen's role following TBI, the bulk of the hormonal data supports a neuroprotective role for both estrogen and progesterone.

The fact that gender may differentially determine TBI incidence, severity, and symptom resolution is a common thread of discussion in experimental neurology, but less well known in neuropsychology. There are considerable gender differences in the neural anatomy and physiology, cerebrovascular organization, and cellular response to concussive stimuli. For example, cortical neuronal densities are greater in males, while the number of neuronal processes is greater in females (de Courten-Myers, 1999). Females also exhibit greater blood flow rates and higher basal rates of glucose metabolism (Andreason, Zametkin, Guo, Baldwin, & Cohen, 1994; Esposito, Van Horn, Weinberger, & Berman, 1996). To the extent that female brains may have higher cortical metabolic demands, the typical decrease in cerebral blood flow along with the increased glycemic demands caused by TBI may interact with the already high gendered demands and result in greater impairment in females than in males.

## *Acute Effect of Concussion History*

In addition to the high rate of injury within sports, mounting evidence has also suggested that the rate of re-injury is higher in athletes who have experienced a prior concussion. For example, Guskiewicz et al. (2003) found that once a concussion is sustained, athletes are four to six times more likely to experience a second concussion, even if the second blow is relatively mild. Along similar lines, athletes with a history of multiple concussions have a greater risk of experiencing more severe symptoms at the time of their next concussive injury (Collins, Lovell, Iverson, Cantu, Maroon, & Field, 2002; Colvin et al., 2009). Subtle but significant, prolonged cognitive effects of concussion also have been demonstrated in "normal" asymptomatic high school athletes who suffered two or more concussions in the past, when compared to youth who reported only one or none (Moser, Schatz, & Jordan, 2005). In addition to the potential long-term morbidity associated with concussion, second impact syndrome, a rare but nonetheless devastating and usually fatal medical event, has been identified as a risk in athletes 21 years old and younger (Cantu, 1998). Second-impact syndrome is characterized by rapid brain swelling after the athlete suffers a second impact to the brain before they have fully recovered from the first insult. The mechanism for this catastrophic injury has been modeled in animal studies and is linked to the changes in brain metabolism following trauma (Giza & Hovda, 2001).

## *Physical Forces That Produce Concussion*

Barth and colleagues have suggested that severity of injury and subsequent neurocognitive impairment can be estimated by the acceleration-deceleration forces acting on the brain (Barth et al., 2001). Since many studies have been conducted with animals, and since animals and humans vary greatly in their ability to withstand impact and accelerative forces on the head, much of the literature is difficult to integrate. In general terms, it is clear that when peak decelerative forces occur over a very brief duration the risk of brain injury greatly increases. Naunheim, Standeven, Richter, and Lewis (2000) indicated in their review that a score in excess of 1,500 on the Gadd Severity Index, or above 1,000 on the Head Injury Criterion (HIC), or a peak accelerative force of 200 g should be considered thresholds for single impacts likely to "cause a significant brain injury" in adult humans. These values were estimated based upon animal studies and observations of accident outcomes in humans. Naunheim et al. (2000) also measured peak accelerative forces in athletic competition by using an accelerometer embedded in helmets worn by soccer, football, and ice hockey players. They recorded *no* impacts that approached the 200 g level, but also observed no events that were correlated with reports of concussion. Although this study does not shed light on the force–concussion relationship it does suggest that concussion-generating forces occur with merciful infrequency in these sports.

Children differ from adults in critical aspects of neural development such that the child's brain may be more vulnerable to injury from forces that would not seem problematic with adults. For example, Schneider and Zernicke (1988) studied concussion risk in soccer heading via a computer simulation model, within which the characteristics of the human participant along with the ball factors (acceleration, vector, and mass) were varied. After first calculating typical accelerative forces in players and nonplayers who were participating in a moderate heading drill, they applied the obtained acceleration, mass ratio, and duration values to the model. They reported that unsafe values of the HIC (>1,000) occurred when *children* were modeled in both translational and rotational acceleration conditions, and for adults in the rotational condition. Because the outcomes with children suggested an interaction between the mass of the individual with the mass of the ball as a critical variable in the equation, Schneider and Zernicke (1988) recommended the use of small soccer balls in contexts in which children might be heading.

## Sport as a Laboratory Assessment Model: The Gold Standard for Studying Sport Concussion

Barth's study of sport-related concussion spurred the evolution of sports neuropsychology. In the early 1980s, Barth and colleagues, including Macciocchi, Alves, Rimel, and Jane and Nelson, began studying college football players who suffered a concussion (Barth et al., 1989; Macciocchi, Barth, & Littlefield, 1998; Macciocchi, Barth, Alves, Rimel, & Jane, 1996). Realizing the improbability of multiple prospective participants for the study of brain injury in the general population, Barth identified college football players as individuals at a significantly high risk of brain injury. Neuropsychological tests were administered before the playing season began, and were repeated for those players who suffered concussion as well as for a non-concussed control group. From a medical, individual, and social perspective, the results were optimistic in that they portrayed the typical sport concussion in football as an event with transient neurocognitive impact. Much more enduring in importance, however, the methodology of that study established for the future a standard that has shaped the discipline. Specifically, Barth's approach of using the sport setting as a laboratory to study mild traumatic brain injury (sport as a laboratory assessment model – SLAM) established prospective, longitudinal methodology as the gold standard in the field (Barth, Harvey, Freeman, & Broshek, 2010). When athletes engage in rough, physical play there is an inevitability of injury, including head injury. The notion of establishing baselines of neurocognitive performance against which post-head injury performance could be compared represented a monumental improvement over the group, normative comparisons that otherwise were the only choice. Moreover, along with pre-injury neurocognitive testing, researchers also could collect information on premorbid physical and cognitive symptomatology. Thus, the baseline assessment model greatly diminished the variance inherent in making group normative comparisons. The remaining variance associated with repeated testing, history, and maturation could be understood better within the individual context. Though trained in using inferential statistics to analyze group data, Barth's training as a clinician, who concentrates on individual behavior, led him to recognize early on that both scientific and applied advances would occur only if an elaborated single-subject methodology was employed. The enormity of his undertaking must be understood in the context of early 1980s neuropsychology. There were no computerized tests. Rather, the process of neuropsychological testing was elaborate and time consuming, necessitating hours of one-on-one interaction. The difficulty of convincing high-level athletes and their coaches to dedicate hours of time *before any injury had occurred* cannot be overestimated. If wagers were placed upon the future of this approach, the smart money would have predicted that baseline assessment of sufficient depth undertaken with entire teams would be a very transient, self-limiting phenomenon. Nonetheless, Barth and his colleagues persevered long enough for the results of their early studies to be published. The first comprehensive report in 1989 (Barth et al., 1989) created a storm of interest that empowered the continuation of the prospective, baseline approach to concussion management. Fortunately also, the 1990s saw the development of the first computerized neurocognitive screening measures (to be discussed shortly), which removed the luxury label from baseline measurement and made the methodology more widely applicable.

What has not been eliminated – indeed it has been enhanced – is the finding of considerable individual differences in such critical and basic areas as (a) differences in the severity of outcome between individuals who receive apparently similar head insults, (b) differences between individuals in duration of recovery from concussions of apparently similar magnitude, (c) differences between individuals in ultimate recovery from concussion such that they can resume their previous activities, (d) effects of recurrent concussions on neurocognitive performance, and (e) effects of sub-concussive blows on neurocognitive performance (Webbe & Barth, 2003).

## Management Programs for Sport-Related Concussion

### Baseline Testing

Best practice calls for preseason neurocognitive baseline testing to establish a player's premorbid level of functioning. Most professional leagues have implemented such testing. For example, in the National Football League (NFL) and National Hockey League (NHL), such testing is mandatory. Following several horror stories of the recent past, neuropsychologists such as Mark Lovell, Mickey Collins, and Ruben Echemendia have been successful in creating an entire network of qualified practitioners who are ready and accessible to test players who have suffered a head injury (Lovell, Echemendia, & Burke, 2004). Common neuropsychological tests employed to assess baseline cognitive performance are shown in Table 11.4.

### Trauma Testing

In sport-related concussion management, neuropsychological assessments are usually given within 24–48 h after the traumatic event to document acute effects of the head injury and to compare level and pattern of performance to baseline. Assessments are repeated 3–5 days later and again at 7–10 days. If

**Table 11.4** Common neuropsychological tests used in sports neuropsychology

| Test category | Test |
|---|---|
| Learning and memory: verbal/auditory | California verbal learning test<br>Hopkins verbal learning test<br>Rey auditory verbal learning test |
| Learning and memory: visual | Brief visuospatial memory test-revised (BVMT-R) |
| Processing speed | Symbol digit modalities test<br>Trail making test<br>Controlled oral word association test<br>Paced auditory serial addition test<br>Wais-III digit symbol test |
| Executive function | Stroop color word test<br>Tower of London–Drexel |
| Attention | WAIS-III digit span |
| Word fluency | Controlled oral word association test (COWAT) |

neuropsychological measures do not indicate a return to baseline functioning within 10 days, further observations may be conducted at weekly intervals thereafter. A new baseline is then collected a minimum of 2 weeks following full recovery (Webbe & Barth, 2003). With children, longer-term assessments may be needed to determine whether mild head injury results in significant impairment in children's social or academic functioning as well (Yeates & Taylor, 2005).

Because of the large number of athletes who may have to be tested and the limitations on hours of availability, neuropsychological batteries used in sports neuropsychology are generally briefer than might be used in normal clinical practice. Forty-five minutes to an hour is the typical time frame. The batteries consist of tests that measure critical domains of functioning known to be at risk for impairment following TBI. Thus, processing speed, memory, and executive functioning have priority for assessment (Gronwall, 1989).

Measures of effort often are required in non-sport settings to insure validity of outcome. Effort has generally not been considered a critical factor with athlete examinees (Lovell et al., 2004). Instead, faking good is the more likely outcome since most athletes aim to return to play as soon as possible. Thus, even with nonstandard testing conditions, motivation is high. Nonetheless, with the advent of high profile sport-concussion injuries and the undoubted potential for liability claims, good practice suggests that assessment of effort (either through direct testing or a process approach) should become commonplace in the sport neuropsychology setting. A greater historic problem in the post-concussion testing is that of repeated measurement. Following a suspected concussion, anywhere from one to five assessments may occur within a 2-week time frame. Thus, it is most important to understand the re-test validity of the measures selected, and to make provision for positive change as a function of testing. As an example, simply scoring near the baseline level in post-trauma follow-up testing may represent impaired performance once the expected improvement due to practice is factored into the equation. Sport neuropsychology researchers have contributed considerably to studies of reliable change in computerized testing and laid the groundwork for clinical interpretation of repeated tests (Parsons, Notebaert, Shields, & Guskiewicz, 2009).

## *Computerized Instruments for Concussion Management*

Computer-based and Web-based neurocognitive assessments, such as Immediate Measurement of Performance and Cognitive Testing (ImPACT; Maroon et al., 2000), Automated Neuropsychological Assessment Metrics (ANAM; Reeves, Kane, & Winter, 1995; Reeves, Thorne, Winter, & Hegge, 1989), CogSport (Collie, Darby, & Maruff, 2001), and the Concussion Resolution Index (CRI; Erlanger et al., 2001), have made possible the baseline approach with entire teams and leagues. Computerized assessments sample domains of brain functioning such as reaction time, speed of processing information, attention and concentration, memory, and cognitive flexibility. Computerized testing allows examiners to assess common sequelae of concussion, including subtle changes in processing speed to the millisecond. Computerized measures also reduce the impact of practice effects by providing multiple equivalent forms of the test. The reliability and validity of these tests for use in the concussed athlete have been established (Schatz & Zillmer, 2003). The complicated task for the sport neuropsychologist is determining whether current measures of performance represent deviation from baseline, and with children, whether the measures are within a normal range for a developing brain.

## Resolution of Symptoms: The Normal Recovery Curve and Complications

### *Length of Recovery*

Barth et al. (1989) showed that the majority of college-aged individuals who suffered mild head injury showed complete resolution of cognitive symptoms after 5–10 days. However, individuals who had sustained multiple concussive or even sub-concussive blows had a slower recovery from post-concussive symptoms. In a follow-up study, Alves (1992) indicated that physical symptoms of concussion usually diminished with time, and completely resolved by 3–6 months post injury. Most studies in the ensuing 20 years have supported the original Barth et al. (1989) findings, suggesting that 85% or so of concussed athletes likely recover cognitively within 1–2 weeks (Webbe & Barth, 2003). Nonetheless, the 15–30% or more of individuals who take longer to recovery represent a significant minority, and frequently this group may be forgotten within the usual generalization (Ruff, Camenzuli, & Mueller, 1996; Sterr, Herron, Hayward, & Montaldi, 2006). For children, the picture is even cloudier. Moser & Schatz (2002) showed that post-concussive symptoms persisted for weeks or months in some youth athletes who had suffered multiple concussive or sub-concussive blows.

The factors that predict which athlete will have a quick versus long symptom resolution have not been identified clearly and unambiguously. Two athletes who suffer similar mild head trauma may differ widely in their recovery and return to play despite no obvious differences in injury mechanics, diagnostic imaging, and sideline symptoms including presence or absence of LOC and PTA. Some of the factors that have been identified as important in understanding duration of recovery and (development and resolution of post-concussion syndrome) include (a) history of previous concussions (Moser et al., 2005), (b) premorbid learning disorders (Collins et al., 1999), (c) psychological and emotional distress (Bailey, Samples, Broshek, Freeman, & Barth, 2010; Hutchison, Mainwaring, Comper, Richards, & Bisschop, 2009; Ruff et al., 1996), (d) genetic characteristics such as the APoE-e4 allele (Kutner, Erlanger, Tsai, Jordan, & Relkin, 2000), and (e) number and recency of previous concussions (Erlanger, Kutner, Barth, & Barnes, 1999; Guskiewicz et al., 2003; Macciocchi, Barth, Littlefield, & Cantu, 2001). In the absence of clear physical data, the severity and duration of symptom involvement remains the clearest estimate of severity.

## *Return to Play*

Severity of concussion is often a post hoc determination based upon the persistence of concussion-related symptoms. The earliest definitions and conceptualizations of concussion concluded that recovery was quite rapid. The vestige of that concept remains in sport when players attempt to reenter games as quickly as possible or deny any recurring symptoms that might persuade others to keep them from returning to play. Similarly, coaches want their players to resume training and playing as soon after concussion as possible. Studies of athletic head injuries most typically report on immediate, short-term, and long-term outcomes for recovery of normal cognitive function and resolution of physical symptoms such as headache and nausea. Assuming that an immediate, sideline judgment has been made that a player suffered a concussion, then subsequent neurocognitive assessments are typically initiated within 24 h in this model. If symptoms still are present, then additional measurement is likely after 3–5 days, and again at 7–10 days. If symptoms and/or cognitive functions have not returned to normal within 10 days, it would be common to make further observations at regular intervals until symptoms have resolved and the player returns to his/her baseline neurocognitive function. The somatic symptoms that predominate during these times are headache, confusion or disorientation (often called fogginess), which are reported by about 50–75% of the athletes (Barth et al., 1989; Macciocchi et al., 1996; McCrea et al., 2003). Thus, what remains to be fine-tuned is to correlate the underlying functional and/or structural changes with recovery from concussion. Although it is tempting to speculate, for example, that hypometabolic alterations are responsible for symptoms in the short-term, and that lasting cytoarchitectural alterations and/or cellular morbidity controls more

**Table 11.5** Zurich conference consensus recommendations for graduated return to play protocol (McCrory et al., 2009)

| Rehabilitation stage | Functional exercise at each stage of rehabilitation | Objective of each stage |
| --- | --- | --- |
| 1. No activity | Complete physical and cognitive rest | Recovery |
| 2. Light aerobic exercise | Walking, swimming or stationary cycling keeping intensity 70% MPHR; no resistance training | Increase HR |
| 3. Sport-specific exercise | Skating drills in ice hockey, running drills in soccer; no head impact activities | Add movement |
| 4. Non-contact training drills | Progression to more complex training drills, e.g., passing drills in football and ice hockey; may start progressive resistance training | Exercise, coordination, and cognitive load |
| 5. Full contact practice | Following medical clearance, participate in normal training activities | Restore confidence and assess functional skills by coaching staff |
| 6. Return to play | Normal game play | |

persisting symptoms, data from human studies still are insufficient to support such conclusions.

So, when should athletes return to play? The conservative approach is the most followed, which dictates, (a) resolution of physical symptoms as determined by self-report and informant observation, (b) clear neurological examination results, (c) neurocognitive test data showing return to or maintenance of premorbid functioning, and (d) balance testing and additional other protocols showing baseline performance. The Zurich Conference in 2007 also provided the following guidelines and objectives, shown in Table 11.5, for a graduated return-to-play once the above conditions are met. Previous return-to-play guidelines such as those described alongside and including ratings of concussion severity (Cantu, 1986, 2001; Kelly & Rosenberg, 1997) combined the severity grade with previous concussion history and resolution of symptoms to determine when it was safe to return. The main problem with those earlier systems was that loss of consciousness was a primary factor in determining severity or grade of concussion. More recent studies have demonstrated that LOC occurs in fewer than 10% of the instances of sport-related concussion (Sosin et al., 1996), and that LOC is not overly related to severity, or predictive of symptom resolution (Lovell, Iverson, Collins, McKeag, & Maroon, 1999; McCrea, Kelly, Randolph, Cisler, & Berger, 2002).

## Effects of Repetitive Head Trauma

With alarming frequency over the past several years, reports of cumulative effects of repetitive sub-concussive and concussive events in current and former athletes have been headline news. In 2007, the professional wrestler Chris Benoit murdered his wife and son and then hanged himself. In 2006, 12 years after retiring from professional football, defensive back Andre Waters shot himself in the head. Twenty-one-year-old University of Pennsylvania linebacker Owen Thomas was found dead on April 27, 2010, another suicide victim. Hall of fame center Mike Webster died homeless in 2002, a victim of progressive dementia before he was 50. Former English Premier League soccer player Jeff Astle died in January of 2002 at age 59. "Astle couldn't remember anything about the game he loved, or even the names of his grandchildren. A coroner ruled: 'it was heading the soccer ball that had killed him'" (Wallace, 2002). What may link the tragic end of all these athletes was a history of repetitive head trauma. This link cannot determine that brain injury was responsible for the abnormal behavior, but the likelihood of a link appears more than hypothetical.

McKee, Stern, and colleagues at Boston University, the Bedford Veterans Administration Medical Center, and the Sports Legacy Institute, have reported a part of the data from their developing brain bank of athletes from contact sports (including Benoit, Waters, and Thomas). The outcomes that they have reported have been surprising and disturbing. First was the report that former professional athletes, primarily from football, exhibited a brain pathology, chronic traumatic encephalopathy (CTE), that was consistent with that seen in former boxers and others who had known histories of repetitive head injuries (McKee et al., 2009). As the brain bank grew, these findings were extended to a few athletes who had competed only in college football as well as to other professionals from the sports of wrestling, hockey, and soccer. Even more recently, newer analyses have reported that a majority of these subjects also had a proteinopathy distributed widely in their brains, which further involved spinal cord and brain stem motor neurons, and which correlated with the symptoms of primary progressive motor neuron diseases such as amyotrophic lateral sclerosis (ALS; McKee et al., 2010). McKee, Stern, and their colleagues point to the repetitive brain trauma suffered by these athletes as the likely cause of the brain pathologies. Although there are a smattering of athletes representing sports other than ice hockey and American football, only those two sports have sufficient participants in the brain bank for preliminary conclusions to be drawn. Moreover, the self-selection bias present both in volunteers and in postmortem donations by family members must be accounted for ultimately with better-controlled methodologies. Even accounting for selection bias, however, the consistency of findings clearly raises alarms regarding repetitive head insults and their life changing potentiality. Much is yet to be learned about the extent of such pathological changes, for example, when they begin, if they are common to all participants in sports where the brain is constantly banged around, and if there are genetic or other idiopathic interactions. However, enough appears to be known to issue caution to participants to possibly alter their style of play, and to administrators to consider changing rules of play. Assisting athletes in actually changing their playing behavior is a difficult and complex task since pathogenic behavior may also be behavior that produces success on the field or court.

## Educational Approaches in Sport Neuropsychology

In its "Heads Up" series, the Centers for Disease Control (CDC; 2010) have led the way in stimulating education on concussion for sport participants, parents, physicians, and youth/high school coaches. More recently, the National Academy of Neuropsychology and the National Athletic Trainers Association (NATA) have taken the lead among professional organizations in devoting time and resources to public education on concussion in general, and sport-related concussion in particular. In both written materials and in educational DVDs, these organizations, with the sponsorship of the NHL, the NHL Players Association, and the NFL have carried this educational message to youth, adult, and professional players, coaches, trainers, team management, and the general public (NAN, 2009). Such efforts are critical to increasing the recognition of concussions when they occur, and also in recognizing and preventing conditions that produce concussions. These efforts also are key in bringing the discussion and the science down to amateur and youth levels, the least regulated and loosest organized sport entities. Moreover, although the impact of concussive brain injuries on children may often be more pronounced than in adults, with longer times to recovery (e.g., Moser & Schatz, 2002), guidelines for returning youth athletes to play are mostly nonexistent (Moser et al., 2007).

In addition to actual and proposed governmental legislation, key athletic organizations and associations also have begun proaction in the area of concussion in sport. Both the NFL and the NHL have ramped up their existing concussion monitoring programs. The NFL, in particular, has adopted a new attitude whereby concussion is not a topic to be mentioned in whispers. Locker room posters, informational literature for players and families, and stricter policies on removal and return-to-play have all appeared in 2010. Similarly, the National Collegiate Athletic Association (NCAA) now has mandated that its member institutions develop concussion management plans that include preseason baseline testing for sports where concussion risk is significant, documented return-to-play guidelines in the event of a concussion, and a mandatory education program for student-athletes and coaches (NCAA, 2010).

These public policy changes are both exciting and gratifying for neuropsychologists who have been publicizing the possible downside of playing contact sports without proper safeguards and monitoring of participants. However, in the vein of being careful of what one wishes for, there now may be more pressure on the neuropsychology discipline not only to provide the testing services required by these policies, but to demonstrate their worth. A very real opportunity for enhancing education and prevention of concussion is readily available at the level of youth sports. Youth organization administrators would benefit from education about the prevention of head injuries so that they would understand the importance of allocating funding toward acquiring qualified trainers to monitor youth games in the event that concussions take place. Due to the limited availability of athletic trainers at youth games currently, referees and game officials are frequently relied upon to identify injuries. Unfortunately, concussion has many subtle signs and symptoms that officials may not be aware of; therefore, they may not stop game play or appropriately remove these youth from play. Thus, education and training specific to concussion should be targeted at youth referees. Safety information would also extend to the environment in which these youth athletes are playing in order to ensure that equipment and other hazards are taken out of the sports arena.

Because children may report many different symptoms after a head injury, it is important for neuropsychologists to also educate coaches and parents about concussion-like symptoms in order to be alert for an early identification of injury. Parents and coaches may have an incomplete knowledge of common post-concussion symptoms, expecting only self-evident problems such as amnesia, confusion, headache, and dizziness. It is also important to explain emotional reactivity and other more subtle symptoms that may arise from rather mild head impacts such as heading a soccer ball as well as other more serious injury sources. This is critical as McLeod, Schwartz, and Bay (2007) highlighted several misconceptions that youth coaches have regarding sports-related concussion. They found that 42% of coaches in their sample ($N = 250$) believed that loss of consciousness was needed for a concussion to have happened, 32% did not believe that a Grade 1 concussion required removal from a game, and 26% reported that they would let a symptomatic athlete return to play. The *CDC's Heads Up in Youth Sports* toolkit mentioned earlier is a free resource provided by the CDC that is useful in disseminating concussion related information to parents, players, and coaches. It includes educational materials such as a video, wallet card listing signs/symptoms, posters, fact sheets, and other concussion-related resources.

## References

Alves, W. (1992). Natural history of post-concussive signs and symptoms. *Physical Medicine and Rehabilitation: State of the Arts Reviews, 6*, 21–32.

Andreason, P. J., Zametkin, A. J., Guo, A. C., Baldwin, P., & Cohen, R. M. (1994). Gender-related differences in regional cerebral glucose metabolism and normal volunteers. *Psychiatry Research, 51*, 175–183.

Bailey, C. M., Samples, H. L., Broshek, D. K., Freeman, J. R., & Barth, J. T. (2010). The relationship between psychological distress and baseline sports-related concussion testing. *Clinical Journal of Sport Medicine, 20*, 272–277.

Barth, J. T., Alves, W. M., Ryan, T. V., Macciocchi, S. N., Rimel, R. W., Jane, J. A., et al. (1989). Mild head injuries in sports: Neuropsychological sequelae and recovery of function. In H. Levin, H. Eisenberg, & A. Benton (Eds.), *Mild head injury* (pp. 257–77). New York: Oxford University Press.

Barth, J. T., Freeman, J. R., Broshek, D. K., & Varney, R. N. (2001). Acceleration-deceleration sport-related concussion: The gravity of it all. *Journal of Athletic Training, 36*, 253–256.

Barth, J. T., Harvey, D. J., Freeman, J., & Broshek, D. K. (2010). Sports as a laboratory assessment model. In F. M. Webbe (Ed.), *Handbook of sport neuropsychology* (pp. 75–89). New York: Springer Publishing.

Bigler, E. D., & Orrison, W. W. (2004). Neuroimaging in sports-related brain injury. In M. R. Lovell, R. J. Echemendia, J. T. Barth, & M. W. Collins (Eds.), *Traumatic brain injury in sports* (pp. 71–93). Lisse, The Netherlands: Swets & Zeitlinger.

Broshek, D. K., Kaushik, T., Freeman, J. R., Erlanger, D., Webbe, F. M., & Barth, J. T. (2005). Gender differences in outcome from sports-related concussion. *Journal of Neurosurgery, 102*, 856–863.

Cantu, R. C. (1986). Guidelines for return to contact sports after a cerebral concussion. *The Physician and Sportsmedicine, 14*, 76–79.

Cantu, R. C. (1998). Second-impact Syndrome. *Clinics in Sports Medicine, 17*, 37–44.

Cantu, R. C. (2001). Posttraumatic retrograde and anterograde amnesia: Pathophysiology and implications in grading and safe return to play. *Journal of Athletic Training, 36*, 244–248.

Centers for Disease Control and Prevention (2010). Concussion in sports. Retrieved September 12, 2010, from http://www.cdc.gov/concussion/sports/index.html

Chen, J. K., Johnston, K. M., Collie, A., McCrory, P., & Ptito, A. (2007). A validation of the post-concussion symptom scale in the assessment of complex concussion using cognitive testing and functional MRI. *Journal of Neurolology, Neurosurgery, & Psychiatry, 78*, 1231–1238.

Collie, A., Darby, D., & Maruff, P. (2001). Computerized cognitive assessment of athletes with sports related head injury. *British Journal of Sports Medicine, 35*, 297–302.

Collins, M. W., Grindel, S. H., Lovell, M. R., Dede, D. E., Moser, D. J., Phalin, B. R., et al. (1999). Relationship between concussion and neuropsychological performance in college football players. *Journal of the American Medical Association, 282*, 964–970.

Collins, M. W., Lovell, M. R., Iverson, G. L., Cantu, T. C., Maroon, J. C., & Field, M. (2002). Cumulative effects of concussion in high school athletes. *Neurosurgery, 51*, 1175–1182.

Colvin, A. C., Mullen, J., Lovell, M. R., West, R. V., Collins, M. W., & Groh, M. (2009). The role of concussion history and gender in recovery from soccer-related concussion. *American Journal of Sports Medicine, 37*, 699–1704.

CPSC (2007). *National Electronic Injury Surveillance System (NEISS) On-line*. Retrieved November 24, 2008, from http://www.cpsc.gov/LIBRARY/neiss.html

de Courten-Myers, G. M. (1999). The human cerebral cortex: Gender differences in structure and function. *Journal of Neuropathology and Experimental Neurology, 58*, 217–226.

Delaney, S., Lacroix, V. J., Leclerc, S., & Johnston, K. M. (2002). Concussions among university football and soccer players. *Clinical Journal of Sport Medicine, 12*, 331–338.

Dick, R. W. (2009). Is there a gender difference in concussion incidence and outcomes? *British Journal of Sports Medicine, 43*, i46–i50.

Echemendia, R. J., & Julian, L. J. (2001). Mild traumatic brain injury in sports: Neuropsychology's contribution to a developing field. *Neuropsychology Review, 11*, 69–88.

Erlanger, D. M., Kutner, K. C., Barth, J. T., & Barnes, R. (1999). Neuropsychology of sports-related head injury: Dementia pugilistica to post concussion syndrome. *The Clinical Neuropsychologist, 13*, 193–209.

Erlanger, D. M., Saliba, E., Barth, J., Almquist, J., Webright, W., & Freeman, J. (2001). Monitoring resolution of post-concussion symptoms in athletes: Preliminary results of a web-based neuropsychological test protocol. *Journal of Athletic Training, 36*, 280–287.

Esposito, G., Van Horn, J. D., Weinberger, D. R., & Berman, K. F. (1996). Gender differences in cerebral blood flow as a function of cognitive state with PET. *The Journal of Nuclear Medicine, 37*, 559–564.

Gerberich, S. G., Priest, J. D., Boen, J. R., Straub, C. P., & Maxwell, R. E. (1983). Concussion incidences and severity in secondary school varsity football players. *American Journal of Public Health, 73*, 1370–1375.

Giza, C. C., & Hovda, D. A. (2001). The neurometabolic cascade of concussion. *Journal of Athletic Training, 36*, 228–235.

Goodman, D., Gaetz, M., & Meichenbaum, D. (2001). Concussions in hockey: There is cause for concern. *Medicine and. Science in Sports and Exercise, 33*, 2004–2009.

Gronwall, D. (1989). Cumulative and persisting effects of concussion on attention and cognition. In H. S. Levin, H. M. Eisenberg, & A. L. Benton (Eds.), *Mild head injury* (pp. 153–162). New York: Oxford University Press.

Guskiewicz, K. M., McCrea, M., Marshall, S. W., Cantu, R. C., Randolph, C., Barr, W., et al. (2003). Cumulative effects associated with recurrent concussion in collegiate football players. *Journal of the American Medical Association, 290*, 2549–2555.

Hovda, D. A., Prins, M., Becker, D. P., Lee, S., Bergsneider, M., & Martin, N. A. (1999). Neurobiology of concussion. In J. E. Bailes, M. R. Lovell, & J. C. Maroon (Eds.), *Sports-related concussion* (pp. 12–51). St. Louis, MO: Quality Medical Publishing, Inc.

Hutchison, M., Mainwaring, L. M., Comper, P., Richards, D. W., & Bisschop, S. M. (2009). Differential emotional responses of varsity athletes to concussion and musculoskeletal injuries. *Clinical Journal of Sport Medicine, 19*, 13–19.

Johnston, K. M., Ptito, A., Chankowsky, J., & Chen, J. K. (2001). New frontiers in diagnostic imaging in concussive head injury. *Clinical Journal of Sport Medicine, 11*, 166–175.

Kelly, J. P., & Rosenberg, J. H. (1997). Practice parameter: The management of concussion in sports (summary statement). Report of the quality standards subcommittee. *Neurology, 4*, 581–585.

Kutner, K., Erlanger, D. M., Tsai, J., Jordan, B., & Relkin, N. R. (2000). Lower cognitive performance of older football players possessing apolipoprotein E e4. *Neurosurgery, 47*, 651–658.

Lezak, M. (1983). *Neuropsychological assessment* (2nd ed.). New York: Oxford University Press.

Lovell, M. R., Echemendia, R. J., & Burke, C. J. (2004). Professional ice hockey. In M. R. Lovell, R. J. Echemendia, J. T. Barth, & M. W. Collins (Eds.), *Traumatic brain injury in sports* (pp. 221–229). Lisse, The Netherlands: Swets & Zeitlinger Publishers.

Lovell, M. R., Iverson, G. L., Collins, M. W., McKeag, D., & Maroon, J. C. (1999). Does loss of consciousness predict neuropsychological decrements after concussion? *Clinical Journal of Sport Medicine, 9*, 193–198.

Lovell, M. R., Iverson, G. L., Collins, M. W., Podell, K., Johnston, K. M., Pardini, D., et al. (2006). Measurement of symptoms following sports-related concussion: Reliability and normative data for the post-concussion scale. *Applied Neuropsychology, 143*, 166–174.

Macciocchi, S. N., Barth, J. T., Alves, W., Rimel, R. W., & Jane, J. A. (1996). Neuropsychological functioning and recovery after mild head injury in college athletes. *Neurosurgery, 39*, 510–514.

Macciocchi, S. N., Barth, J. T., & Littlefield, L. M. (1998). Neurologic athletic head and neck injuries. *Clinics in Sports Medicine, 17*(1), 27–37.

Macciocchi, S. N., Barth, J. T., Littlefield, L., & Cantu, R. C. (2001). Multiple concussions and neuropsychological functioning in collegiate football players. *Journal of Athletic Training, 36*, 303–306.

Maroon, J. C., Lovell, M. R., Norwig, J., Podell, K., Powell, J. W., & Hartl, R. (2000). Cerebral concussion in athletes: Evaluation and neuropsychological testing. *Neurosurgery, 47*, 659–672.

McCrea, M., Guskiewicz, K. M., Marshall, S. W., Barr, W., Randolph, C., Cantu, R. C., et al. (2003). Acute effects and recovery time following concussion in collegiate football players. *Journal of the American Medical Association, 290*, 2556–2563.

McCrea, M., Hammeke, T., Olsen, G., Leo, P., & Guskiewicz, K. (2004). Unreported concussion in high school football players: Implications for prevention. *Clinical Journal of Sport Medicine, 14*, 13–17.

McCrea, M., Kelly, J. P., Randolph, C., Cisler, R., & Berger, L. (2002). Immediate neurocognitive effects of concussion. *Neurosurgery, 50*, 1032–1042.

McCrory, P., Meeuwisse, W., Johnston, K., Dvorak, J., Aubry, M., Molloy, M., et al. (2009). Consensus statement on concussion in sport 3rd international conference on concussion in sport held in Zurich, november 2008. *Clinical Journal of Sport Medicine, 19*, 85–200.

McKee, A. C., Cantu, R. C., Nowinski, A. B., Hedley-Whyte, T., Gavett, B. E., Budson, A. E., et al. (2009). Chronic traumatic encephalopathy in athletes: Progressive tauopathy after repetitive head injury. *Journal of Neuropathology and Experimental Neurology, 68*, 709–735.

McKee, A. C., Gavett, B. E., Stern, R. A., Nowinski, C. J., Cantu, R. C., Kowall, N. W., et al. (2010). TDP-43 proteinopathy and motor neuron disease in chronic traumatic encephalopathy. *Journal of Neuropathology & Experimental Neurology, 69*, 918–929.

McLeod, T. C. V., Schwartz, C., & Bay, C. (2007). Sport-related concussion misunderstandings among youth coaches. *Clinical Journal of Sport Medicine, 17*, 140–142.

Moser, R. S., Iverson, G. L., Echemendia, R., Lovell, M., Schatz, P., Webbe, F. M., et al. (2007). Neuropsychological testing in the diagnosis and management of sports-related concussion. *Archives of Clinical Neuropsychology, 22*, 909–916.

Moser, R. S., & Schatz, P. (2002). Enduring effects of concussion in youth athletes. *Archives of Clinical Neuropsychology, 17*, 91–100.

Moser, R. S., Schatz, P., & Jordan, B. D. (2005). Prolonged effects of concussion in high school athletes. *Neurosurgery, 57*, 300–306.

NAN (2009). Raising Concussion Awareness Educational DVD. Accessed August 17, 2010, from http://www.nanonline.org/NAN/Home/Home/HockeyVideo.aspx

Naunheim, R. S., Standeven, J., Richter, C., & Lewis, L. M. (2000). Comparison of impact data in hockey, football, and soccer. *The Journal of Trauma, 48*, 938–941.

NCAA (2004). 1981-82 – 2002-03 *NCAA sports sponsorship and participation rates report*. Indianapolis, IN: National Collegiate Athletic Association.

NCAA (2010). Legislative Requirement—Concussion Management Plan—Effective August 16, 2010. http://web1.ncaa.org/web_files/DII_MC_PC/Miscellaneous/Concussion%20Management%20Memorandum.pdf. Accessed August 17, 2010.

NCYS (2001). National Report on Trends and Participation in Organized Youth Sports. Retrieved November 17, 2008, from http://www.ncys.org/pdf/marketResearch.pdf.

NFHS (2005). 2004-05 *NFHS high school athletics participation survey*. Indianapolis, IN: National Federation of State High School Associations.

Parsons, T. D., Notebaert, A. J., Shields, E. W., & Guskiewicz, K. M. (2009). Application of reliable change indices to computerized neuropsychological measures of concussion. *International Journal of Neuroscience, 119*, 492–507.

Powell, J. W. (2001). Cerebral concussion: Causes, effects, and risks in sports. *Journal of Athletic Training, 36*, 307–311.

Reeves, D., Kane, R., Winter, K., et al. (1995). *Automated neuropsychological assessment metrics (ANAM): Test administration manual (Version 3.11)*. St. Louis, MO: Missouri Institute of Mental Health.

Reeves, D., Thorne, R., Winter, S., & Hegge, F. (1989). *Cognitive Performance Assessment Battery (UTC-PAB). Report 89-1*. San Diego, CA: Naval Aerospace Medical Research Laboratory and Walter Reed Army Institute of Research.

Roof, R. L., Duvdevani, R., & Stein, D. G. (1993). Gender influences outcome of brain injury: Progesterone plays a protective role. *Brain Research, 607*, 333–336.

Roof, R. L., & Hall, E. D. (2000). Gender differences in acute CNS trauma and stroke: Neuroprotective effects of estrogen and progesterone. *Journal of Neurotrauma, 17*, 367–388.

Ruff, R. M., Camenzuli, L., & Mueller, J. (1996). Miserable minority: Emotional risk factors that influence the outcome of a mild traumatic brain injury. *Brain Injury, 10*, 551–565.

Schatz, P., & Zillmer, E. A. (2003). Computer-based assessment of sports-related concussion. *Applied Neuropsychology, 10*, 42–47.

Schneider, K., & Zernicke, R. F. (1988). Computer simulation of head impact: Estimation of head-injury risk during soccer heading. *International Journal of Sport Biomechanics, 4*, 358–371.

Sosin, D. M., Sniezek, J. E., & Thurman, D. J. (1996). Incidence of mild and moderate brain injury in the United States, 1991. *Brain Injury, 10*, 47–54.

Sterr, A., Herron, K., Hayward, C., & Montaldi, D. (2006). Are mild head injuries as mild as we think? Neurobehavioral concomitants of chronic post-concussion syndrome. *BMC Neurology, 6*, 7.

Webbe, F. M. (2006). Definition, physiology, and severity of cerebral concussion. In R. J. Echemendia (Ed.), *Sports neuropsychology: Assessment and management of traumatic brain injury* (pp. 45–70). New York: The Guilford Press.

Webbe, F. M., & Barth, J. T. (2003). Short-term and long-term outcome of athletic closed head injuries. *Clinics in Sports Medicine, 22*, 577–592.

Weinberg, R. S., & Gould, D. (2007). *Foundations of sport and exercise psychology* (4th ed.). Champaign, IL: Human Kinetics.

West, M., Parkinson, D., & Havlicek, V. (1982). Spectral analysis of the electroencephalographic response to experimental concussion in the rat. *Clinical Neurophysiology, 53*, 192–200.

Williamson, I. J. S., & Goodman, D. (2006). Converging evidence for the under-reporting of concussions in youth ice hockey. *British Journal of Sports Medicine, 40*, 128–132.

Wallace, W. (2002, December 22). Death awakens soccer world. The Los Angeles Times. Retrieved from http://articles.latimes.com/2002/dec/27/sports/sp-headers27.

Yeates, K. O., & Taylor, G. (2005). Neurobehavioural outcomes of mild head injury in children and adolescents. *Pediatric Rehabilitation, 8*, 5–16.

# Chapter 12
# Aggression in Competitive Sports: Using Direct Observation to Evaluate Incidence and Prevention Focused Intervention

Chris J. Gee

The term *aggression* has developed into something of an umbrella construct, in both its social and academic applications (Widmeyer, Dorsch, Bray, & McGuire, 2002). For example, pushy and persistent salespeople are often referred to as aggressive, as are baseball players who run the bases exceptionally hard and sacrifice their bodies for the betterment of their teams. Unfortunately, neither of these examples reflects the academic conceptualization of the term. As such, before moving further into this chapter, I want to clarify the meaning of aggression within the context of the behavioral sciences.

Within the sport psychology literature, aggressive behavior is defined as "any overt act (verbal or physical) that has the capacity to cause psychological or physical injury to another. The act must be purposeful (non-accidental) and chosen with the intent of causing harm" (Stephens, 1998, p. 277). These behaviors for the most part fall outside of the formal rulebook (as most sports penalize intentionally harmful behavior), meaning that tackling in rugby and football, and body-checking in ice hockey, are not the primary behaviors of interest. Rather, aggressive behaviors reflect those actions that go above and beyond the strategic physical contact allowed by many sports and are reflected in those behaviors in which the transgressor intentionally tries to harm their opponent.

Apropos the preceding discussion, ice hockey is frequently heralded as the gold standard sport through which sport-specific aggression is studied and understood. Yet despite numerous and multidisciplinary research endeavors concerned with hockey aggression, our current understanding of the etiology of these behaviors is still incomplete and unreliable (Coulomb & Pfister, 1998; Gee & Sullivan, 2006; Gee, 2010a; Kirker, Tenenbaum, & Mattson, 2000; Stephens, 1998). Many of the criticisms directed toward the sport aggression literature have been methodological in nature and have subsequently forced academics to reevaluate the utility and validity of how aggressive behavior is currently being operationalized. This process of critical reflection has spawned several methodological alternatives that address many of these perceived limitations.

C.J. Gee (✉)
Department of Exercise Sciences, University of Toronto, Toronto, ON, Canada M9W 5Z8
e-mail: chris.gee@utoronto.ca

As is indicated by the title of this chapter, behavioral observation is useful for studying sport-related aggressive behavior. In the following sections, I review observational methodologies for studying sport-specific aggression and comment about their strengths and contribution to behavioral sport psychology.

## Previous Methodologies Employed to Study Sport-Specific Aggression

Overwhelmingly, research concerned with the etiology of aggressive behavior in sport has been carried out using one of two methodologies: self-report or archival (penalty records). Both methodologies have strengths as well as limitations.

### *Self-Report Methodology*

Studies utilizing self-report instruments (i.e., questionnaires) have predominantly been concerned with assessing athletes' attitudes and legitimacy perceptions as they relate to the use of aggressive behavior in sport (Stephens, 1998). Some of the most widely used instruments are (1) Sport Behavior Inventory (SBI; Conroy, Silva, Newcomer, Walker, & Johnson, 2001), (2) Judgments About Moral Behavior in Youth Sport Questionnaire (JAMBYSQ; Stephens, Bredemeier, & Shields, 1997), and (3) Bredemeier Athletic Aggression Inventory (BAAGI; Bredemeier, 1978). The implicit assumption underpinning self-report research on aggressive behavior is that an athlete's responses on these assessments reflect validly how they would actually behave during competition. Unfortunately, this assumption is not supported empirically, as many of these instruments have never been tested for construct validity (Gee, 2010b; Stephens, 1998). In those few instances where a valid measure of within-competition behavior has been included (e.g., penalty records), researchers have reported weak, and even negative, correlations between athletes' self-reported aggressive tendencies and their actual within-competition behaviors (Gee, 2010b; Loughead & Leith, 2001; Worrell & Harris, 1986). Consequently, the validity of employing self-report instruments to study aggressive behavior in sport, especially as the sole dependent variable, has been routinely questioned and criticized (Gee & Sullivan, 2004; Gee & Sullivan, 2006; Kirker et al., 2000; Sheldon & Aimar, 2001; Stephens, 1998).

Poor ecological validity associated with self-report instruments may explain why there is a disconnect between athlete's self-report scores and their actual overt behavior (Bredemeier & Shields, 1984, 1986a, 1986b; Gee & Sullivan, 2006; Stephens, 1998). Predominantly, these research studies have queried athletes about their aggressive beliefs and/or attitudes at home or during a practice situation, as to not interfere with a team's competitive preparation. However, as Bredemeier and Shields (1986a) state, "patterns of moral reasoning in sport differ from the patterns of moral reasoning that are used in most other aspects of life. Movement into the sport world involves a transformation of moral meaning" (p. 20).

These authors speculate that the normative moral code present within competitive hockey, and other competitive sports, coupled with other stimuli that are specific to this social context (e.g., emphasis on athletic competence, "win-at-all-costs" mentality, hypermasculine ideals), are all determinants of sport-specific aggressive behavior and cannot validly be replicated in other environments. As a result, it is quickly becoming consensus within the academic community that studies concerned with the etiology of aggressive behavior must include these and other ecological influences in order to obtain a valid and reliable assessment of a particular athlete's competitive deportment (Gee & Sullivan, 2006; Gee, 2010a, 2010b; Kirker et al., 2000). As such, studies that continue to employ self-report assessments as the sole dependent measure should, at the very least, have participants complete the assessment within the context of interest. From a best practices perspective, self-report assessments should be included as part of a mixed methods approach whereby they are used to assess attitudinal and perceptual constructs, but are not the dependent proxy measure of aggression.

In summary, self-report instruments allow for large populations to be assessed expeditiously, and they provide researchers with insight into the aggressive thoughts, attitudes, and perceptions of athletes. Unfortunately, due to the unique climate of competitive sport, self-report data by athletes outside of this context may not accurately reflect their overt aggressive behavior. Accordingly, when self-report data are used as a proxy dependent measure of sport-specific aggression, the validity and reliability of the research findings must be questioned.

## *Archival Methodology*

By far the most widely employed methodology for studying sport-specific aggression has been official penalty records during games. Aggressive behaviors within this framework are operationalized as those acts that violate the formal rules of the game and are subsequently punished by trained game officials. Using this approach, an athlete's actual within-competition behaviors are now being directly measured, which subsequently reduces concerns about the ecological or external validity of the results as compared to self-report data. This final point is extremely important because of the comments made earlier about the unique contributing factors present within the context of competitive sport. Consequently, because competitive sport is such a unique social context, it is important that the behavioral criterion of interest be observed and extrapolated directly from this environment (Russell & Russell, 1984; Vokey & Russell, 1992).

Studies that have relied on archival penalty records have also been heavily critiqued on ecological grounds (Gee & Sullivan, 2004; Kirker et al., 2000; Sheldon & Aimar, 2001). However, unlike self-report studies that have been criticized based on the generalizability of the research context, archival designs have been targeted for a different violation of ecological validity (Schmuckler, 2001). For example, because of the speed of competitive sports such as ice hockey, coupled with the multiple responsibilities allocated to each game official (e.g., issue penalties, line infractions, judge legitimacy of goals), it has been widely argued that a large proportion of aggressive behaviors go unnoticed during a competitive contest (Bar-Eli & Tenenbaum, 1989; Gee & Sullivan, 2006; Kirker et al., 2000; Mark, Bryant, & Lehman, 1983; Sheldon & Aimar, 2001). Moreover, it has also been suggested that a game official's decisions to penalize particular behaviors may be influenced by such factors as the game location, score differential, crowd reaction, and time remaining in the contest (Greer, 1983; Jones, Bray, & Olivier, 2005; Nevill, Balmer, & Williams, 2002). It is not uncommon, for instance, to hear that the refs have "put away their whistles" or that they "are letting the teams play" when an important game is close in score. In such situations, game officials do not want to become the deciding factor, and therefore, they penalize only those behaviors that are flagrant or potentially injurious (Gee & Sullivan, 2006). Nevertheless, several behaviors that adhere to the conceptual definition of aggression (e.g., possess the intent to cause harm) occur during these periods of non-penalization, which subsequently detracts from the representativeness of the sample of behaviors collected using archival methodology.

In contrast, certain acts of aggression are volitionally overlooked by game officials, as they are considered "typical" within the sport and part of the "unwritten rulebook." As an example, in ice hockey a player who digs for the puck once the goalie has it covered will routinely be pushed or punched by several defensive players after the whistle. Such reciprocation has become part of the game and has come to be expected as punishment for poking at a team's goalie.

When combined, the result of missed and overlooked infractions by game officials has the potential to significantly distort our understanding of the frequency and distribution of aggressive behavior in sport. As an illustration, Gee and Sullivan (2006) found that 69% of the infractions among Junior B (15–18 years old) hockey players met the operational criteria in a study of aggressive behavior but ultimately went unsanctioned by game officials. So when two-thirds of the observations comprising the dependent variable fail to be accounted for, one has to be highly critical of the validity and reliability of the eventual findings. In effect, very different conclusions could be drawn from a competitive sport event depending upon the methodology that was used to collect the behavioral data.

## Direct Observation as Method for Obtaining a Valid Measure of Aggressive Behavior

In an attempt to overcome the limitations cited in the previous section, researchers have sought viable methodological alternatives. Behavioral observation is one method that has received recent empirical attention. It is a descriptive technique in which participants' behaviors are observed and coded within their natural setting (Thomas & Nelson, 2001). With respect to aggression, Kirker et al. (2000) stated, "the observation of game behavior in real time and the context in which it occurs provides the best opportunities to understand the dynamics of aggressive behavior in sport" (p. 376). Consequently, direct observation has several features for capturing valid, reliable, and ecologically valid behavioral data.

First, direct observation can be conducted from videotape, allowing researchers to stop, rewind, and pause the competitive action and isolate specific behaviors. This more static, thorough, and objective process has the potential to significantly add to the validity of the overall assessment process and thus to the comprehensiveness of the overall sample of behaviors measured. Many direct observation techniques within sport have actually opted to use multiple cameras in order to investigate several influential factors simultaneously (Gee & Sullivan, 2003; Kirker et al., 2000; Teipel, Gerisch, & Busse, 1983), as well as having multiple coders analyze the data. This methodology has the potential of giving a more holistic account of aggression during competition. Furthermore, it permits researchers to assess interrater agreement, a feature not present within previous archival research (Gee, 2010a). By having multiple independent coders analyzing the data through video analysis, behavioral observation can more effectively document the high frequency of missed and overlooked calls that currently plague the archival approach.

One of the most dramatic improvements in measuring aggressive behavior with direct observation is its ability to encompass all aggressive infractions, especially those that have become part of the "unwritten rulebook." As several of these actions adhere to the conceptual and operational criteria of aggression, including them is necessary for ensuring the validity of the dependent measure. The ability for the researcher to code the aggressive behaviors outside of the competitive atmosphere certainly aids in this pursuit. As was mentioned earlier, some of the concerns surrounding the accuracy of archival data pertain to the pressures and environmental influences that often impact game officials' decisions. Referencing Gee and Sullivan (2006) again, their research found that a large number of aggressive behaviors during ice hockey games were overlooked when the score differential was relatively small (e.g., teams are one or two goals apart), presumably because the game officials did not want to be the deciding factor in the competitive contest. Moreover, game officials must also consider the potential crowd reaction to their within-game decisions and thus balance adherence to the rulebook with overall game and crowd control. Finally, a practical concern for game officials is that they must stop the game in order to assess a particular penalty infraction. Consequently, if a game official was to penalize all behaviors that violated the formal rulebook, it is plausible that some sporting events would take days, rather than hours, to complete. This simple reality introduces a source of motivation to avoid calling infractions and could detract from the validity of the sample of behaviors collected. Direct observation allows researchers to be more objective about whether or not a certain infraction should be included, as they do not face the same consequences or environmental factors as do game officials. Overall, when aggressive behaviors are recorded through videotaped observation, the sample of behaviors should be more valid and generalizable (Gee & Sullivan, 2006; Gee, 2010a).

Another methodological advantage of direct observation is being able to analyze and incorporate verbal aggression. As Kirker et al. (2000) concluded in their observational study of men's basketball and ice hockey, negative verbalizations directed toward opponents and game officials are the most frequent form of within-competition aggressive conduct. Verbal aggression, in fact, may act as a catalyst for more severe, overt acts of aggression routinely observed within competitive sport. Previous methodologies have not included verbal aggression, making such assessment a fruitful line of research for the future. Consequently, a comprehensive understanding of verbal aggression within the competitive environment is desirable.

Overall then, there are two primary advantages associated with the direct observation of sport-related aggression. First, researchers can assess athletes' aggressive behavior within the unique social context of competitive sport. Doing so maximizes ecological validity. Second, direct observation has the potential to yield a more valid and reliable measure of aggression.

## *Behavioral Observation and Measuring "Intent"*

As was mentioned in the introduction, the defining characteristic of an aggressive infraction is the transgressor's "intent to harm." Previous methodologies have failed to properly measure an athlete's intent, opting instead to infer intent through other cognitive or behavioral measures. Intent is obviously a cognitive construct, and therefore, it cannot be readily observed by a third party. As such, similar to criticisms levied against the archival approach (Kirker et al., 2000; Sheldon & Aimar, 2001), current observation methodologies also possess an inherent inferential bias. Nevertheless, there are adjunct methodologies that, when employed as part of a mixed methods approach alongside behavioral observation, could synergistically address this limitation in the future.

First, direct observation allows the researcher to follow particular players across the span of a game. In doing so, researchers become privy to circumstances and incidents within the game that provide insight into or context to events that transpire later in the game (Katorji & Cahoon, 1992). This feature is particularly important as Widmeyer et al. (2002) suggest that provocation and rivalries are two important determinants of athlete aggression. This contextual information can reveal a player's behavioral intentions, when understood and evaluated within the context of the larger game. This strategy is not a comprehensive solution to measuring intent, but it highlights how direct observation moves us closer to this pursuit.

Secondly, researchers have recently begun to use retrospective stimulated recall interviews following observational assessments in an attempt to directly assess athletes' intent (Kirker et al., 2000; Shapcott, Bloom, & Loughead, 2007). Players are shown a clip of their aggressive behavior and asked to explain why they engaged in the particular act. This approach advances the study of aggressive behavior and reflects yet another advantage associated with using a videotaped observation methodology. Notably, stimulated recall interviews will be especially beneficial with "gray area" infractions where an athlete's intent cannot be readily inferred from his/her overt actions.

Finally, creating customized lists of athletes' self-reported aggressive behaviors is an adjunct strategy worthy of future attention (Gee, 2010b). Similar to the methods employed by Widmeyer and Birch (1984) and Widmeyer and McGuire (1997), where coaches, referees, and players were asked to list the behaviors that they employed with the intent to harm an opponent, researchers could undertake a similar process at the level of the individual athlete. When combined with direct observation, researchers could assess each player's within-game deportment, while only including those infractions that the athlete reported as aggressive (see Widmeyer & Birch, 1984, for a more detailed description of this a priori methodology). As with all of the previously cited strategies, some degree of error exists in trying to control for intent. Ultimately, however, methods and future designs should strive toward accounting for and controlling for this error whenever possible.

## *Direct Observation as a Method for Studying the Acquisition of Aggressive Behavior*

Up to this point I have primarily discussed behavioral observation as a data collection tool for capturing within-competition incidents of aggressive behavior. However, the unique methodological properties and rich qualitative insight of behavioral observation also make it a strong choice when attempting to address broader lines of research concerned with the acquisition of aggressive behavior. In this section, I review how direct observation can be used to study the socialization of aggressive behavior and how researchers can address perceived barriers to obtaining valid information from parents and sport coaches.

A primary line of research in the study of sport-specific aggression is how athletes learn and ultimately exhibit such behavior. By focusing on an athlete's primary social group within the athletic domain (i.e., parents, coaches, teammates), researchers have sought to establish how these important socializing agents transmit information about aggressive behavior and subsequently how athletes behave accordingly. Research to date suggests that many athletes believe that their parents and coaches approve of aggressive conduct within the context of competitive sport (Faulkner, 1974; Smith, 1979; Vaz & Thomas, 1974). However, this research has not explained how these perceptions are ultimately formed. Unfortunately, we do not fully understand how and why parents and coaches teach athletes to be aggressive (both inside and outside of the sporting domain) and, subsequently, how and why they reinforce persistent aggressive behavior.

I believe that in order to answer the aforementioned questions, a candid look inside the dressing room, behind the bench, in the stands, and in the car ride home is likely required (Gee, 2010b). Michael Smith, a prominent scholar in Canada, undertook a large-scale qualitative study into the etiology of aggressive behavior in Canadian youth ice hockey in the late 1970s. Through this project Dr. Smith was able to gain access to several of these "behind the scene" areas and was subsequently privy to the types of conversations believed to be central to our understanding of the socialization process. For example, Smith (1979) overheard a bantam-level (13–14-year-olds) hockey coach state the following:

Look, if this character starts anything, take him out early. We can't have him charging around hammering people. Somebody's going to have to straighten him out. Just remember, get the gloves off and do it in a fair fight. If you shake him up early he can't keep it up. Besides, it's best to take penalties early in the game before we get too tired to kill them effectively (p. 108).

While in the lobby after another youth hockey game, Smith (1979) overheard one parent say to another, "Boy! little Ian isn't afraid to hit" (p. 80). When little Ian emerged from the dressing room, his father remarked, "looks like we have a little Tiger Williams on our hands" (p. 80). Unfortunately, Smith's research was predominantly qualitative, and therefore, even though it provided great insight into the content of these behind-the-scene messages, it failed to examine their effect over athletes' actual within-competition behavior. Consequently, future research should study the actions and verbalizations of these primary socializing agents, but do so in conjunction with other key intrapersonal factors and ultimately against athletes' within-competition use of aggression.

One of the distinct advantages that observation methodologies have in the above pursuit, especially if they are conducted without the participants' knowledge, is overcoming social desirability. Previous investigations concerned with the influence of coaches and parents on athletes' aggressive behavior have frequently reported results contrary to common hypotheses. These findings, or the lack thereof, are believed to reflect the tendency for adult participants queried about aggressive behavior to give "appropriate" responses (Gee, 2010b; Givvin, 2001; White, 2007). With the negative media stereotypes depicting the "crazed sporting parent" and the "win-at-all-costs coach," it is understandable why these adult participants might respond in a self-effacing manner. Nevertheless, this source of error makes it difficult to obtain valid and reliable data from these groups. I recommend that direct observation should focus on how parents and coaches behave within the competitive context, especially prior to and following aggressive transgressions.

## The Role of Behavioral Observation in Prevention-Based Intervention

This final section describes how behavioral observation can inform future prevention-based intervention, including recommendations for parents, coaches, game officials, and athletes.

### *Coaches/Parents*

Currently within amateur sport, there are initiatives directed toward parents/coaches aimed at curbing aggressive conduct. These initiatives oftentimes revolve around educating parents and coaches about their influence on young athletes' behavior. In many cases, parents and coaches are mandated to attend educational seminars before the season and asked to sign "Good Behavior" contracts. Unfortunately, as I stated earlier, there appears to be a disconnect between what parents and coaches say they will do and what actually transpires when the competitive whistle blows. In line with Bredemeier and Shields's (1986a) assertion around the contextual nature of morality, parents and coaches often denounce aggressive conduct when queried about it in a classroom setting, yet send very different messages about the legitimacy of aggressive behavior when immersed within the competitive climate (Goldstein & Iso-Ahola, 2008). Again, there appears to be something quite unique about competition (e.g., emotion, competition, different norms, and moral code) that causes parents and coaches to reinforce and legitimize behaviors that they would not otherwise reinforce in other circumstances (Bryant, 1989; Bryant, Zillman, & Raney, 1998; Raney, 2006). To reiterate, these behaviors should be measured directly within the social context of interest. This, of course, is where an observational method could prove to be effective. All of us have seen ourselves on camera and thought "Is that how I behave/sound/look like to other people"? This reflective process can affect the way people see themselves and ultimately their future behavior, especially if the images caught on tape are less than flattering (Tice & Wallace, 2003). Therefore, by employing video surveillance during youth sporting events, sporting administrators would have not only a method for monitoring spectator and coach behavior, but also a methodology for addressing incidents post hoc with those individuals involved. Using actual camera footage of the incident could have a substantial impact on the learning and eventual behavioral change that takes place following a particular incident. Moreover, having actual footage of the incident would remove any of the hearsay and ambiguity that potentially cloud the reprisal process. The cameras would clearly show what transpired, making the punitive process much more "cut and dry." Placing cameras at youth sporting events would also likely serve as a deterrent, forcing spectators and coaches to be more cognizant of their behavior when attending these events. Similar observational methodologies have been employed with coaches in the past; however, these tapes were subsequently used for coaching development purposes (Trudel, Cote, & Danz, 1996). Nevertheless, the individualized nature of the approach has advantages when it comes to changing future behavior.

## *Game Officials*

Observational methodologies may also have a place in educating game officials. Actual game tapes could be used to exemplify particular circumstances or trends that have been shown to facilitate violent or aggressive episodes, allowing officials to see in real time how these events transpire. Moreover, similar to the process employed in many professional sports, videotape analysis can be used to show individual game officials where certain mistakes were made throughout the game. In accordance with the statements made in the previous subsection, having these events presented in a video format removes much of the hearsay involved with these situations and can often facilitate quick and long-lasting behavioral changes. Previous research into the etiology of aggressive behavior has identified the quality and consistency of officiating as a potential determinant of aggressive behavior (Pascall, 2000). It is hypothesized that game officials have the ability to set the tone for the game, but can also introduce unwanted frustration and emotion into the competitive contest by being inconsistent in the way they penalize infractions. Including video analysis may help ensure consistency in the way penalties are called and can also be used for educational purposes at the individual level.

## *Athletes*

Direct observation may also play an important role in curbing the use of aggressive behavior at the level of the athlete. For example, in the early 2000s, in response to a perceived spike in spinal cord and neck injuries among Canadian youth hockey players, a large-scale educational campaign was launched to remove the proposed determinants of these injuries (e.g., dangerous body checks from behind). A primary component of this campaign was mandatory educational sessions for all athletes, which included both on- and off-ice materials. Off-ice materials included video analysis of what constitutes a legal and illegal check moving forward, leaving very little in the way of ambiguity. These lessons were subsequently reinforced during the on-ice sessions through practical demonstrations. The literature suggests that athletes often do not understand what is "too much" or illegal within their sport, in part because officials call penalties inconsistently. As Gee and Potwarka (2007) suggest, "a line between what is acceptable and what is not needs to be clearly defined ... [and] athletes need to understand that there is an upper limit to what is acceptable within the confines of the competitive atmosphere." Consequently, video analysis could be used as an educational tool to help athletes clearly understand what is acceptable and unacceptable deportment. Moreover, if these parameters are consistently reinforced by game officials, and the negative consequences associated with rule violations are severe enough, profound behavioral changes would be projected to follow. Such procedures have been used by professional sports when new rule changes have been introduced during the off-season.

## Summary and Conclusions

Direct observation, used for data collection and intervention planning, addresses many concerns previously encountered in the study of sport-specific aggression. Specifically, direct observation overcomes limitations with an archival approach, including the large number of infractions that go unseen or uncalled by game officials. Consequently, by offering the opportunity to slow down, rewind, and pause the competition action, while also allowing multiple independent coders to assess the content, observation produces a more valid sample of aggressive behavior. Moreover, direct observation gives researchers the opportunity to assess the competitive climate in a more holistic fashion, assessing spectator, coach, and player variables simultaneously. The ability to move the study of aggressive behavior from the micro to the macro, as well as from the artificial to the ecological, represents a significant step forward for this area of inquiry.

# References

Bar-Eli, M., & Tenenbaum, G. (1989). Observations of behavioral violations as crisis indicators in competition. *The Sport Psychologist, 3*, 237–244.

Bredemeier, B. (1978). The assessment of reactive and instrumental aggression. In *Proceedings of the international symposium of psychological assessment in sport* (pp. 136–145). Netanya, Israel: Wingate Institute for Physical Education and Sport.

Bredemeier, B., & Shields, D. (1984). Divergence in moral reasoning about sport and everyday life. *Sociology of Sport Journal, 1*, 304–318.

Bredemeier, B., & Shields, D. (1986a). Athletic aggression: An issue of contextual morality. *Sociology of Sport Journal, 3*, 15–28.

Bredemeier, B., & Shields, D. (1986b). Game reasoning and interactional morality. *Journal of Genetic Psychology, 147*, 257–275.

Bryant, J. (1989). Viewer's enjoyments of televised sports violence. In L. A. Wenner (Ed.), *Media sports and society* (pp. 270–289). Newbury Park, CA: Sage.

Bryant, J., Zillman, D., & Raney, A. A. (1998). Violence and the enjoyment of media sports. In L. A. Wenner (Ed.), *Media sport* (pp. 252–265). London: Routledge.

Conroy, D. E., Silva, J. M., Newcomer, R. R., Walker, B. W., & Johnson, M. S. (2001). Personal and participatory influences on the socialization of aggressive sport behavior. *Aggressive Behavior, 27*, 405–418.

Coulomb, G., & Pfister, R. (1998). Aggressive behavior in soccer as a function of competitive level and time: A field study. *Journal of Sport Behavior, 21*, 222–232.

Faulkner, R. R. (1974). Making violence by doing work: Selves, situations, and the world of professional hockey. *Sociology of Work and Occupations, 1*, 288–312.

Gee, C. J. (2010a). Using a direct observation methodology to study aggressive behavior in ice hockey: The good, the bad, and the ugly. *Journal of Behavioral Health and Medicine, 1*, 79–90.

Gee, C. J. (2010b). *Predicting the use of aggressive behavior among Canadian amateur hockey players: A psychosocial examination*. Unpublished doctoral dissertation, University of Toronto, Toronto, Ontario, Canada.

Gee, C. J., & Potwarka, L. R. (2007). The impact of introducing legal punishment on the frequency of aggressive behaviour in professional ice hockey: Using the Todd Bertuzzi incident as an ecological case study. *Athletic Insight, 9*(3). http://www.athleticinsight.com/Vol9Iss3/LegalPunishment.htm.

Gee, C. J., & Sullivan, P. J. (2003, October 18). *The direct observation of aggressive behavior in hockey*. Presented at the Canadian Society for Psychomotor Learning and Sport Psychology conference (SCAPPS), Hamilton, ON.

Gee, C.J., & Sullivan, P. J. (2004). Aggression and coaching in sport. *Coaches Report, 10*(3), 25–27.

Gee, C. J., & Sullivan, P. J. (2006). Using a direct observation approach to study aggressive behavior in ice hockey: Some preliminary findings. *Athletic Insight, 8*. http://www.athleticinsight.com/Vol8Iss1/DirectObservation.htm.

Givvin, K. B. (2001). Goal orientations of adolescents, coaches, and parents: Is there a convergence of beliefs? *Journal of Early Adolescence, 21*, 227–247.

Goldstein, J. D., & Iso-Ahola, S. E. (2008). Determinants of parents' sideline-rage emotions and behaviors at youth soccer games. *Journal of Applied Social Psychology, 38*, 1442–1462.

Greer, D. L. (1983). Spectator booing and the home advantage: Study of social influence in the basketball arena. *Social Psychology Quarterly, 46*, 252–261.

Jones, M. V., Bray, S. R., & Olivier, S. (2005). Game location and aggression in rugby. *Journal of Sport Science, 23*, 387–393.

Katorji, K., & Cahoon, M. A. (1992). *The relationship between aggression and injury in Junior "B" hockey*. Unpublished manuscript, University of Waterloo, Waterloo, Ontario, Canada.

Kirker, B., Tenenbaum, G., & Mattson, J. (2000). An investigation of the dynamics of aggression: Direct observation in ice hockey and basketball. *Research Quarterly for Exercise and Sport, 71*, 373–386.

Loughead, T. M., & Leith, L. M. (2001). Hockey coaches' and players' perceptions of aggression and the aggressive behavior of players. *Journal of Sport Behavior, 24*, 394–407.

Mark, M. M., Bryant, F. B., & Lehman, D. R. (1983). Perceived injustice and sports violence. In J. H. Goldstein (Ed.), *Sports violence* (pp. 83–109). New York: Springer.

Nevill, A. M., Balmer, N. J., & Williams, A. M. (2002). The influence of crowd noise and experience upon referring decisions in football. *Psychology of Sport and Exercise, 3*, 261–272.

Pascall, B. (2000, May). *Violence in hockey*. Report to the honourable Ian G. Waddell, British Columbia Ministry of Small Business, Tourism, and Culture.

Raney, A. A. (2006). Why we watch and enjoy mediated sports. In A. A. Raney & J. Bryant (Eds.), *Handbook of sports and media* (pp. 313–330). New York: Lawrence Earlbaum Associates.

Russell, G. W., & Russell, A. M. (1984). Sport penalties: An alternative means of measuring aggression. *Social Behavior and Personality: An International Journal, 12*, 69–74.

Schmuckler, M. A. (2001). What is ecological validity? A dimensional analysis. *Infancy, 2*, 419–436.

Shapcott, K. M., Bloom, G. A., & Loughead, T. M. (2007). Factors influencing aggressive and assertive intentions of women ice hockey players. *International Journal of Sport Psychology, 38*, 145–162.

Sheldon, J. P., & Aimar, C. M. (2001). The role aggression plays in successful and unsuccessful ice hockey behaviors. *Research Quarterly for Exercise and Sport, 72*, 304–309.

Smith, M. D. (1979). Towards an explanation of hockey violence: A reference other approach. *Canadian Journal of Sociology, 4*, 105–123.

Stephens, D. E. (1998). Aggression. In J. L. Duda (Ed.), *Advances in sport and exercise psychology measurement* (pp. 277–294). Morgantown, WV: Fitness Information Technology.

Stephens, D. E., Bredemeier, B., & Shields, D. L. (1997). Construction of a measure designed to assess players' description and prescription of moral behavior in youth sport soccer. *International Journal of Sport Psychology, 28*, 370–390.

Teipel, D., Gerisch, G., & Busse, M. (1983). Evaluation of aggressive behavior in football. *International Journal of Sport Psychology, 14*, 228–242.

Thomas, J. R., & Nelson, J. K. (2001). *Research methods in physical activity*. Champaign, IL: Human Kinetics.

Tice, D. M., & Wallace, H. M. (2003). The reflected self: Creating yourself as you think others see you. In M. R. Leary & J. P. Tangney (Eds.), *Handbook of self and identity* (pp. 91–105). New York: Guilford Press.

Trudel, P., Cote, J., & Danz, B. (1996). Systematic observation of youth ice hockey coaches during games. *Journal of Sport Behavior, 19*, 50–65.

Vaz, E., & Thomas, D. (1974). What price is victory? An analysis of minor hockey league player attitudes towards winning. *International Review of Sport Sociology, 2*, 33–53.

Vokey, J. R., & Russell, G. W. (1992). On penalties in sport as a measure of aggression. *Social Behavior and Personality: An International Journal, 20*, 219–225.

White, S. A. (2007). Parent-created motivational climate. In S. Jowett & D. Lavallee (Eds.), *Social psychology of sport* (pp. 132–143). Champaign, IL: Human Kinetics.

Widmeyer, W. N., & Birch, J. S. (1984). Aggression in professional ice hockey: A strategy for success or reaction to failure? *Journal of Psychology, 117*, 77–84.

Widmeyer, W. N., Dorsch, K. D., Bray, S. R., & McGuire, E. J. (2002). The nature, prevalence, and consequence of aggression in sport. In J. M. Silva & D. E. Stevens (Eds.), *Psychological foundations of sport* (pp. 328–351). Boston: Allyn & Bacon.

Widmeyer, W. N., & McGuire, E. J. (1997). Frequency of competition and aggression in professional ice hockey. *International Journal of Sport Psychology, 28*, 57–66.

Worrell, G. L., & Harris, D. V. (1986). The relationship of perceived and observed aggression of ice hockey players. *International Journal of Sport Psychology, 17*, 34–40.

# Chapter 13
# Behavioral Effects of Sport Nutritional Supplements: Fact or Fiction?

**Stephen Ray Flora**

The pages of fitness, health, sport, and sport enthusiast (biking, running, bodybuilding, etc.) magazines are filled with advertisements for various nutritional supplements, all claiming to significantly improve the athletic performance of the supplement user. These advertisements often include dramatic "before and after" pictures showing greatly changed (improved) physiques that supposedly occurred as a result of taking the advertised supplement. The advertisements may also include pictures of individuals with impressively muscled physiques or pictures of famous athletes who claim to have achieved great results with the advertised supplement. However, "before and after" pictures are often altered. In some cases the pictures may even be taken on the same day and then altered on the computer (widening of the chest and shoulders, narrowing of the waist, airbrushing; Bell, 2008). In advertisements, muscular models might take the advertised supplement, but they also may ingest illegal steroids, use other products, and engage in other physique-altering activities (Bell, 2008). Furthermore, athletes providing testimonials for products are likely to be taking other nutritional supplements as well as participating in other performance-enhancing activities (physical training, getting proper rest) that may account more for performance outcomes than does taking the advertised supplement.

Deceptive advertising practices such as airbrushing pictures, and confounds including effects of other consumed supplements, training habits, and nutritional practices of athletes taking supplements, make it difficult to evaluate the effectiveness, if any, of most nutritional supplements. A particular supplement *might* enhance performance, have no effect, or in fact contribute to performance decrements. Without controlled experimental analysis of the questioned supplement's effect on performance, it is impossible to know what effect, if any, the supplement has on performance.

Another difficulty in evaluating the possible effectiveness of supplements is that many of them contain ingredients and "proprietary blends," making it nearly impossible to ascertain which, if any, of the ingredients in a supplement have a

---

S.R. Flora (✉)
Youngstown State University, Youngstown, OH, USA
e-mail: srflora@ysu.edu

performance-enhancing effect. Products use the cover of "proprietary blends" both to hide the exact mixes and amounts of ingredients from potential copycat product competitors and to blind consumers to the often miniscule amounts of the ingredients actually used. A general rule for the consumer of supplements is to avoid any supplement that lists a "proprietary blend," and if supplements are consumed, take only supplements that list *exact amounts* of *all* ingredients that are purchased from a reputable source.

The ability to ascertain the effects of supplements is further hampered in the United States as a result of the Dietary Supplement Health and Education Act of 1994 (DSHEA). The DAHEA put supplements in a separate category, limited the Food and Drug Administration (FDA)'s ability to regulate supplements, gave supplement companies wide latitude in the (often unsubstantiated) claims that could be made about products, and exempted manufactures from having to submit safety information before marketing products (Barrett, 2007). Furthermore, since products are called "dietary supplements" rather than "drugs," the FDA cannot guarantee that the products are safe, much less effective. "Despite their sometimes-potent pharmacological effects, dietary supplements are now classified as foods and are presumed to be safe unless the government can prove otherwise. Drugs, on the other hand, must be proven safe by the manufacturers before going on the market" (Mencimer, 2001, p. 5). The DSHEA allows manufactures of dietary supplements to advertise "statements of support" that claim benefit and describe well-being that occurs from taking the products without any objective way to evaluate the claims (Barrett, 2007).

The free rein given to producers of dietary supplements by the DSHEA occurred primarily as the result of the work of U.S. senator Orrin Hatch from Utah, who was the "chief architect and sponsor" of the DSHEA (Mencimer, 2001). Not surprisingly, supplement manufactures are the largest political contributors to Hatch, and his home state of Utah accounts for about 20% of the nation's multi-billion dollar supplement business. Despite the Hatch-supported, industry-friendly DSHEA, many of Hatch's supplement manufacturer donors including Nu Skin, Herbalife, Rexall Sundown, and Sunrider have nevertheless violated federal and state regulations of various sorts (Mencimer, 2001).

A marginally regulated supplement industry is not without consequence. Many deaths have resulted from taking dietary supplements that contained powerfully harmful ingredients. Note, too, that Olympic athletes who did not take steroids have tested positive for steroids because they took "dietary supplements" that, while not technically steroids, nevertheless physiologically functioned as steroids and produced the metabolic profile of steroid ingestion and a positive steroid blood test (Barrett, 2007; Mencimer, 2001). A minor improvement for public protection came with the 2006 passage of the Dietary Supplement and Nonprescription Drug Consumer Protection Act. "However, public protection is only slightly increased because other parts of DSHEA make it very cumbersome for the FDA to ban dietary supplements and herbs" (Barrett, 2007).

## Behavioral Effects of Sport Nutritional Supplements: General Considerations

The athlete, trainer, or coach cannot rely on the product manufacturer or on the government for accurate information about the effectiveness or safety of any supplement. Instead, they must rely on science, on objective experimentation, to evaluate such supplements. Unfortunately, such information is often lacking, the outlets (e.g., peer-reviewed scientific journals) of the science may be unavailable, or the reader might not know how to evaluate and analyze the methodology and results of such reports. Nonbiased scientific research on conditioning factors such as training regimens and diet is often lacking. Additionally, the research that does exist typically compares only the difference between large group averages of multiple athletes recorded at one point in time. But as Kinugasa, Cerin, and Hooper (2004) advised, "at the elite level, applied conditioning research requires a focus on an individual athlete rather than on groups of 'average' athletes to make a confident assessment of the effect of an intervention (e.g., a specific training method [or a specific nutritional supplement]) on the performance of an individual athlete" (p. 1036). In fact, many sports scientists have called for an increase in behavioral, single-subject research in sports science:

> "applied conditioning research would greatly benefit from single-subject research designs. Single-subject research designs allow us to find out the extent to which a specific conditioning regimen [or supplement] works for a specific athlete... Sports scientists should use single-subject research designs in applied conditioning research to understand how well an intervention (e.g., a training method [or supplement]) works and to predict performance for a particular athlete" (Kinugasa et al., 2004, p. 1035).

Chapter 4 in this book should be referenced for an overview of single-case evaluation designs in behavioral sport psychology.

In sum, despite the existence of scientifically effective methodological techniques and research designs, the evaluation of supplements with behavioral research designs is hampered by a relative lack of behavioral research on supplement effectiveness. Another constraint is that some elite athletes may refuse to participate in potentially meaningful behavioral research. Lastly, the often shadowy world of supplement manufactures does not lend itself to evaluation. Indeed, many supplement producers have a financial stake in *not* having their products objectively evaluated least they be found to be ineffective and unsafe.

I noted previously that the definitions of, and distinctions between, drugs, dietary supplements, and nutritional supplements are vague and overlapping. If a product is labeled a *drug*, it falls under FDA regulations, but if the same product (or a functionally equivalent product) is called a *dietary supplement*, then it is subject only to the DSHEA. Confusing the matter further, how, or if, a product is isolated and concentrated may affect its label. Caffeine, for example, occurs naturally in coffee and cocoa beans (chocolate), tea leaves, and many other natural plants. Caffeine is also isolated, concentrated, and sold in drugstores, and may be added to other products as part of pills and powders for pain relief or as an ingredient in diet products. So is caffeine a drug, a dietary supplement, a naturally occurring compound, all of these, or none? You get the point: How caffeine is defined depends on who is selling it and who is buying it.

As referenced in this chapter, a *drug* will be considered to be any product that is either artificially created by humans or isolated and concentrated by humans to strengths seldom seen in nature and that when introduced internally to the physiological organism (via ingestion, intravenously, subcutaneously, or otherwise) affects either physiological functioning or behavior by mechanisms other than the typical manner by which water and foodstuffs affect functioning or development. Use of performance-enhancing drugs is generally illegal in competitive sports (either by national state governments or by governing bodies of sport), and, with the exception of caffeine, they are not recommended. A *dietary supplement* is something that is added to complete or strengthen one's diet, and a *nutritional supplement* is a supplement that *nourishes*, where *nourish* refers to the Latin *nutrire*, to nurse, to provide material necessary for growth and sustenance. While all these definitions overlap, it is difficult to state that a drug nourishes, and a nutritional supplement is a dietary supplement, but a dietary supplement, such as a diuretic, may not nourish.

## Behavioral Effects of Sport Nutritional Supplements: Research Support

Despite the many regulatory, research and definitional problems with evaluating supplements, there exists sufficient evidence to make recommendations for several sport supplements that have been extensively researched. Research-supported recommended supplements include sports drinks, whey protein, creatine, and caffeine. Nonsupported sport-enhancing supplements include antioxidant vitamin supplements and testosterone prohormones. The following discussion will focus on behavioral effects of sport nutritional supplements and be as nontechnical as possible.

*Sports drinks.* An athlete must be well hydrated and have sufficient energy for optimal performance. Dehydration degrades performance. Exercise requires energy and generates metabolic heat that must be dissipated to maintain body temperature within narrow limits. Heat is dissipated primarily through sweat (even in cool temperatures), resulting in fluid and sodium (Na) loss and, to a much lesser degree, potassium (K) loss. Increased blood flow to the skin may also assist in vital heat dissipation. Dehydration not only compromises the body's ability to cool, but also lowers blood plasma volume, making it more difficult to transport vital nutrients and oxygen to working muscles and organs. Extreme dehydration can result in disability or death (Shirreffs, Armstrong, & Cheuvront, 2004).

Even fluid losses as small as 1–2% of body weight can dramatically hurt performance. For example, "A 1% reduction in body weight due to water loss may evoke an undue stress on the cardiovascular system accompanied by increases in heart rate and inadequate heat transfer to the skin and the environment, increase plasma osmolality, decrease plasma volume, and may affect the intracellular and extracellular electrolyte balance" (von Duvillard, Braun, Markofski, Beneke, & Leithauser, 2004, p. 651). In track races of distances of 1.5, 5, and 10 km, a dehydrating 2% body weight fluid loss (via a diuretic) increased times by 3.4, 6.6, and 6.7%, respectively (Armstrong, Costill, & Fink, 1985). This decline in performance is dramatic considering that in highly competitive races, an increased time of less than one-half of 1% can be the difference between winning and finishing last. "It is well documented that even small body water deficits, incurred before or during exercise can significantly impair exercise performance, especially in the heat" (Shirreffs, Armstrong & Cheuvront, 2004, p. 57).

Drinks containing between 4% and 10% carbohydrate (and a smaller portion of protein) and sodium (the critical ingredients in sport drinks) consumed during exercise help prevent dehydration and prevent performance declines. But *consuming plain water does not prevent performance declines* and does not prevent dehydration as well as sports drinks.

In a well-controlled experiment by Dougherty, Baker, Chow, and Kenney (2006), elite adolescent male basketball players first exercised (treadmill and stationary cycling) for 2 h in bouts of 15 min in a warm environment to result in either a 2% weight loss (dehydration) or consumed either water to prevent fluid weight loss or a 6% carbohydrate–sodium sport drink to prevent dehydration. Each player participated in each condition in random order separated by 1 week. Following a 1-h recovery period, players completed basketball drills to stimulate game performances. At the end of the "game" when the players were either dehydrated or hydrated with water, they felt more lightheaded and fatigued compared to when they were hydrated with sports drink. Shooting percentage and sprint times were significantly impaired by dehydration and significantly improved by sports drink hydration compared to water hydration. Dougherty et al. (2006) concluded, "This degree of improvement [achieved by drinking a sports drink] is important in a sport where subtle changes in skill performance could be the difference between winning and losing" (p. 1657). Other studies have found that compared to hydration with water, ingestion of a carbohydrate–sodium sports drink "has been shown to improve tennis stroke performance at the end of prolonged play, results in faster 20-m sprint times, increases the number of sprints performed during a soccer game, delays time to fatigue during intermittent, high-intensity cycling, and improves endurance-running capacity during prolonged intermittent exercise" (Dougherty et al., 2006, p. 1657). In short, "development of sports drinks with appropriate and adequate concentrations of electrolytes [Na] and CHOs [carbohydrates] promotes maintenance of homeostasis, prevents injuries, and maintains optimal performance" (von Duvillard et al., 2004, p. 651).

Carbohydrates are necessary both to provide energy – glucose in the blood stream, stored as glycogen in the liver – and to promote hydration. According to UK researcher R. J. Maughan (1998, p. 16, emphasis added):

> Carbohydrate ingested during exercise will enter the blood glucose pool ... [and] exercise capacity *should be improved* when carbohydrate is consumed. Several studies have shown that the ingestion of glucose during prolonged intense exercise will prevent the development

of hypoglycemia by maintaining or raising the circulating glucose concentration ... A substantial part of the carbohydrate ingested during exercise is available for oxidation [energy], but there appears to be an upper limit of about 1 g/min to the rate at which ingested carbohydrate can be oxidized, even when larger amounts are ingested ... As well as providing an energy substrate for the working muscles, *the addition of carbohydrate in ingested drinks will promote water absorption in the small intestine.*

High concentrations of carbohydrate are not only unnecessary because there is a limit to the rate at which they can be utilized, but also can actually be counterproductive, delaying gastric emptying. In fact, "if the concentration is high enough ... net secretion of water into the intestine will result, and this will actually increase the danger of dehydration" (Maughan, 1998, p. 17). Despite advertisement claims promoting various formulations of carbohydrates in sports drinks, with the possible exception of fructose, which is more likely to cause gastrointestinal upset, the form(s) of carbohydrate in sports drinks – glucose, sucrose, long-chain glucose polymers, maltodextrins – does not matter (Coombes & Hamilton, 2000; Maughan, 1998).

In addition to glucose, sodium (Na) is the other critical component in sports drinks for events lasting 1 h or more, and even more vital for events lasting over 4 h. In addition to water, Na is lost in sweat (and to a lesser degree K). Na is vital to every organ in the body, including every muscle cell and every neuron in the nervous system. If large amounts of Na are lost through sweat, Na will leave cells to equalize osmotic pressure resulting in intracellular dehydration, a dangerous situation slowing down cellular processes. Therefore, Na lost during sweat must be replaced. Additionally, "Na will stimulate sugar and water uptake in the small intestine and will help maintain extracellular fluid volume" (Maughan, 1998, p. 18). Consumption of carbohydrate and Na sports drink after dehydration results in greater blood volume restoration and greater hydration than does consumption of water alone (e.g., Costill & Sparks, 1973; Gonzalez-Alonso, Heaps, & Coyle, 1992). While there is a very small amount of K lost during sweat, in events lasting less than 4 h, evidence does not support the need for it to be added to sports drinks.

Assuming the athlete is well hydrated, well nourished, or "glycogen sufficient" before exercise, research (for example, Coombes & Hamilton, 2000) supports the following *generalizations and recommendations.* First, if the athlete is well hydrated and glycogen sufficient, then there is no need to drink a sports drink prior to exercise or competition. However, because many athletes and fitness participants are in a state of mild dehydration prior to exercising, consuming approximately 0.5 l of sports drink 1 h prior to exercising may provide "insurance" against premature exercise-induced performance-degrading dehydration. For moderate exercise lasting 1 h or less, consuming sports drinks is not necessary. For intense exercise lasting 1 h or less, the evidence is mixed as to whether or not a sports drink will be beneficial. In the case of prolonged intermittent exercise, "studies strongly suggest that consumption of a carbohydrate beverage can improve performance during intermittent exercise" (Coombes & Hamilton, 2000, p. 192). For prolonged exercise lasting between 1 and 4 h, 23 of 36 studies reported "significant ergogenic benefit" of consuming a sports drink during exercise (Coombes & Hamilton, 2000, p. 192). When prolonged exercise lasts more than 4 h, consuming fluid, carbohydrates, and Na (the critical ingredients of sports drinks) is vital for performance. In fact, depending on the temperature and exercise-generated heat, additional Na supplementation, beyond that of sports drinks, may be necessary.

*Protein in sport drinks?* Some studies have found that the addition of 1 part protein to 4 parts carbohydrate in sports drinks consumed during exercise improves performance beyond the benefit from consuming carbohydrate-only sports drinks. For example, male cyclists cycling to exhaustion cycled 40% longer when consuming a carbohydrate–protein drink every 15 min than they did when drinking a carbohydrate beverage at the same rate (Saunders, Kane, & Todd, 2004). However, the carbohydrate–protein drink contained more calories. When a carbohydrate–protein drink was compared to a carbohydrate-only drink having equal calories, times to exhaustion were not different (Van Essen & Gibala, 2006).

While additional follow-up studies failed to find that consumption of the carbohydrate–protein beverage during exercise improved performance to a level of statistical significance over the effects of consuming a carbohydrate-only beverage, the average time to exhaustion was *several minutes longer* in the carbohydrate–protein condition. Consuming either beverage significantly improved endurance compared to consuming a placebo (noncaloric) beverage (Romano-Ely, Todd, Saunders, & St. Laurent, 2006; Valentine, Saunders, Todd, & St. Laurent, 2008). Furthermore, indices of muscle damage (e.g., creatine kinase) were lower in the carbohydrate–protein condition, and post-exercise leg extensions (a measure of muscle strength) 24 h later were greater after consuming carbohydrate–protein drink than after consuming the carbohydrate drink (Valentine et al., 2008). These results suggest that consuming a carbohydrate–protein sports drink instead of a carbohydrate sports drink (both would contain Na) during exercise may not improve performance during that exercise session much, or at all. Nevertheless, consuming a carbohydrate–protein drink during exercise sessions instead of a carbohydrate-only sports drink may increase performance over many exercise sessions.

In sum, the research suggests that a person should consume approximately 100 ml (4 ounces) sports drink containing 6–10% carbohydrate, Na, and 1 part protein for 4 parts carbohydrate every 15–20 min for intense exercise and all exercise sessions lasting 1 h or longer. Any commercially available sports drink will work. For sports drinks that do not contain protein, a small amount of whey protein may be mixed into the drink. In fact, effective sports drinks can be made with ingredients that are common to almost every kitchen (except whey protein, which is widely available). For every 100 ml (just under 4 ounces) of water, add 8 g (approximately 1/2 tablespoon) of sugar, 57 mg (a pinch) of salt, and 2 g (1/4 tablespoon) of whey protein and add flavoring if desired (a few drops of lemon juice). For a 16 oz drink, multiply portions by 4.

*Recovery drinks.* Without going into excessive physiological detail, if nutrients, particularly protein and carbohydrate, are consumed as soon as possible after exercise (ideally within half an hour), glycogen synthesis, muscle repair, and strengthening will be maximized. Consequently, as compared to the effects of consuming these nutrients at other times, future athletic performances and fitness will be much greater if these nutrients are consumed immediately after exercise: "The resynthesis of glycogen between training sessions occurs most rapidly if carbohydrates are consumed within 30 min to 1 h after exercise" (Karp et al., 2006, p. 78).

In a review of the available research, Manninen (2006) concluded that post-exercise consumption of easily digested, high-glycemic carbohydrate and high-quality and easily digested protein is vastly superior to consumption of carbohydrates alone (which is vastly superior to consumption of water alone). For example, after cycling for 2 h, male cyclists consumed either a carbohydrate sports drink or a carbohydrate–protein recovery drink and then 4 h later cycled to exhaustion. The cyclists rode 55% longer if they consumed the carbohydrate–protein drink (Williams, Raven, Fogt, & Ivy, 2003). Drinking the carbohydrate–protein beverage also resulted in a 17% greater plasma glucose response, a 92% greater insulin response (responsible for muscle cells taking in glucose and protein that maximizes recovery and strengthening), and 128% greater storage of muscle glycogen compared to the effects of a carbohydrate sports drink.

Again, timing is critical. Elderly men (average age 74 years) who took protein immediately after resistance training for 10 weeks saw increases in muscle fiber, but those who consumed the protein drink 2 h after resistance training, did not. Additionally, isokinetic strength increased by 46% in the immediate protein intake condition but increased only 15% in the 2-h post-workout protein intake condition (Esmarck et al., 2001). According to Manninen (2006):

> ... post-exercise recovery drinks containing these nutrients [quality protein and simple carbohydrates] in conjunction with appropriate resistance training may lead to increased skeletal muscle hypertrophy (growth) and strength. If so, such post-exercise supplements would be of considerable benefit not only to athletes but also to anyone who has lost muscle function through disease – for example, Duchenne muscular dystrophy (p. 904).

Just as sports drinks can be made with common kitchen ingredients, an effective carbohydrate–protein recovery drink is available in most kitchens in the form of milk or, particularly, low-fat chocolate milk. Plain milk has a fairly high fat content that is not necessary, but low-fat chocolate milk has less fat and more simple sugars. Both have sufficient Na, and both have been shown to be fairly effective recovery drinks (e.g., Karp et al., 2006; Shirreffs, Watson, & Maughan, 2007).

*Whey protein.* While milk or low-fat chocolate milk may function as effective low-cost, post-exercise recovery drinks (assuming one is not lactose intolerant), whey protein (a milk by-product) has conclusively been shown to be a highly effective sports nutritional supplement. The Romano-Ely et al. (2006) and Valentine et al. (2008) carbohydrate–protein supplement studies on cycling performance (discussed previously in this chapter) used whey protein as the protein source. Any athlete attempting to gain maximum physical performance should consume a small amount of whey protein prior to exercising and larger amounts immediately after exercise. Compared to other sources of protein (egg, soy, red meat, poultry, fish), whey is the most easily digestible and complete protein available. Moreover, it is one of the best sources of essential amino acids (the protein molecules that the human body cannot form on its own, so must be obtained from food) and branched-chain amino acids (BCAA – the amino acids that are the most responsible for rapid muscle synthesis). Consumption of whey not only has been found to increase lean muscle mass, but may also assist in weight loss (Baer et al., 2006).

Young men exercised one leg and rested the other and then consumed either a whey protein–carbohydrate beverage (containing 10 g of whey) or a carbohydrate beverage. Muscle protein synthesis was greater in the exercised legs than in the rested legs, and the rate of muscle protein synthesis was greater in the whey condition than in the carbohydrate condition (Tang et al., 2007). Compared to carbohydrate or placebo consumption, pre- and post-exercise whey supplementation increases muscle size and strength by several methods, including increasing skeletal muscle glycogen recovery, maximizing muscle protein synthesis, activating key enzymes (Morifuji, Kanda, Koga, Kawanaka, & Higuchi, 2010), and possibly altering gene expression (Humi, Kovanen, Selanne, & Mero, 2008).

Whey is widely available in many products and sold separately in health food stores, grocery stores, and in "big box" department stores. There is no advantage of consuming higher priced name brand whey. In fact, at least one "big box" brand of whey is packaged in the same size and colored package as a more expensive name brand whey, and its label states it is produced in the same town with the same zip code as the more expensive brand. This suggests that two products are identical with the only difference being a different label and higher price for the name brand whey.

*Creatine.* Like whey, any athlete attempting to gain maximum physical performance should consume creatine. The liver and kidneys produce about 2 g of creatine each day, and some creatine is obtained from food sources (primarily meat). Creatine was initially popular, and still is, with bodybuilders who found that creatine supplementation could increase muscle size. Early myths about creatine supplementation included beliefs that while it might increase muscle size, it did not increase muscle strength, that it caused bloating and water retention, that it would cause dehydration and/or cramps in endurance athletes, and that it could cause kidney damage. Research has shown all of the myths to be unfounded (similar myths about whey protein are also unfounded). In reality, the safety and efficacy of creatine have been so well established that it has been recommended as a "training enhancer" by the popular *Bicycling* magazine (June 2006, p. 121), and *The Center for Science in the Public Interest* has recommended it, particularly for seniors, in its *Nutrition Action Healthletter* (Schardt, 2009). Among other evidence, the newsletter cited research that found that, compared to 70-year male men who resistance trained three times a week for 12 weeks and drank a placebo beverage, those elderly men who resistance trained and consumed creatine had greater increases in strength, endurance, and average power (Chrusch, Chilibeck, Chad, Shawn, & Burke, 2001). Creatine supplementation has been shown to increase strength, power, and functional performance in older women as well (Gotshalk, Kraemer, Mendoca et al., 2008).

Of course, creatine is not just for seniors. In an earlier study, men trained for 12 weeks during which time they took either creatine supplements or a placebo. After 12 weeks, compared to the placebo group, the men taking creatine had significant increases in bench press strength, squat strength, and much greater increases in both fast-twitch (strength) and slow-twitch (endurance) muscle fibers (Volek, Duncan, & Mazzetti, 1999).

Inside the individual muscle cell, at the molecular level, energy lasting a few seconds is produced when adenosine triphosphate (ATP) loses a phosphate molecule, becoming adenosine diphosphate (ADP). Creatine phosphate gives its phosphate molecule to ADP, changing it back into ATP. In short, more creatine phosphate results in more ATP, which gives the muscle more potential energy and the potential to work harder. Creatine supplementation greatly increases levels of creatine phosphate in the muscle.

In a review of over 500 studies on the effects of creatine supplementation on physiology and/or performance, Kreider (2003, p. 89) concludes,

> ... supplementation has typically been reported to increase total creatine content by 10–30% and phosphocreatine stores by 10–40%. Of the approximately 300 studies that have evaluated the potential ergogenic [performance enhancing] value of creatine supplementation, about 70% of these studies report statistically significant results while remaining studies generally report non-significant gains in performance. No study reports a statistically significant ergolytic [performance degrading] effect.

Along with gains in other areas, particularly high-intensity exercise, supplementation increases maximal power 5–15%, improves single sprint performance 1–5%, and improves repetitive sprint performance 5–15%.

Likewise, in a review of studies published since 1999, Bemben and Lamont (2005) found that "creatine does significantly impact force production regardless of sport, sex or age" and that "when performance is assessed based on intensity and duration of the exercises, there is contradictory evidence relative to both continuous and intermittent endurance activities. However, activities that involve jumping, sprinting or cycling generally show improved sport performance following creatine ingestion" (p. 107).

As with whey, creatine is widely available in many outlets, and similarly, there is no need to by high-priced name brand creatine, which may be spiked with unnecessary additional ingredients. "Big box," department, or grocery store brands work just as well as any other brand.

*Caffeine.* While not a nutritional supplement, caffeine has conclusively been shown to enhance athletic performance. In a recent review, Davis and Green (2009, pp. 813, 814) reported,

> ... recent studies incorporating trained subjects and paradigms specific to intermittent sports activity support the notion that caffeine is ergogenic to an extent with anaerobic exercise. Caffeine seems highly ergogenic for speed endurance exercise ranging in duration form 60 to 180 s ... studies employing sport-specific methodologies (i.e., hockey, rugby, soccer) with shorter duration (i.e., 4–6 s) show caffeine to be ergogenic during high-intensity intermittent exercise.

In a study on caffeine supplementation on multiple sprint running performances, compared to physically active men who took a placebo, men who took a caffeine capsule significantly improved their sprint times compared to baseline showing that "caffeine has ergogenic properties with the potential to benefit performance in both single and multiple sprint sports" (Glaister et al., 2008, p. 1835). Beyond sprint sports, "caffeine improves physical and cognitive performance during exhaustive exercise" (Hogervorst et al., 2008, p. 1841). In randomized counterbalanced order, 24 trained cyclists consumed either a carbohydrate bar, a carbohydrate bar containing caffeine, or a placebo beverage before cycling 2.5 h and again after 55 and 115 min into the exercise, followed by a ride to exhaustion. The cyclists were also given cognitive tests during and after the ride. When they consumed caffeine, they completed the cognitive tests faster with no decline in accuracy compared to the carbohydrate-only condition, which was better than the placebo condition. When the cyclists consumed caffeine, time to exhaustion was longer, relative to the carbohydrate-only condition, which was better than the placebo condition. Thus, caffeine "can significantly improve endurance performance and complex cognitive ability during and after exercise. These effects may be salient for sports performance in which concentration plays a major role" (Hogervorst et al., 2008, p. 1841).

Caffeine affects physiological functioning in several ways, and the physiological mechanisms by which caffeine enhances sport performance is not conclusively known (Davis & Green, 2009). Clearly, caffeine is a central nervous system (CNS) stimulant (primarily as an adenosine inhibitor). Since adenosine is a CNS inhibitor, inhibiting adenosine activates the CNS. Caffeine increases the release of adrenaline, may increase blood glucose, and "from [its] inhibitory effects on adenosine, [it] leads to modified pain perception while sustaining motor unit [muscle cell] firing rates and neuro-excitability. This then is the leading hypothesis for the ergogenic effect of caffeine on performance" (Davis & Green, 2009, p. 823).

There are two caveats when considering caffeine as a sports supplement. First, studies reporting beneficial effects tend to use well-trained athletes. Studies using untrained individuals have more inconsistent results (Davis & Green, 2009). It may be that novice athletes have too many variables affecting their performance and physiological adaptation to training to see any effect of caffeine. Second, ingesting caffeine from coffee does not improve athletic performance. When subjects consumed caffeine capsules and then ran to exhaustion 1 h later, they ran 7.5–10 min longer than when they ran an hour after drinking coffee, drinking decaffeinated coffee, drinking decaffeinated coffee with caffeine added, or after taking a placebo capsule. "Endurance was only increased in the caffeine capsule trial: there were no differences among the other four tests. One cannot extrapolate the effects of caffeine to coffee. There must be a component(s) of coffee that moderates the actions of caffeine" (Graham, Hibbert, & Sathasivam, 1998, p. 883).

Conditioned compensatory responses may be the mechanism that moderates the effect of caffeine in coffee. Conditioned compensatory responses are conditioned responses that counteract the effects of an unconditioned stimulus allowing the organism to maintain a homeostatic state (Siegel, 2005). For example, one unconditioned effect of caffeine is increased salivation, but coffee stimuli produce a compensatory decrease in salivation (Rozin, Reff, Mark, & Schull, 1984). The sight and smell of coffee may function as condition stimuli that also elicit compensatory conditioned responses to counter the stimulatory effects of coffee and eliminate any possible sport-enhancing effect of consuming caffeine in coffee. Regardless, the research suggests that to obtain a sport performance–enhancing effect, caffeine should be consumed in a form other than in coffee. Or more generally, caffeine should be consumed in a form different from the source that the athlete typically gets caffeine from, be it coffee, tea, or so-called energy drinks to avoid conditioned compensatory responses.

*Nonsupported supplements: Antioxidant vitamins.* Free radicals, reactive oxygen species (ROS), may be one component that contributes to muscle damage after exercise. Therefore, it might be expected that supplementation with antioxidant vitamins may minimize this damage and promote recovery. However, in a comprehensive review of the available data, it was found that neither acute, pre-exercise, or post-exercise supplementation of either vitamin C, E, or their combination had any protective effect against muscle damage (McGinley, Shafat, & Donnelly, 2009). McGinley et al. (2009) posit, "Given that antioxidants do not appear to be beneficial in protecting against muscle damage, and that vitamin E in particular may in fact be potentially harmful, the casual use of large doses of antioxidants should be curtailed," and further, "Of greater relevance to athletes and other sports persons, antioxidant supplementation may not only fail to protect against EIMD [exercise induced muscular damage], but could in fact interfere with the cellular signaling functions of ROS. Therefore, in ingesting antioxidant vitamins in an attempt to enhance muscle performance, these individuals may actually be retarding the adaptive processes to exercise" (p. 1029).

*Testosterone prohormone supplements.* High levels of the "male" hormone testosterone (females do produce very small amounts) are associated with strength, power, winning, high social status, and aggression. Testosterone supplementation is illegal. Prohormones are chemical precursors to testosterone – supplementing with them is claimed to increase testosterone and in turn muscular strength and athletic performance. Baseball superstar Mark McGwire said that he used the prohormone androstenedione during the season he broke the major league home run record (subsequent reports from his brother suggest he was using other illegal substances as well). With the passage of the Anabolic Steroid Control Act of 2004 that defined anabolic steroids as "any drug or hormonal substance, chemically and pharmacologically related to testosterone," most prohormones and other steroids are now illegal, including androstenedione (Brown, Vukovich, & King, 2006). Nevertheless, despite their possible illegality these substances or highly similar substances are still heavily advertised in weightlifting and bodybuilding magazines.

In a review of the available scientific research on testosterone prohormone supplements, Brown et al. (2006) concluded, "Contrary to marketing claims, research to date indicates that the use of prohormone nutritional supplements (DHEA, androstenedione, androstenediol, and other steroid hormone supplements) does not produce either anabolic or ergogenic effects in men. Moreover, the use of prohormone nutritional supplements may raise the risk for negative consequences" (p. 1451). Instead of raising testosterone in men, these supplements simply result in "either reduced absorption, enhanced clearance, or enhanced metabolism of the ingested substance" (p. 1452). Generally the research shows that improvements that might occur in men only occur for those with initially low levels of testosterone;

otherwise resistance training with placebo works as well as resistance training with androstenedione. The popular prohormone DHEA works no better: "It appears that DHEA does not promote fat loss or muscle gain or augment adaptations to resistance training in healthy men" (Brown et al., 2006, p. 1547). Furthermore "herbal extracts do not alter the fate of ingested androstenedione" (Brown et al., 2006, p. 1457). Still more concerning is that "many androgenic supplements are contaminated with hormones, caffeine, ephedrine or other banned substances not listed on the product label" (Brown et al., 2006, p. 1458).

While "Intake of 100–200-mg doses of androstenedione or androstenediol, or up to 1,600 mg of DHEA, does not increase serum testosterone concentrations in men ... It is clear that ingesting androstenedione [and chronic intake of DHEA] increases serum testosterone concentrations in women" (Brown et al., 2006, p. 1457). But the potential performance-enhancing effects for women must be weighed against the side effects including "insulin resistance, increased incidence of acne, facial hair, and other symptoms of hirsuitism [excessive hairiness in women]" (Brown et al., 2006, p. 1458).

Testosterone levels may be raised without steroids or prohormone supplements. Both estrogen and testosterone are synthesized in the body from cholesterol. Those wanting to insure that they have sufficient "basic material" for increased testosterone could simply eat a few more eggs (also a good source of quality protein in addition to dietary cholesterol). While excessive cholesterol in the cardiovascular system may not be healthy, it is necessary to consume some cholesterol for hormone production, and it is unclear as to whether high cholesterol intake or high saturated fat intake is responsible for high cardiovascular levels of cholesterol. Additionally, when professional rugby players engaged in a session of resistance training, their testosterone levels rose. When they trained and consumed caffeine, their testosterone levels were higher still. Coupled with the training stimulus, the more caffeine ingested, the greater the rise in the athletes' testosterone levels (Beaven et al., 2008). Testosterone prohormone supplements are neither recommended nor necessary.

## Conclusion

If an athlete eats a balanced diet including plenty of protein, carbohydrates, fruits, and vegetables; gets proper rest; and trains appropriately, then the athlete will have improved performance without taking any supplements. Conversely, if the athlete does not train appropriately, does not have a good diet, or consumes excessive alcohol, then performance gains will be subpar or nonexistent even if the athlete is taking many supplements. Without the proper training stimulus, all supplements are worthless for sport performance. Many supplements, herbs, and aids are advertised without sufficient support for their performance-enhancing claims. Some supplements (e.g., antioxidant vitamins and prohormones) have shown to be ineffective if not dangerous.

Conversely, if consumed at the proper time and in proper amounts, carbohydrate–protein–Na sports drinks, whey protein, creatine, and caffeine all have been shown to be safe performance-enhancing sport supplements. Again, optimal performance can be best achieved with dedicated training, rest, diet, and nutritional supplementation. What further unites these products (sports drinks, whey protein, creatine, and caffeine) is that they are all widely available, not patented, and low cost. Most critical is that their effectiveness and safety as sports supplements have been researched and documented in an open manner at academic research universities across the globe.

## References

Armstrong, L. E., Costill, D. L., & Fink, W. J. (1985). Influence of diuretic-induced dehydration in competitive running performance. *Medicine and Science in Sports and Exercise, 17*, 456–461.
Baer, D. J., Stote, K. S., Clvidence, B. A., Harris, G. K., Paul, D., & Rumpler, W. V. (2006). Whey protein decreases body weight and fat in supplemented overweight and obese adults. *Federation of American Societies for Experimental Biology,* San Francisco.
Barrett, S. (2007). How the Dietary Supplement Health and Education Act of 1994 Weakened the FDA. *Quackwatch.org*. Retrieved April 23, 2010, from http://www.quackwatch.org/02ConsumerProtection/dshea.html
Beaven, C. M., Hopkins, W. G., Hansen, K. T., Wood, M. R., Cronin, J. B., & Lowe, T. E. (2008). Dose effect of caffeine on testosterone and cortisol responses to resistance exercise. *International Journal of Sport Nutrition and Exercise Metabolism, 18*, 131–141.
Bell, C. (2008). Bigger stronger faster. *Magnolia Pictures*. Los Angeles.
Bemben, M. G., & Lamont, H. S. (2005). Creatine supplementation and exercise performance: Recent findings. *Sports Medicine, 35*, 107–125.
Brown, G. A., Vukovich, M., & King, D. S. (2006). Testosterone prohormone supplements. *Medicine and Science in Sports and Exercise, 38*, 1451–1461.
Chrusch, M. J., Chilibeck, P. F., Chad, K. E., Shawn, D. K., & Burke, D. G. (2001). Creatine supplementation combined with resistance training in older men. *Medicine and Science in Sports and Exercise, 33*, 2111–2117.
Coombes, J. S., & Hamilton, K. L. (2000). The effectiveness of commercially available sports drinks. *Sports Medicine, 29*, 181–209.
Costill, D. L., & Sparks, K. E. (1973). Rapid fluid replacement following thermal dehydration. *Journal of Applied Physiology, 34*, 299–303.
Davis, J. K., & Green, J. M. (2009). Caffeine and anaerobic performance. *Sports Medicine, 39*, 813–832.
Dougherty, K. A., Baker, L. B., Chow, M., & Kenney, W. L. (2006). Two percent dehydration impairs and six percent carbohydrate drink improves boys basketball skills. *Medicine and Science in Sport and Exercise, 38*, 1650–1658.
Esmarck, B., Andersen, J. L., Olsen, S., Richter, E. A., Mizuno, M., & Kjaer, M. (2001). Timing of post-exercise protein intake is important for muscle hypertrophy with resistance training in elderly humans. *The Journal of Physiology, 535*, 301–311.
Glaister, M., Howatson, G., Abraham, C. S., Lockey, R. A., Goodwin, J. E., Foley, P., et al. (2008). Caffeine supplementation and multiple sprint running performance. *Medicine and Science in Sports and Exercise, 40*, 1835–1840.
Gonzalez-Alsonso, J., Heaps, C. L., & Coyle, E. F. (1992). Rehydration after exercise with common beverages and water. *International Journal of Sports Medicine, 13*, 399–406.
Gotshalk, L. A., Kraemer, W. J., Mendoca, M. A., Vingren, J. L., Kenny, A. M., Spiering, B. A., et al. (2008). Creatine supplementation improves muscular performance in older women. *European Journal of Applied Physiology, 102*, 223–231.

Graham, T. E., Hibbert, E., & Sathasivam, P. (1998). Metabolic and exercise endurance effects of coffee and caffeine ingestion. *Journal of Applied Physiology, 85*, 883–889.

Hogervorst, E., Bandelow, S., Schmitt, J., Jentjens, R., Oliveira, M., Allgrove, J., et al. (2008). Caffeine improves physical and cognitive performance during exhaustive exercise. *Medicine and Science in Sports and Exercise, 40*, 1841–1851.

Humi, J. J., Kovanen, V., Selanne, H., & Mero, A. A. (2008). The effects of whey protein on myostatin and cell cycle-related gene expression responses to a single heavy resistance exercise bout in trained older men. *European Journal of Applied Physiology, 102*, 205–213.

Karp, J. R., Johnson, J. D., Tecklenburg, S., Mickleborough, T. D., Fly, A. D., & Stager, J. M. (2006). Chocolate milk as a post-exercise recovery aid. *International Journal of Sport Nutritional Metabolism, 16*, 78–91.

Kinugasa, T., Cerin, E., & Hooper, S. (2004). Single-subject research designs and data analysis for assessing elite athletes' conditioning. *Sports Medicine, 34*, 1035–1050.

Kreider, R. B. (2003). Effects of creatine supplementation on performance and training adaptations. *Molecular and Cellular Biochemistry, 244*, 89–94.

Manninen, A. H. (2006). Hyperinsulinaemia, hyperaminoacidaemia and post-exercise muscle anabolism: The search for the optimal recovery drink. *British Journal of Sports Medicine, 40*, 900–905.

Maughan, R. J. (1998). The sports drink as a functional food: Formulations for successful performance. *Proceedings of the Nutrition Society, 57*, 15–23.

McGinley, C., Shafat, A., & Donnelly, A. E. (2009). Does antioxidant vitamin supplementation protect against muscle damage? *Sports Medicine, 39*, 1011–1032.

Mencimer, S. (2001). Scorin' with Orrin: How the gentleman form Utah made it easier for kids to buy steroids, speed, and Spanish fly. *Washington Monthly*. Retrieved April 24, 2010, from http://www.washingtonmonthly.com/features/2001/0109.mencimer2.html

Morifuji, M., Kanda, A., Koga, J., Kawanaka, K., & Higuchi, M. (2010). Post-exercise carbohydrate plus whey protein hydrolysates supplementation increases skeletal muscle glycogen level in rats. *Amino Acids, 38*, 1109–1115.

Romano-Ely, B. C., Todd, M. K., Saunders, M. J., & St. Laurent, T. (2006). Effect of an isocaloric carbohydrate-protein-antioxidant drink on cycling performance. *Medicine and Science in Sport and Exercise, 38*, 1608–1616.

Rozin, P., Reff, D., Mark, M., & Schull, J. (1984). Conditioned opponent responses in human tolerance to caffeine. *Bulletin of the Psychonomic Society, 22*, 117–120.

Saunders, M. J., Kane, M. D., & Todd, M. K. (2004). Effects of a carbohydrate-protein beverage on cycling endurance and muscle damage. *Medicine and Science in Sport and Exercise, 36*, 1233–1238.

Schardt, D. (2009, December issue). Seven facts you may not know about exercise. *Nutrition Action: Health Letter, 36*, 7–10.

Shirreffs, S. M., Armstrong, L. E., & Cheuvront, S. N. (2004). Fluid and electrolyte need for preparation and recovery from training and competition. *Journal of Sports Sciences, 22*, 57–63.

Shirreffs, S. M., Watson, P., & Maughan, R. J. (2007). Milk as an effective post-exercise rehydration drink. *British Journal of Nutriion, 98*, 173–180.

Siegel, S. (2005). Drug tolerance, drug addiction, and drug anticipation. *Current Directions in Psyhological Science, 14*, 296–300.

Tang, J. E., Manolakos, J. J., Kujbida, G. W., Lysecki, P. J., Moore, D. R., & Phillips, S. M. (2007). Minimal why protein with carbohydrate stimulates muscle protein synthesis following resistance exercise in trained young men. *Applied Physiology, Nutrition and Metabolism, 32*, 1132–1138.

Valentine, R. J., Saunders, M. J., Todd, M. K., & St. Laurent, T. G. (2008). Influence of carbohydrate-protein beverage on cycling endurance and indices of muscle disruption. *International Journal of Sport Medicine and Exercise Metabolism, 18*, 363–378.

Van Essen, M., & Gibala, M. J. (2006). Failure of protein to improve time trial performance when added to a sports drink. *Medicine and Science in Sports and Exercise, 38*, 1484–1491.

Volek, J. S., Duncan, N. D., Mazzetti, S. A., et al. (1999). Performance and muscle fiber adaptations to creatine supplementation and heavy resistance training. *Medicine and Science in Sport and Exercise, 31,* 1147–1156.

von Duvillard, S. P., Braun, W. A., Markofski, M., Beneke, R., & Leithauser, R. (2004). Fluids and hydration in prolonged endurance performance. *Nutrition, 20,* 651–656.

Williams, M. B., Raven, P. B., Fogt, D. L., & Ivy, J. L. (2003). Effects of recovery beverages in glycogen restoration and endurance exercise performance. *Journal of Strength and Conditioning Research, 17,* 12–19.

# Chapter 14
# Cognitive–Behavioral Coach Training: A Translational Approach to Theory, Research, and Intervention

Ronald E. Smith and Frank L. Smoll

The science of psychology exists as a sprawling domain within which behavioral phenomena are studied at multiple and complementary levels of analysis in the search for biological, psychological, and environmental causal factors. One consequence of this approach is an increased emphasis on translational research, which involves the application of theories, constructs, measurement approaches, research results, and intervention techniques across psychological domains. For example, Tashiro and Mortensen (2006) have shown how constructs and empirical results from traditional social psychological research might inform the diagnosis, prevention, treatment, and service delivery in clinical psychology and how, in turn, knowledge of mental illness can result in enhanced understanding of social psychological processes.

The most fundamental translational concept is found in the distinction between basic and applied science. Basic science is commonly defined as the development of theories and the discovery of knowledge for its own sake, whereas applied science involves the applications of knowledge derived from basic science for the solution of practical problems. However, this dichotomy begins to blur when we consider relations among theory development and testing, empirical research, and interventions designed to have practical impact. These relations do not simply involve a one-way causal path from knowledge or theory to application. Instead, they involve reciprocal interactions between theory, research, and interventions, meaning that each of the three facets has a causal impact on the others and is, in turn, influenced by them. Thus, our theories deepen our understanding and guide our research, and our research, in turn, is the most important influence on theory development and testing. Our theories also affect the interventions we develop, but the success of these interventions reflects, in part, the adequacy of our theory and may prompt theory revisions. Finally, the link connecting intervention and research is also a reciprocal one. Our research provides leads for intervention, and sound outcome research allows us to assess the efficacy of the interventions and, perhaps, to identify the aspects of the intervention that are responsible for its success. In turn, the nature

R.E. Smith (✉)
University of Washington, Seattle, WA, USA
e-mail: resmith@uw.edu

of the intervention dictates the outcome variables that we focus on and the way the evaluation is conducted. Attending to these three reciprocal linkages helps us ensure that our conceptual frameworks, research, and applied activities will support one another and advance our field as a scientific and applied discipline. Where interventions are concerned, adherence to the model helps ensure that they are based on firm theoretical and research foundations (frequently from other domains of scientific inquiry) and that they will be evaluated in a manner that conforms to standards of scientific accountability.

In this chapter, we describe the evolution of a program of research on coaching behaviors and interventions that has spanned more than three decades and has resulted in an empirically supported coach training program. We describe the manner in which a theoretical model derived from the areas of learning, social and personality psychology, and developmental psychology has helped guide a program of basic and applied research. Research results derived from the basic and applied research has guided the intervention program's development, and research results from basic research and program evaluations address important theoretical issues.

## Phase 1: Basic Research on Coaching Behaviors

### Theoretical Underpinnings

In the early 1970s, recognition of the potential impact of coaches on young athletes' psychological welfare prompted several scientific questions that we felt were worth pursuing. For example, what do coaches do, and how frequently do they engage in such behaviors as encouragement, punishment, instruction, and organization? What are the psychological dimensions that underlie such behaviors? And, finally, how are observable coaching behaviors related to children's reactions to various aspects of their organized athletic experiences? Answers to such questions are not only a first step in describing the behavioral ecology of the youth sport setting, but also provide an empirical basis for the development of psychologically oriented intervention programs, which did not exist at the time.

To begin to answer such questions, we carried out a systematic program of basic research over a period of several years. The project was guided by a mediational model of coach–athlete interactions, the basic elements of which are represented as follows: Coach behaviors → athlete perception and recall → athletes' evaluative reactions. This model, inspired by the "cognitive revolution" that was occurring at the time and the contributions of social cognitive theory (Bandura, 1969; Mischel, 1973), stipulates that the ultimate effects of coaching behaviors are mediated by the meaning that athletes confer on them. We assumed that how the athletes perceive and what they remember about their coach's behaviors affect the way that athletes feel about the coach and evaluate their sport experiences. Furthermore, a complex interaction of cognitive and affective processes is involved at this mediational level. The athletes' perceptions and reactions are likely to be affected not only by the coach's behaviors, but also by other factors, such as the athlete's age, what

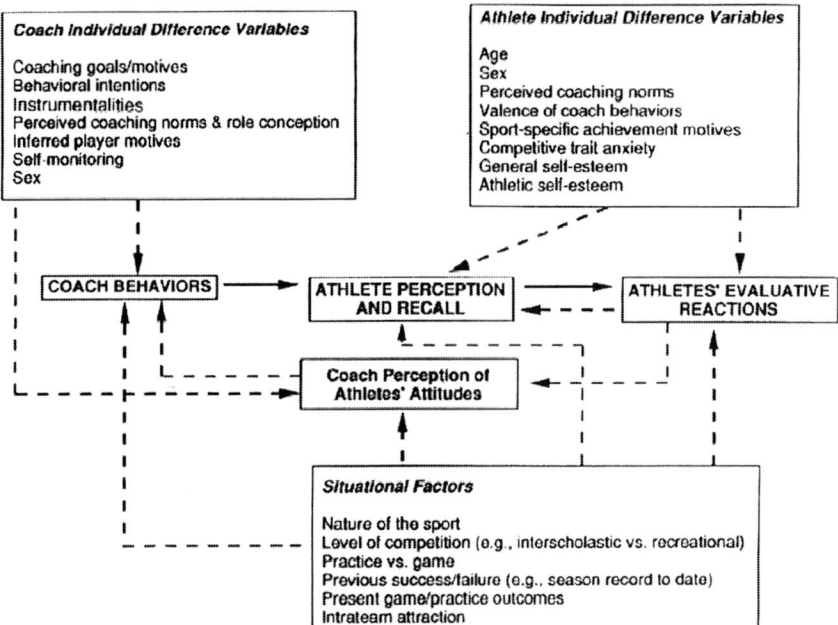

**Fig. 14.1** A model of adult leadership behaviors in sport, showing hypothesized relations among situational, cognitive, behavioral, and individual difference variables (adapted from Smoll & Smith, 1989)

he/she expects of coaches (normative beliefs and expectations), and certain personality variables, such as self-esteem and anxiety. Eventually, the basic three-element model was expanded to reflect these factors (Smoll & Smith, 1989). The elaborated model, shown in Fig. 14.1, specifies a number of situational factors as well as coach and athlete characteristics that could influence coach behaviors and the perceptions and reactions of athletes to them. Using this model as a starting point, we have sought to determine how observed coaching behaviors, athletes' perception and recall of the coach's behaviors, and athlete attitudes are related to one another. We have also explored the manner in which athlete and situational characteristics might serve to affect these relations.

## *Measurement of Coaching Behaviors*

Within behavioral psychology, behavioral assessment techniques were proving to be reliable and valid measures of naturalistic behaviors (Komaki, 1986; White, 1975). In order to measure leadership behaviors, we developed the Coaching Behavior Assessment System (CBAS) to permit the direct observation and coding of coaches' actions during practices and games (Smith, Smoll, & Hunt, 1977). The CBAS contains 12 categories divided into two major classes of behaviors.

Reactive (elicited) behaviors are responses to immediately preceding athlete or team behaviors, while spontaneous (emitted) behaviors are initiated by the coach and are not a response to a discernible preceding event. Reactive behaviors are responses to either desirable performance or effort (Reinforcement, Nonreinforcement), mistakes and errors (Mistake-contingent Encouragement, Mistake-contingent Technical Instruction, Punishment, Punitive Technical Instruction, Ignoring Mistakes), or misbehaviors on the part of athletes (Keeping Control). The spontaneous class includes General Technical Instruction, General Encouragement, Organization, and General Communication (unrelated to the current situation). The system thus involves basic interactions between the situation and the coach's behavior. Use of the CBAS in observing and coding coaching behaviors in a variety of sports by us and by other research teams has shown that (a) the scoring system is sufficiently comprehensive to incorporate the vast majority of overt leader behaviors, (b) high interrater reliability can be obtained, and (c) individual differences in behavioral patterns can be discerned (Smith, Smoll, & Christensen, 1996). Factor analyses of the CBAS have revealed three major factors that account for about 75% of the behavioral variance: supportiveness (comprised of Reinforcement and Mistake-contingent Encouragement), instructiveness (General Technical Instruction and Mistake-contingent Technical Instruction versus General Communication and General Encouragement), and punitiveness (Punishment and Punitive Technical Instruction).

The theoretical model assumes that the effects of coaching behaviors will be mediated by athletes' perceptions and recall of the behaviors. Accordingly, we constructed the CBAS Player-perceived Behavior Scale (CBAS-PBS) on which athletes are given descriptions of each of the CBAS behaviors and asked to indicate on 7-point scales how frequently their coach behaved in that fashion.

## *Behavioral Signatures*

A major advance within social cognitive theory was the demonstration that although behaviors may show marked inconsistency across situations (a finding that at one time was seen as a major challenge to the viability of personality), the consistency implied by a concept of personality is to be found in stable individual differences in situation–behavior relations. These patterns are called behavioral signatures (Shoda, Mischel, & Wright, 1994). The discovery of behavioral signatures in conduct-disordered children prompted us to reanalyze a large body of our behavioral data, and our new analyses revealed that most coaches do indeed show individualized patterns of behavior in response to certain situations, in this case, whether the team was winning, losing, or in a tie game at the time (Smith, Shoda, Cumming, & Smoll, 2009). For example, some coaches consistently responded when losing with an increased rate of punitive behaviors and a reduced rate of instructional behaviors, whereas others decreased in punitiveness and become relatively more supportive or instructive under this situational condition. Moreover, the high-profile stability coefficients (often exceeding 0.90) we discovered indicate that these differences in behavioral patterning occurred consistently in the three classes of situations and were not merely random fluctuations. This demonstration of behavioral signatures in translational research on youth sport coaches thus offers valuable support to the social cognitive theoretical model. Moreover, it advances our understanding of coaching behaviors, for, as we shall see, behavioral signatures are more predictive of athletes' attitudes toward the coach than are the CBAS behaviors considered in isolation.

## Coaching Behaviors and Children's Evaluative Reactions

Following development of the CBAS, a field study was conducted to establish relations between coaching behaviors and several athlete variables specified in the conceptual model (Smith, Smoll, & Curtis, 1978). Fifty-one male Little League Baseball coaches were observed by trained coders during 202 complete games. A total of 57,213 individual coaching behaviors were coded into the 12 categories, and a behavioral profile based on an average of 1,122 behaviors was computed for each coach.

Data from 542 players were collected after the season during individual interviews and questionnaire administrations carried out in the children's homes. Included were measures of their recall and perception of the coach's behaviors (on the same scales as the coaches had rated their own behavior), their liking for the coach and their teammates, the degree of enjoyment they experienced during the season, and their general self-esteem.

Relations between coaches' scores on these behavioral dimensions and player measures indicated that players responded most favorably to coaches who engaged in higher percentages of supportive and instructional behaviors. Players on teams whose coaches created a supportive environment also liked their teammates more. A somewhat surprising finding was that the team's won–lost record was essentially unrelated to how well the players liked the coach and how much they wanted to play for the coach in the future. This finding that coaching behaviors were far more important predictors of liking for the coach than was won–lost record was replicated in another large study involving youth basketball (Cumming, Smoll, Smith, & Grossbard, 2007). It is worth noting, however, that winning assumed greater importance beyond age 12, although it continued to be a less important attitudinal determinant than coaching behaviors.

Another important finding concerns the degree of accuracy with which coaches perceive their own behaviors. Correlations between CBAS observed behaviors and coaches' ratings of how frequently they performed the behaviors were generally low and nonsignificant. The only significant correlation occurred for punishment. Children's ratings on the same perceived behavior scales correlated much more highly with CBAS measures than did the coaches' ratings! It thus appears that coaches have limited awareness of how frequently they engage in particular forms of behavior and that athletes are more accurate perceivers of actual coach behaviors. This finding suggested that any effective intervention would need to increase coaches' self-awareness of their behavior.

## *Situational and Personality Moderators of Behavior–Attitude Relations*

The theoretical model shown in Fig. 14.1 posited a number of situational and individual difference variables that were expected, on theoretical grounds, to moderate relations between coaching behaviors and athletes' evaluative responses to the coach.

*Game situation.* One situational variable shown in the figure involves how successful the team is currently or was in the past. The demonstration of behavioral signatures by Shoda and his coworkers (1994) prompted us to reanalyze our behavioral data, revealing the existence of behavioral signatures. During the baseball study described above, we had coded the score of the game at the end of each half-inning, enabling us to determine how individual coaches behaved when their teams were winning or losing, or when the game was tied or with a one-run differential. We then related factor scores on the supportiveness, punitiveness, and instructiveness dimensions while the team was winning or losing or in a close contest with athletes' liking for the coaches and found substantial differences between the correlations as a function of game situation. Rate of supportive behaviors delivered while the team was winning correlated highly with liking, whereas supportive behaviors while losing bore no relation to liking for the coach. The opposite occurred for punitive behaviors, which were strongly and negatively related to liking when delivered in losing situations, but were only weakly related when given during winning situations. Instructiveness was not differentially affected by the score at the time it occurred (Smith, Shoda et al., 2009). Instructiveness during losing half-innings was negatively related to liking and positively related to athlete liking during winning half-innings, but the correlations were less extreme. These relations became clear when the situation-behavior profiles of the best-liked and least-liked coaches were compared (see Fig. 14.2).

Thus, the nature of the situation in which a class of coaching behaviors occurred moderated the behavior's relation with liking for the coach, particularly for supportive and punitive behaviors. These relations accounted for between 14% and 25% of the variance in athletes' liking for the coach, whereas less than 4% of the variance in liking scores was accounted for by the behaviors when situation was not taken into account. This finding exemplifies the manner in which decontextualized behavior aggregates may mask important relations that appear only when situation-behavior units are analyzed, a key tenet of the social cognitive model (Mischel & Shoda, 1998). From a translational perspective, the results add support from a unique naturalistic setting to laboratory-based results in cognitive psychology that address mood-congruent memory and judgment. One possible explanation for the behavior–attitude relations may be found in previous research on mood congruence (Bower & Forgas, 2000). Attitude data were collected from athletes at the end of the season, so these measures may be regarded at least in part as indirect memory measures reflecting recalled affective responses to the coach during the season. Mood congruence may affect such recall, so that the impact of positively valenced supportive behaviors in an affectively pleasant winning situation may be

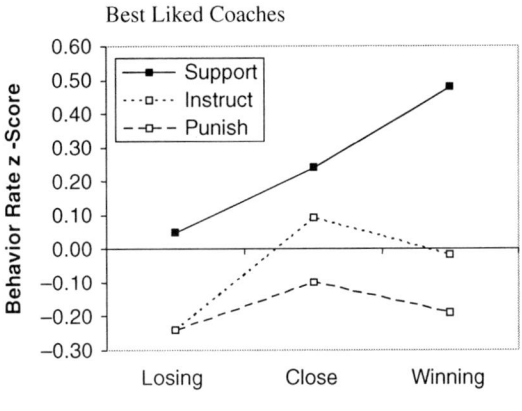
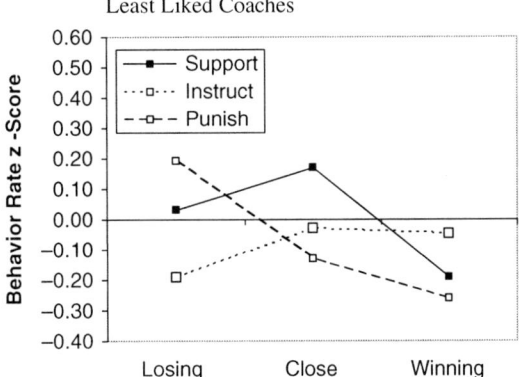

**Fig. 14.2** Intraindividual behavioral signatures of best-liked and least-liked youth sport coaches across three game situations, showing situation-specific patterning of supportive, instructive, and punitive behaviors (Smith, Shoda et al., 2009)

better encoded and later remembered. In like fashion, negatively valenced punitive behaviors that occurred during losing situations while the athletes were feeling bad may have been encoded more deeply and affected retrospective recall about how the athletes felt about their coach during the season. Such encoding could well influence global postseason attitudes toward the coach.

*Motivational climate.* Achievement goal theory has had a major influence on sport psychology over the past two decades (Duda, 2005; Roberts, Treasure, & Conroy, 2007). Achievement goal theory focuses on understanding the function and meaning of goal-directed actions, based on how participants define success and how they judge whether or not they have demonstrated competence (Ames, 1992b; Dweck, 1999). The two central constructs in the theory are individual goal orientations that guide achievement perceptions and behavior, and the motivational climate created within adult-controlled achievement settings. In a mastery motivational climate, success is self-referenced, defined in terms of giving maximum effort, enjoyment of the activity, and personal improvement. An ego-oriented climate defines success in social-comparison terms, emphasizing outperforming others, winning, and those who perform best get special attention.

A large body of research indicates that in sports, as in other achievement settings, mastery achievement goals and a mastery-oriented motivational climate are associated with salutary effects on athletes (Chi, 2004). Compared with ego-oriented students and athletes, those high in mastery orientation report higher feelings of competence, greater enjoyment of the activity, and higher intrinsic motivation and effort (Duda, 2005). A mastery orientation (particularly in combination with a low ego orientation) is also related to lower levels of cognitive trait anxiety and pre-event state anxiety (Newton & Duda, 1999; Papaioannou & Kouli, 1999). Finally, a mastery goal orientation is related to a variety of adaptive achievement behaviors, such as exerting consistent effort, persistence in the face of setbacks, and sustained and improved performance (Ames, 1992a; Dweck, 1999). Although an ego orientation has at times been linked to high levels of achievement, it also has a number of less-desirable correlates, such as inconsistent effort, higher levels of performance anxiety, reduced persistence or withdrawal in the face of failure, decreased intrinsic motivation for sport involvement, and a willingness to use deception and illegal methods in order to win (Duda, 2005; Roberts et al., 2007).

A mastery motivational climate counters the "win at all costs" philosophy that is all too common in youth sports. In such a climate, students and athletes tend to adopt adaptive achievement strategies such as selecting challenging tasks, giving maximum effort, persisting in the face of setbacks, and taking pride in personal improvement. In contrast, an ego-involving climate promotes social comparison as a basis for success judgments. When coaches create an ego climate, they tend to give differential attention and positive reinforcement to athletes who are most competent and instrumental to winning, and skill development is deemed more important to winning than it is to personal improvement and self-realization. They are also more likely to respond to mistakes and poor performance with punitive responses. Several studies conducted in physical education classes have shown that motivational climate is a stronger predictor of such outcomes as intrinsic motivation and voluntary activity participation than are students' achievement goal orientations (Roberts et al., 2007). Within youth sports, a mastery climate is associated with more positive attitudes toward the coach, whereas an ego climate is negatively associated with athletes' attitudes toward the coach. Moreover, won–lost percentage accounts for far less attitudinal variance than does the motivational climate created by the coach (Cumming et al., 2007).

Our research has shown that coach-initiated motivational climate has an effect on athletes' achievement goal orientation over the course of a sport season. In a longitudinal study involving 50 youth basketball teams, we used a motivational climate scale created for young athletes to predict changes in young athletes' achievement goal orientations over the course of a season. Coach-initiated mastery climate scores predicted increases in mastery goal orientation and decreases in ego orientation. Ego motivational climate scores were associated with increases in ego goal orientation (Smith, Smoll, & Cumming, 2009).

*An individual difference factor: Athlete self-esteem.* The conceptual model shown in Fig. 14.1 also specifies coach and athlete individual difference variables that are hypothesized to influence coaching behaviors and their effects. Originating within humanistic conceptions of personality (James, 1890; Rogers, 1959), self-esteem has

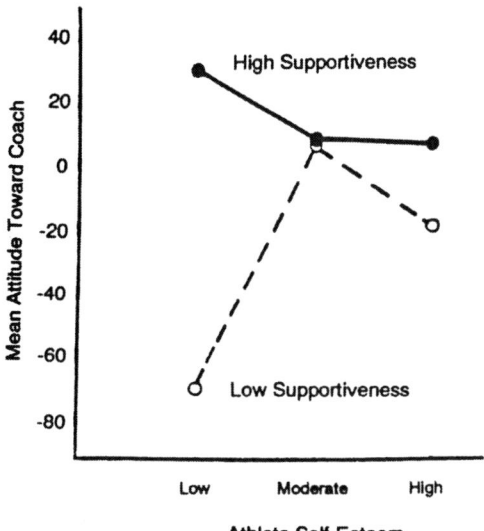

Fig. 14.3 Mean evaluations of coaches by athletes as a function of athletes' self-esteem and supportiveness of the coach (Smith & Smoll, 1990)

proven to be a personality variable of major importance (Brown, 1998). Of particular interest within our research program, how people feel about themselves influences how they respond to the behaviors of other people (Brown, 1998). We therefore hypothesized that level of self-esteem would moderate relations between coaching behaviors and children's attitudes toward themselves, the coach, and other aspects of their sport experience. In the Little League Baseball study described above, analysis of the children's attraction responses toward the coaches revealed a significant interaction between coach supportiveness (the tendency to reinforce desirable performance and effort and to respond to mistakes with encouragement) and athletes' level of self-esteem (Smith & Smoll, 1990). As shown in Fig. 14.3, children with low self-esteem were especially responsive to variations in supportiveness in a manner consistent with a self-enhancement model of self-esteem (Swann, 1990). This finding is consistent with the results of other studies that, collectively, suggest that self-enhancement motivation causes people who are low in self-esteem to be especially responsive to variations in supportiveness because of their greater need for positive feedback from others (Tesser & Campbell, 1983). We therefore concluded that children who are low in self-esteem are especially in need of a positive sport experience and that coaches can help provide that experience.

## Phase 2: Translating Basic Research Findings into a Coach Intervention

Data from our basic research indicated clear relations between coaching behaviors and the reactions of youngsters to their athletic experience. Along with findings from research inspired by achievement goal theory, these relations provided a foundation for developing a set of coaching guidelines that formed the basis for an intervention that was initially called Coach Effectiveness Training (Smith, Smoll, & Curtis, 1979). With the later emergence of achievement goal theory and the wealth of research it inspired, we incorporated its principles into an evolved program called the Mastery Approach to Coaching (MAC) that explicitly focuses on the development of a mastery motivational climate. This emphasis is highly consistent with principles (particularly our conception of success as doing one's best and striving to maximize one's potential) that have been emphasized in CET from the beginning.

The MAC program incorporates information on goal orientations and motivational climate and includes specific guidelines on how to create a mastery climate. An overview of MAC content and procedures for its implementation is now presented. A more comprehensive discussion of cognitive–behavioral principles and techniques used in conducting psychologically-oriented coach training programs appears elsewhere (Smoll & Smith, 2010).

Five key principles are emphasized in a MAC workshop, and behavioral guidelines are presented for implementing each principle (see Smith & Smoll, 2002). The empirically derived guidelines (i.e., coaching *do's* and *don'ts*) serve two important functions: (a) they allow us to conduct MAC as an information-sharing rather than speculative enterprise, and (b) the scientific origin of the guidelines increases their credibility with coaches. By presenting a workshop as informational in nature, we can play to coaches' desire to provide the best possible experience for youngsters (the prevailing motivation for most volunteer coaches). We are not telling them what they "should do," but rather what research has shown to be effective in helping them meet their goals and how they can incorporate these findings into their own coaching style. We have always found coaches receptive to this approach.

The first MAC principle deals with a developmentally oriented philosophy of winning. Coaches are urged to focus on athletes' effort and enjoyment rather than on success as measured by statistics or scoreboards. They are encouraged to emphasize "doing your best," "getting better," and "having fun" as opposed to a "win at all costs" orientation (Smoll & Smith, 1981). This principle attempts to reduce the ultimate importance of winning relative to other prized participation motives (e.g., skill development and affiliation with teammates) and takes into account the inverse relation between enjoyment and competitive anxiety (Scanlan & Lewthwaite, 1984; Scanlan & Passer, 1978, 1979). Moreover, coaches are instructed to help promote separation of athletes' feelings of self-worth from game outcomes or won–lost records. Although formulated prior to the emergence of achievement goal theory, this principle is clearly consistent with the procedures designed by Ames (1992a, 1992b), Dweck (1999), and Epstein (1988, 1989) to create a mastery learning climate in the classroom.

Our second principle emphasizes a "positive approach" to coaching (see Smith, 2010). In such an approach, coach–athlete interactions are characterized by the liberal use of positive reinforcement, encouragement, and sound technical instruction that help create high levels of interpersonal attraction between coaches and athletes. Punitive and hostile responses are strongly discouraged as they have been shown to create a negative team climate and to promote fear of failure in athletes. We emphasize that reinforcement should not be restricted to the learning and performance of sport skills. Rather, it should also be liberally applied to strengthen desirable responses (e.g., mastery attempts and persistence, teamwork, leadership, sportsmanship). MAC also includes several "positive approach" guidelines pertaining to the appropriate use of technical instruction. For example, when giving instruction, we encourage coaches to emphasize the good things that will happen if athletes execute correctly rather than focusing on the negative things that will occur if they do not. This approach is designed to motivate athletes to make desirable things happen (i.e., helps develop a positive achievement orientation) rather than building fear of making mistakes.

The third coaching principle is to establish norms that emphasize athletes' mutual obligations to help and support one another. Such norms increase social support and attraction among teammates and thereby enhance cohesion and commitment to the team, and they are most likely to develop when coaches (a) are themselves supportive models and (b) reinforce athlete behaviors that promote team unity. We also instruct coaches in how to develop a "we're in this together" group norm. This norm can play an important role in building team cohesion, particularly if the coach frequently reinforces athletes' demonstrations of mutual supportiveness.

A fourth principle is that compliance with rules of conduct is most effectively achieved by involving athletes in decisions regarding team rules and by reinforcing compliance with them rather than by using punitive measures to punish noncompliance, a principle consistent with guidelines for shared decisional responsibility in the mastery-oriented motivational climate of the classroom (Ames, 1992a, 1992b; Dweck, 1999; Epstein, 1988, 1989). By setting explicit guidelines that the athletes help formulate and by using positive reinforcement to strengthen desirable responses, coaches can foster self-discipline and often prevent athlete misbehaviors from occurring.

A fifth principle is that coaches should become more aware of their own behavior and its consequences. To enhance awareness, MAC coaches are taught the use of behavioral feedback and self-monitoring, which are described below.

During a 75-min MAC workshop, behavioral guidelines are presented verbally with the aid of animated PowerPoint slides and cartoons illustrating important points. Additionally, a mastery climate is explicitly described, its creation is strongly recommended, and a list of established salutary effects derived from research is presented. The didactic presentation of MAC principles is augmented by modeling both desirable and undesirable methods of responding to specific situations (e.g., athlete mistakes, reinforcing good performance and effort). Coaches are also invited to role play desired responses.

To reinforce the didactic portions of the workshop, coaches are given a 34-page booklet, which highlights the advantages of a mastery motivational climate and provides behavioral guidelines for creating one (Smoll & Smith, 2008). It also supplements the guidelines with concrete suggestions for communicating effectively with young athletes, gaining their respect, and relating effectively to their parents.

A notable finding from our basic research was that coaches had very limited awareness of how often they behaved, as indicated by low correlations between observed and coach-rated behaviors (Smith et al., 1978). Similar findings occurred in another youth sport observational study (Burton & Tannehill, 1987). Thus, an important goal of MAC is to increase coaches' awareness of what they are doing, for no change is likely to occur without it. MAC coaches are taught the use of two proven behavioral-change techniques, namely, behavioral feedback (Edelstein & Eisler, 1976; Huberman & O'Brien, 1999) and self-monitoring (Crews, Lochbaum, & Karoly, 2001; Kanfer & Gaelick-Buys, 1991). To obtain feedback, coaches are encouraged to work with their assistants as a team and share descriptions of each other's behaviors. Another feedback procedure involves coaches soliciting input directly from their athletes.

With respect to self-monitoring, the workshop manual contains a brief Coach Self-Report Form, containing nine items related to the behavioral guidelines (see Smoll & Smith, 2008, p. 24). On the form, coaches are asked how often they engaged in the recommended behaviors in relevant situations. For example, "When athletes gave good effort (regardless of the outcome), what percent of the time did you respond with reinforcement?" MAC coaches are instructed to complete the form immediately after practices and games, and they are encouraged to engage in self-monitoring on a regular basis in order to achieve optimal results.

MAC also includes discussion of coach–parent relationships and provides instructions on how to organize and conduct a sport orientation meeting with parents. Some purposes of the meeting are to inform parents about their responsibilities for contributing to the success of the sport program and to guide them toward working cooperatively and productively with the coach (see Smoll & Cumming, 2006).

## Phase 3: Outcome Research

We now summarize the results of five CET and MAC outcome studies conducted by our research group, by Conroy and Coatsworth (2004), and by Sousa, Smith, and Cruz (2008). Collectively, these studies have assessed the effects of the intervention on a host of behavioral, attitudinal, motivational, and personality variables.

### *Coaching Behaviors*

The CET/MAC intervention is designed to influence observed and athlete-perceived coaching behaviors, and these changes, in turn, are thought to mediate other effects of the training on young athletes. A major goal of the intervention is to increase supportive behaviors and reduce aversive coach behaviors to create a more positive and enjoyable sport experience for young athletes.

Because of the labor-intensive demands of CBAS training and data collection, observable coaching behaviors have served as outcome variables in only three studies. In the first randomized trial of CET, we compared 18 trained Little League Baseball coaches with 13 untrained coaches, collecting a total of 26,413 behaviors over four games, an average of 813 behaviors per coach (Smith et al., 1979).

A stepwise discriminant analysis of the behavioral differences indicated that in accordance with the CET behavioral guidelines, the trained coaches exhibited more reinforcement and mistake-contingent encouragement behaviors and fewer punitive and control-keeping responses. However, the group difference was significant only in the case of positive reinforcement. Positive reinforcement differences were also reported by Conroy and Coatsworth (2004) in a smaller study involving four swimming coaches trained in CET principles and three untreated control coaches. However, the small scope of the study precluded a meaningful test of statistical significance. Finally, a replicated single-subject approach was used by Sousa et al. (2008) to assess the effects of coach training on four youth soccer coaches. CBAS data were collected on the coaches at baseline, and the coaches were then exposed to CET principles via a DVD. They were provided with behavioral profiles of their baseline CBAS behaviors and allowed to set individual goals for behaviors they wanted to increase or decrease. Although the specific behavioral goals varied, the coaches uniformly wanted to become more supportive and/or less punitive in their behaviors. Follow-up CBAS observations showed that two of the coaches achieved positive changes in all three of their target behaviors, and a third coach improved on two of the targeted behaviors. The fourth coach showed no change. Although more research is needed, it does appear that the intervention produces changes in observed coaching behaviors that are consistent with the behavioral guidelines.

Athlete-perceived behavioral ratings also provide strong evidence for positive behavioral differences linked to the CET intervention. In two large-scale outcome studies, athletes who played for CET-trained coaches reported that their coaches were more highly and consistently reinforcing and encouraging rather than punitive in response to mistakes, and gave higher levels of instruction than did untrained coaches (Smith et al., 1979; Smoll, Smith, Barnett, & Everett, 1993). The intervention thus promotes both observed and athlete-perceived behaviors that are in accordance with the CET/MAC principles and behavioral guidelines.

## *Athlete Attitudes*

The positive behaviors encouraged by the CET/MAC research-derived guidelines would be expected to be reflected in more positive attitudes on the part of athletes to their coaches and other aspects of their sport experience. Significant differences in athlete attitudes favoring trained coaches have been found in two large experimental studies involving 49 youth baseball coaches, and 477 athletes have shown significant postseason differences in liking for the coach, increased liking for the coach over the course of the season, enjoyment of their sport experience, liking for teammates, evaluation of the coach's teaching ability, and desire to play for the coach in the future (Smith et al., 1979; Smith, Smoll, & Barnett, 1995). These differences cannot be attributed to differences in won–lost records. In the latter study, the athletes also believed that their trained coaches liked them more. In neither study did they increase their liking for the sport itself. Unfortunately, Conroy and Coatsworth (2004) did not assess athlete attitudes in their study. To this point, however, it appears that the training program is associated with positive differences both in coaching behaviors and in athletes' evaluative responses to the coach and other aspects of their sport experience.

## *Self-Esteem*

We have been interested in self-esteem as both a moderator of athletes' responses to their coaches and to the effects of the intervention on athletes' feelings of self-worth. Our expectation (based in part on the moderator effect shown in the basic research phase) was that children low in self-esteem are particularly in need of a positive sport experience and that the supportive and instructive behaviors recommended by the behavioral guidelines would be especially well received by them. This hypothesis was strongly supported in the first experimental trial (Smith et al., 1979), where a significant main effect of training status on athletes' overall evaluation of the coach was qualified by a significant interaction involving level of self-esteem. As in the basic research, effects of the intervention were especially large for children with low self-esteem.

We have also assessed the effects of the intervention on changes in self-esteem. Specifically, we found that children who played for the trained coaches showed a significant increase in global self-esteem from the previous year to the end of the season following training, whereas the control group athletes showed no change (Smith et al., 1979). In a later study tracking self-esteem from the beginning of the season to the end, positive changes in self-esteem occurred for children who were below the median self-esteem score at preseason (Smoll et al., 1993). The magnitude of the increase in self-esteem moved the average low-esteem child who played for a trained coach from approximately the 25th to the 50th percentile of the preseason distribution. This change could not be attributed to regression to the mean, for the low-self-esteem children who played for an attention-placebo control group showed no increase in self-esteem scores.

## *Achievement Goal Orientation*

Both the MAC and its historical CET predecessor are explicitly designed to produce a coach-initiated mastery climate and to discourage a "win at all costs" ego climate. A major effect of a mastery climate is to promote the development of a mastery achievement goal orientation in young athletes. A mastery goal orientation has a wide range of salutary effects identified in achievement goal theory research in both sport and educational settings (see Ames, 1992b; Roberts et al., 2007).

The effects of the MAC intervention on achievement goal orientations was assessed in a study involving 37 basketball teams with 225 boys and girls (Smoll, Smith, & Cumming, 2007a). Coach-initiated motivational climate was assessed using the Motivational Climate Scale for Youth Sports (MCSYS; Smith, Cumming, & Smoll, 2008). Mastery and ego goal orientations were measured at the

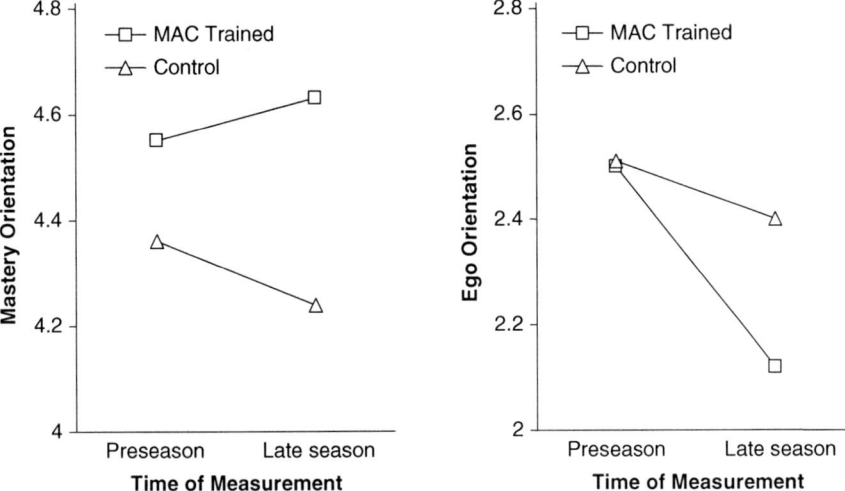

**Fig. 14.4** Changes in AGSYS achievement goal orientation scores from preseason to late-season in children who played for either MAC-trained coaches or untrained coaches (Smoll et al., 2007a)

beginning and end of the season using the Achievement Goal Scale for Youth Sports (AGSYS; Cumming, Smith, Smoll, Standage, & Grossbard, 2008). Both measures have fourth-grade reading levels that make them appropriate for athletes down to ages 8–9 years. The MAC intervention resulted in significantly higher mastery-climate scores and lower ego-climate scores compared with the control condition. Moreover, multilevel analyses revealed that athletes who played for the trained coaches exhibited significant increases in mastery goal orientation scores and significant decreases in ego-orientation scores across the season, whereas control group participants did not (see Fig. 14.4). These results applied to both boys and girls teams. Although additional experimental trials are needed, this study indicates that the MAC intervention has its intended impact on both coach-initiated motivational climate and athletes' achievement goal orientations.

## Performance Anxiety

Our initial interest in developing a coach intervention was stimulated by concerns that adult-organized youth sports can place inappropriate pressures on children, thereby promoting needless stress and anxiety. The behavioral guidelines of the original CET intervention were designed to create a positive athletic environment that would enhance enjoyment and promote positive psychosocial consequences of participation. The emphasis on a mastery climate promotion in both CET and MAC programs that evolved over time also is consistent with the negative relations found between anxiety and both mastery climate and mastery goal orientation (Chi, 2004).

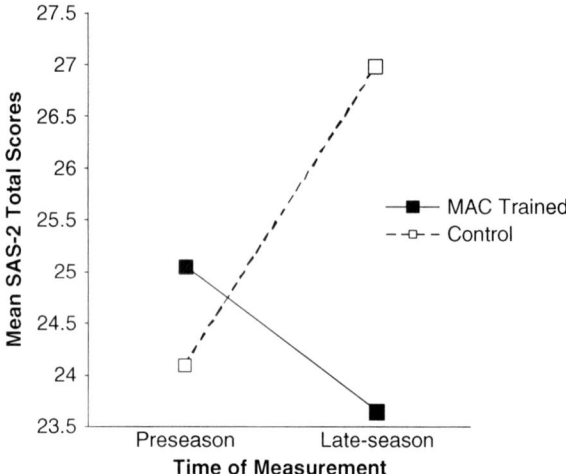

**Fig. 14.5** Changes in SAS-2 performance trait anxiety scores from preseason to late-season in children who played for either MAC-trained coaches or untrained coaches (Smith et al., 2007)

Two studies provide evidence that the CET/MAC intervention helps reduce anxiety. In a study of youth baseball teams, we found that children who played for CET-trained coaches showed a significant decrease in two different trait measures of sport performance anxiety, whereas children who played for coaches in an attention-placebo condition exhibited no change in anxiety (Smith et al., 1995). In the more recent MAC-evaluation study cited above in relation to achievement goal orientation, the children were also administered the revised Sport Anxiety Scale-2 (SAS-2; Smith, Smoll, Cumming, & Grossbard, 2006), which has a fourth-grade reading level that makes it more appropriate for youth sport research than the measures used in the 1995 study. As shown in the significant multilevel groups × time interaction presented in Fig. 14.5, children who played for the untrained coaches exhibited an increase in SAS-2 total score as competitive pressures increased over the course of the season, whereas those whose coaches received the MAC intervention showed a decrease in anxiety. This pattern was also exhibited on the somatic anxiety, worry, and concentration disruption subscales of the SAS-2 (Smith, Smoll, & Cumming, 2007).

## *Dropout Rate*

Attrition is a major problem in youth sport programs, where approximately 35% of athletes drop out each year (Gould, 1987). Sport attrition research shows that a major reason why children say they drop out of programs is aversive coaching behaviors and pressures to win. If children who play for trained coaches like their coach and teammates more, feel more positively about themselves, and have more positive and adaptive mastery achievement goals, they should be more likely to continue their sport participation. Barnett, Smoll, and Smith (1992) followed up children who had played for trained and untrained coaches to assess attrition (defined as total withdrawal from sports participation the following year). They found that 26% of the children who had played for untrained coaches had dropped out of sport, compared with only 5% of those who played for coaches trained in CET/MAC principles.

## *Conclusion*

Although more research is clearly needed, particularly by other investigators, evidence for the efficacy of the CET and MAC interventions has been provided by three different research groups. Our research group has done three large-scale experimental outcome studies, plus a smaller MAC intervention study within an inner-city African American basketball program that also produced a significant increase in mastery goal orientation scores and a significant decrease in ego-orientation scores on the AGSYS relative to a control condition (Smith, Smoll, Cumming, & DeCano, 2006). It appears that the empirically derived behavioral principles can be readily applied by coaches and that their application has salutary effects on a range of psychosocial outcome variables in boys, girls, and minority populations.

## Phase 4: Dissemination

Given the ever-expanding nature of organized athletics for children and adolescents, the need for effective coach training programs is obvious. Likewise, the large coach turnover from year to year creates a continuing demand for intervention. Our experience in offering coaching workshops has shown that youth sport coaches are committed to providing a positive experience for youngsters. It is also reassuring to note that coaches are willing to spend time to acquire additional information, and they do take advantage of the availability of workshops. Indeed, more than 25,000 coaches have participated in some 500 CET and MAC workshops in the United States and Canada. Workshops have been presented to volunteer coaches in a variety of sport-specific organizations (e.g., Little League Baseball, US Soccer Federation, Minnesota Hockey) and multisport organizations (e.g., Catholic Youth Organization, YMCA, community recreation departments). The program has also been offered as in-service training for physical education teachers and coaches in public school districts.

The need for effective dissemination of evidence-based treatments has been recognized within the fields of medicine (Institute of Medicine, 2001) and clinical psychology (McHugh & Barlow, 2010). But the impact of an intervention, no matter how promising, is limited if a means cannot be found to make it accessible to its target population. Given the body of evidence that has accumulated for the efficacious and economical MAC intervention, we believe that it is ready for widespread dissemination to youth sport organizations.

There are obvious limitations in the number of workshops that can be conducted by the program's developers, indicating the need for a mechanism to provide wider dissemination. In order to maximize the distribution of MAC, we have transformed the workshop into a self-instructional format, consisting of a DVD and a 32-page manual, the content of which is linked to the DVD (Smoll & Smith, 2009a, 2009b). This provides a fully-integrated instructional package. The 66-min DVD presents video-recorded segments of a live workshop and incorporates several educational procedures (lecture, dynamic interaction, modeling, and role playing). It is specifically designed to teach the mastery-oriented principles with the aid of animated coach–athlete cartoons, photos, and embedded videos. Additionally, a 12-min video has been produced that presents an overview of the DVD content. The demonstration video can be viewed on our Youth Enrichment in Sports project website (www.y-e-sports.com).

In recognition of the importance of educating youth sport parents as well as coaches, we have also developed a 1-h workshop titled the Mastery Approach to Parenting in Sports (MAPS). Similar to our coach training intervention, MAPS applies positive influence and mastery climate principles to parenting young athletes. This allows both coaches and parents to be "on the same page" in the sport experiences that they provide. An initial experimental study presenting the MAC and MAPS workshops in a youth basketball league resulted in significant reductions in athletes' performance anxiety over the course of the season, whereas a no-treatment control condition was associated with increased anxiety (Smoll, Smith, & Cumming, 2007b). As for MAC, we have transformed the companion sport–parent workshop into self-instructional DVD format (Smoll & Smith, 2009c). A description of the 45-min MAPS DVD and a 12-min video preview of it are available on our project website.

Given a product that is appropriate in content and format to widespread dissemination, how is this to be accomplished? We do not believe that direct sales to individual coaches and parents would result in the desired level of dissemination. Therefore, we are currently working to find corporate and foundation sponsors to deliver the training – free of charge – to youth sport organizations nationwide (Munsey, 2010). Hopefully, sponsors will financially support production of significant quantities of the MAC and MAPS programs, and they will be shipped to youth sport organizations on behalf of the sponsors. The organizations will then distribute the educational materials to their coaches and parents at no cost.

## General Conclusion

Our translational approach has drawn upon methods, constructs, and the research literature in a variety of fields to develop a conceptual model of coaching behaviors that has guided our basic research. The basic research, in turn, has provided an empirical basis for the development of behavioral guidelines that have proven their efficacy in program evaluation studies. Finally, a number of our basic and applied research results have definite translational value for other domains of psychology, such as personality and social psychology and cognitive psychology.

Coach training has become a large-scale commercial enterprise in the United States – most notably the American Coaching Effectiveness Program, the National Youth Sports Coaches Association, and the Positive Coaching Alliance. Unfortunately, however, virtually nothing is known about what effects these programs have on coaches and athletes and how well they achieve their objectives. The absence of empirical attention is understandable, as developers of existing programs have been focused primarily on development and dissemination, rather than evaluation, and they have not had the benefit of research grant support to guide their work. Yet evaluation research is not only desirable but also essential. In the words of Lipsey and Cordray (2000), "... the overarching goal of the program evaluation enterprise is to contribute to the improvement of social conditions by providing scientifically credible information and balanced judgment to legitimate social agents about the effectiveness of interventions intended to produce social benefits" (p. 346). In concluding this chapter, it is appropriate to state our firm belief that efforts to improve the quality and value of coach training programs are best achieved by means of well-conceived and properly conducted evaluation research.

**Acknowledgments** Preparation of this chapter and much of the research reported herein was supported in part by Grant #1529 from the William T. Grant Foundation. Early phases of the research program were supported by Grant RO1 MH24248 from the National Institute of Mental Health.

# References

Ames, C. (1992a). Classrooms: Goals, structures, and student motivation. *Journal of Educational Psychology, 84*, 261–271.

Ames, C. (1992b). Achievement goals and adaptive motivational patterns: The role of the environment. In G. C. Roberts (Ed.), *Motivation in sport and exercise* (pp. 161–176). Champaign, IL: Human Kinetics.

Bandura, A. (1969). *Principles of behavior modification*. New York: Holt, Rinehart, & Winston.

Barnett, N. P., Smoll, F. L., & Smith, R. E. (1992). Effects of enhancing coach-athlete relationships on youth sport attrition. *The Sport Psychologist, 6*, 111–127.

Bower, G. H., & Forgas, J. P. (2000). Affect, memory, and social cognition. In E. Eich, J. F. Kihlstrom, G. H. Bower, J. P. Forgas, & P. M. Niedenthal (Eds.), *Cognition and emotion* (pp. 87–168). New York: Oxford University Press.

Brown, J. D. (1998). *The self*. New York: McGraw-Hill.

Burton, D., & Tannehill, D. (1987, April). *Developing better youth sport coaches: An evaluation of the American Coaching Effectiveness Program (ACEP) Level 1 training*. Paper presented at the meeting of the American Alliance of Health, Physical Education, Recreation and Dance, Las Vegas, NV.

Chi, L. (2004). Achievement goal theory. In T. Morris & J. Summers (Eds.), *Sport psychology: Theory, applications, and issues* (2nd ed., pp. 152–174). Milton, Australia: Wiley.

Conroy, D. E., & Coatsworth, J. D. (2004). The effects of coach training on fear of failure in youth swimmers: A latent growth curve analysis from a randomized, controlled trial. *Journal of Applied Developmental Psychology, 25*, 193–214.

Crews, D. J., Lochbaum, M. R., & Karoly, P. (2001). Self-regulation: Concepts, methods and strategies in sport and exercise. In R. N. Singer, H. A. Hausenblaus, & C. M. Janelle (Eds.), *Handbook of research on sport psychology* (2nd ed., pp. 566–584). New York: Wiley.

Cumming, S. P., Smith, R. E., Smoll, F. L., Standage, M., & Grossbard, J. R. (2008). Development and validation of the Achievement Goal Scale for Youth Sports. *Psychology of Sport and Exercise, 9*, 686–703.

Cumming, S. P., Smoll, F. L., Smith, R. E., & Grossbard, J. R. (2007). Is winning everything? The relative contributions of motivational climate and won-lost percentage in youth sports. *Journal of Applied Sport Psychology, 19*, 322–336.

Duda, J. L. (2005). Motivation in sport: The relevance of competence and achievement goals. In A. J. Elliot & C. S. Dweck (Eds.), *Handbook of competence and motivation* (pp. 318–335). New York: Guildford Publications.

Dweck, C. S. (1999). *Self-theories and goals: Their role in motivation, personality, and development*. Philadelphia: Taylor & Francis.

Edelstein, B. A., & Eisler, R. M. (1976). Effects of modeling and modeling with instructions and feedback on the behavioral components of social skills. *Behavior Therapy, 7*, 382–389.

Epstein, J. (1988). Effective schools or effective students? Dealing with diversity. In R. Haskins & B. MacRae (Eds.), *Policies for America's schools* (pp. 89–126). Norwood, NJ: Ablex.

Epstein, J. (1989). Family structures and students motivation: A developmental perspective. In C. Ames & R. Ames (Eds.), *Research on motivation in education: Vol. 3. Goals and cognitions* (pp. 259–295). New York: Academic.

Gould, D. (1987). Understanding attrition in children's sport. In D. Gould & M. R. Weiss (Eds.), *Advances in pediatric sport sciences* (pp. 61–85). Champaign, IL: Human Kinetics.

Huberman, W. L., & O'Brien, R. M. (1999). Improving therapist and patient performance in chronic psychiatric group homes through goal-setting, feedback, and positive reinforcement. *Journal of Organizational Behavior Management, 19*, 13–36.

Institute of Medicine (2001). *Crossing the quality chasm: A new health system for the 21st century*. Washington, DC: Author.

James, W. (1890). *Principles of psychology*. New York: Holt.

Kanfer, F. H., & Gaelick-Buys, L. (1991). Self-management methods. In F. H. Kanfer & A. P. fGoldstein (Eds.), *Helping people change: A textbook of methods* (4th ed., pp. 305–360). New York: Pergamon.

Komaki, J. L. (1986). Toward effective supervision: An operant analysis and comparison of managers at work. *Journal of Applied Psychology, 71*, 270–279.

Lipsey, M. W., & Cordray, D. S. (2000). Evaluation methods for social intervention. *Annual Review of Psychology, 51*, 345–376.

McHugh, R. K., & Barlow, D. H. (2010). The dissemination and implementation of evidence-based psychological treatments. *American Psychologist, 65*, 73–84.

Mischel, W. (1973). Toward a cognitive social learning reconceptualization of personality. *Psychological Rreview, 80*, 252–283.

Mischel, W., & Shoda, Y. (1998). Reconciling processing dynamics and personality dispositions. *Annual Review of Psychology, 49*, 229–258.

Munsey, C. (2010, April). Coaching the coaches: Promoting a "mastery climate" motivates young athletes to do their best, says this scientist-practitioner team. *Monitor on Psychology, 41*, 58–61.

Newton, M. L., & Duda, J. L. (1999). The interaction of motivational climate, dispositional goal orientation and perceived ability in predicting indices of motivation. *International Journal of Sport Psychology, 30*, 63–82.

Papaioannou, A., & Kouli, O. (1999). The effect of task structure, perceived motivational climate and goal orientations on students' task involvement and anxiety. *Journal of Applied Sport Psychology, 11*, 51–71.

Roberts, G. C., Treasure, D. C., & Conroy, D. E. (2007). Understanding the dynamics of motivation in sport and physical activity: An achievement goal interpretation. In G. Tenenbaum & R. C. Eklund (Eds.), *Handbook of sport psychology* (3rd ed., pp. 3–30). New York: Wiley.

Rogers, C. R. (1959). A theory of therapy, personality, and interpersonal relationships, as developed within the client-centered framework. In S., Koch (Ed.), *Psychology: A study of a science* (Vol. 3, pp. 184–266). New York: McGraw-Hill.

Scanlan, T. K., & Lewthwaite, R. (1984). Social psychological aspects of competition for male youth sport participants: I. Predictors of competitive stress. *Journal of Sport Psychology, 6*, 208–226.

Scanlan, T. K., & Passer, M. W. (1978). Factors related to competitive stress among male youth sport participants. *Medicine and Science in Sports, 10*, 103–108.

Scanlan, T. K., & Passer, M. W. (1979). Sources of competitive stress in young female athletes. *Journal of Sport Psychology, 1*, 151–159.

Shoda, Y., Mischel, W., & Wright, J. C. (1994). Intraindividual stability in the organization and patterning of behavior: Incorporating psychological situations into the idiographic analysis of personality. *Journal of Personality and Social Psychology, 67*, 674–687.

Smith, R. E. (2010). A positive approach to coaching effectiveness and performance enhancement. In J. M. Williams (Ed.), *Applied sport psychology: Personal growth to peak performance* (6th ed., pp. 42–58). Boston: McGraw-Hill.

Smith, R. E., Cumming, S. P., & Smoll, F. L. (2008). Development and validation of the Motivational Climate Scale for Youth Sports. *Journal of Applied Sport Psychology, 20*, 116–136.

Smith, R. E., Shoda, Y., Cumming, S. P., & Smoll, F. L. (2009). Behavioral signatures at the ballpark: Intraindividual consistency of adults' situation-behavior patterns and their interpersonal consequences. *Journal of Research in Personality, 43*, 187–195.

Smith, R. E., & Smoll, F. L. (1990). Self-esteem and children's reactions to youth sport coaching behaviors: A field study of Self-enhancement processes. *Developmental Psychology, 26*, 987–993.

Smith, R. E., & Smoll, F. L. (2002). *Way to go, coach! A scientifically-proven approach to coaching effectiveness* (2nd ed.). Portola Valley, CA: Warde.

Smith, R. E., Smoll, F. L., & Barnett, N. P. (1995). Reduction of children's sport performance anxiety through social support and stress-reduction training for coaches. *Journal of Applied Developmental Psychology, 16*, 125–142.

Smith, R. E., Smoll, F. L., & Christensen, D. S. (1996). Behavioral assessment and intervention in youth sports. *Behavior Modification, 20*, 3–44.

Smith, R. E., Smoll, F. L., & Cumming, S. P. (2007). Effects of a motivational climate intervention for coaches on children's sport performance anxiety. *Journal of Sport & Exercise Psychology, 29*, 39–59.

Smith, R. E., Smoll, F. L., & Cumming, S. P. (2009). Motivational climate and changes in young athletes' achievement goal orientations. *Motivation and Emotion, 33*, 173–183.

Smith, R. E., Smoll, F. L., Cumming, S. P., & DeCano, P. (2006). *Effects of the Mastery Approach to Coaching program within an African American population*. Unpublished data, University of Washington, Seattle, WA.

Smith, R. E., Smoll, F. L., Cumming, S. P., & Grossbard, J. R. (2006). Measurement of multidimensional sport performance anxiety in children and adults: The Sport Anxiety Scale-2. *Journal of Sport & Exercise Psychology, 28*, 479–501.

Smith, R. E., Smoll, F. L., & Curtis, B. (1978). Coaching behaviors in Little League Baseball. In F. L. Smoll & R. E. Smith (Eds.), *Psychological perspectives in youth sports* (pp. 173–201). Washington, DC: Hemisphere.

Smith, R. E., Smoll, F. L., & Curtis, B. (1979). Coach effectiveness training: A cognitive-behavioral approach to enhancing relationship skills in youth sport coaches. *Journal of Sport Psychology, 1*, 59–75.

Smith, R. E., Smoll, F. L., & Hunt, E. B. (1977). A system for the behavioral assessment of athletic coaches. *Research Quarterly, 48*, 401–407.

Smoll, F. L., & Cumming, S. P. (2006). Enhancing coach-parent relationships in youth sports: Increasing harmony and minimizing hassle. In J. M. Williams(Ed.), *Applied sport psychology: Personal growth to peak performance* (5th ed., pp. 192–204). Boston: McGraw-Hill.

Smoll, F. L., & Smith, R. E. (1981). Developing a healthy philosophy of winning. In V. Seefeldt, F. L. Smoll, R. E. Smith, & D. Gould(Eds.), *A winning philosophy for youth sports programs* (pp. 17–24). East Lansing, MI: Institute for the Study of Youth Sports.

Smoll, F. L., & Smith, R. E. (1989). Leadership behaviors in sport: A theoretical model and research paradigm. *Journal of Applied Social Psychology, 19*, 1522–1551.

Smoll, F. L., & Smith, R. E. (2008). *Coaches who never lose: Making sure athletes win, no matter what the score* (3rd ed.). Palo Alto, CA: Warde.

Smoll, F. L., & Smith, R. E. (Producers). (2009a). *Mastery approach to coaching: A self-instruction program for youth sport coaches [DVD]*. Seattle, WA: Youth Enrichment in Sports.

Smoll, F. L., & Smith, R. E. (2009b). *Mastery approach to coaching: A leadership guide for youth sports*. Seattle, WA: Youth Enrichment in Sports.

Smoll, F. L., & Smith, R. E. (Producers). (2009c). *Mastery approach to parenting in sports: A self-instruction program for youth sport parents [DVD]*. Seattle, WA: Youth Enrichment in Sports.

Smoll, F. L., & Smith, R. E. (2010). Conducting psychologically oriented coach-training programs: A social-cognitive approach. In J. M. Williams (Ed.), *Applied sport psychology: Personal growth to peak performance* (6th ed., pp. 392–416). Boston: McGraw-Hill.

Smoll, F. L., Smith, R. E., Barnett, N. P., & Everett, J. J. (1993). Enhancement of children's self-esteem through social support training for youth sport coaches. *Journal of Applied Psychology, 78*, 602–610.

Smoll, F. L., Smith, R. E., & Cumming, S. P. (2007a). Effects of a psychoeducational intervention for coaches on changes in child athletes' achievement goal orientations. *Journal of Clinical Sport Psychology, 1*, 23–46.

Smoll, F. L., Smith, R. E., & Cumming, S. P. (2007b). Effects of coach and parent training on performance anxiety in young athletes: A systemic approach. *Journal of Youth Development, 2*, Article 0701FA002. http://www.nae4ha.org/directory/jyd/index.htmlSummer

Sousa, C., Smith, R. E., & Cruz, J. (2008). An individualized behavioral goal-setting program for coaches: Impact on observed, athlete-perceived, and coach-perceived behaviors. *Journal of Clinical Sport Psychology, 2*, 258–277.

Swann, W. B. (1990). To be known or to be adored? The interplay of self-enhancement and self-verification. In R. M. Sorrentino & E. T. Higgins (Eds.), *Handbook of motivation and cognition: Foundations of social behavior* (Vol. 2, pp. 408–488). New York: Guilford Press.

Tashiro, T., & Mortensen, L. (2006). Translational research: How social psychology can improve psychotherapy. *American Psychologist, 61*, 959–966.

Tesser, A., & Campbell, J. (1983). Self-definition and self-evaluation maintenance. In J. Suls & A. G. Greewald (Eds.), *Psychological perspectives on the self* (Vol. 2, pp. 1–32). Hillsdale, NJ: Erlbaum.

White, M. A. (1975). Natural rates of teacher approval and disapproval in the classroom. *Journal of Applied Behavior Analysis, 8*, 367–372.

# Chapter 15
# Conclusions and Recommendations: Toward a Comprehensive Framework of Evidenced-Based Practice with Performers

**Gershon Tenenbaum and Lael Gershgoren**

In the search of laws, which govern human behavior, Skinner (1969) wrote "Science is, of course, more than a set of attitudes. It is a search for order, for uniformities, for lawful relations among the events in nature. It begins, as we begin, by observing single episodes, but it quickly passes on to the general rule, to scientific law. If we could not find some uniformity in the world, our conduct would remain haphazard and ineffective" (p. 13). Our intent in this concluding chapter is to summarize chapters in the book by identifying several salient themes that impact behavioral sport psychology assessment, intervention, and research. In doing so, we present a framework of evidence-based practice and associated recommendations that expand upon many of the suggestions offered by chapter authors.

## Measurement Issues

Research regarded as scientific must start with the smallest unit of analysis. Consequently, the initial method of searching for truth and laws in human behavior was termed *Single Subject Research* (SSR) and is also termed single case, intensive, within-subject, repeated measures, and time series experimental design (Eldar, 2005, p. 543). Martin and Thomson (Chapter 1), referring specifically to sport psychology, state that *behavioral sport psychology* relies on the principles of behavior analysis and techniques, which are aimed at enhancing performance and satisfaction. Briefly, they state that a target behavior must be articulated and then reliably measured as prerequisite to examining the efficacy of any intervention. Thus, when one seeks an evidenced-based practice, the behavior must be well defined, and the tools should measure it as reliably as possible. They then assume that the treatment or intervention follows the principles of Pavlovian and operant conditioning, and state that cognition is involved in the entire process. From a practical perspective, an intervention must be socially validated in that both coaches (and parents

---

G. Tenenbaum (✉)
Florida State University, Tallahassee, FL, USA
e-mail: gtenenbaum@fsu.edu

if necessary) and athletes must share their thoughts about meeting goals, quality of the intervention, and its consequences. To satisfy these requirements (e.g., identification of target behaviors, identification of causes to behaviors, selection of interventions, and evaluating interventions' outcomes; Martin & Pear, 2011), Martin and Thomson recommend using common inventories (or checklists) for measuring general and sport-specific inventories, which have proved to be both valid and reliable. Furthermore, these requirements can be satisfied by self-instructional manuals that can be used without the involvement of an expert, though more research is needed to test the utility and effectiveness of these sport-specific, "easy to use" measures.

Measuring overt and, especially, covert behaviors presents a major challenge to scientists and practitioners alike. Nonetheless, we propose that the *psychology of performance* must share the same accountability that the *biology and physiology of performance* do. To what degree do the measures advocated by Martin and Thomson in the first chapter of this book provide sufficient data on the performer's psychological state? How confident can the practitioner and the scientist be in the performer's response to these introspective measures? If evidenced-based practice is indeed a requirement in the application of behavioral analysis and applications, then a robust approach must be applied to the measurement component within the practice of performance psychology.

We strive to use psychological measures that provide the practitioner with reliable indicators of the performer's status in relation to his or her qualities before any intervention was applied. We wish to have a *yard-stick* that consists of three basic requirements: an *origin* (i.e., a *zero point*), a consistent *unit of measurement*, and a *linear continuum*. In the absence of these requirements, the measures we use to elicit quantities of variables such as anxiety, confidence, and goal orientation among performers pre- and post-intervention are of limited value, and, thus, their accountability is questionable at best.

An additional concern in the measurement of psychological *state testing* is the inability to measure athletes' thoughts and feelings during their performance, thus relying mainly on retrospective measures, reflections, and observations post performance. Tryon (Chapter 2) mentions devices such as touch-pads designed for swimmers or high-speed cameras for analyzing movements and decision-making, as well as counting energy expenditure. These are objective methods, which are used to operationalize *overt behaviors*. Heart rate monitors and core temperature are used as indirect measures of energy expenditure. Other measures of energy expenditure consist of drinking water laced with stable isotopes of hydrogen and oxygen, and measuring the loss of these isotopes over time from saliva, urine, or blood – a gold standard that is directly proportional to activity level. Tryon further describes pedometers and actigraphs as direct measures of energy expenditures but states, "It is important to know how much variability is associated with efforts that people make to reproduce behaviors in the same way, because this level of variability limits our ability to detect change such as improvements due to training." All instrumented measures of human activity level in applied contexts such as sports necessarily confound instrument unreliability with human biomechanical, neural, and psychological limits and will necessarily be more variable than instrument reliability suggests. It is important for trainers and athletes to repeatedly measure performances that they feel are the same and compare them with measurements of behaviors that they feel are different.

Direct measurement of critical behaviors is at the heart of single-case evaluation design according to Luiselli (see Chapter 4). Performance measures must be defined in behavior-specific terms so that they can be recorded accurately and not be influenced by observer bias. He further states, "Behaviors selected for intervention also must change in a desirable direction, with minimal variability, and at a level that is clinically significant. One of the standard guidelines when conducting a single-case evaluation design is changing only one independent variable at a time per intervention phase." He advocates using video technology to increase the reliability of the measured variable.

The assessment of cognitive processes is also a concern for Donohue, Dickens, and Del Vecchio in Chapter 5. They recommend *in vivo* assessment for better remembering cognitions that may be triggered in specific locations where a performance is expected to occur. This kind of an assessment allows an "on-going examination of cognitive restructuring exercises that are often assigned during intervention phases. When in vivo cognitive assessment is not possible, we encourage clients to bring videos of their performance to the office, and subsequently instruct them to report cognitions they remember having during key events and activities." Assessment in their view is dependent on an interview that precedes the applied measurement process. "Once the initial target cognitions are identified, we utilize behavioral observation procedures to more specifically examine how thoughts are related to actions in performance scenarios. Observations should occur in both competitive and practice settings. Structured self-monitoring exercises may assist in gaining an accurate representation of problems interfering with performance… Athletes may be instructed to record the frequency of cognitions that occur within a prescribed time frame (e.g., number of positive self-evaluation statements during a 2-h block) and setting (e.g., practice, game, team launch). Alternatively, specific thoughts and ratings of intensity can be recorded during critical points of performance. As in behavioral observation, the antecedent stimuli (e.g., being criticized) and consequences (e.g., threw ball away) of monitored thoughts should be recorded to assist in understanding etiological factors maintaining the respective cognitions. Incorporating measurement and observations are functional in that these determine which environmental stimuli and thought pattern affect behaviors in real-life situations eliciting perceptions of pressure, and possibly negative emotions, which are not necessarily facilitative. Soliciting evidence from the performer's close environment is an additional step to assure accountability."

As one can notice, behavioral researchers, practitioners, and analysts draw much attention to the measurement and assessment tools they use. No less important is the reliance on several sources of observations and the use of various methods required to elicit a reliable observation of the performer's state to ensure that the *change in behavior* is attributable to the intervention process (e.g., *true variance*) and not to measurement unreliability (e.g., *error variance*). The concern of long and short introspective measures, however, remains problematic. It is commonly believed that introspective measures must contain many items that represent the variable we intend to quantify. The psychometric literature is overloaded with procedures describing methods of reliability and validity, which are needed to produce sufficient measure. Surprisingly enough, the measures that share the highest ecological validity are *one-item scales* such as the ones designed to measure self-efficacy (Bandura, 2006), and rate of perceived exertion (RPE; Borg, 1998). Short and well-defined one-item scales have been found to be easier to use and of high predictive validity in situations where rapid changes occur, such as momentum shifts, high stakes events, and other situations and conditions performers encounter. Long introspective measures can be effective for measuring traits and dispositions. However, when one wishes to measure changes in state of either cognitive, perceptual, or emotional states, short single-item measures are preferable (see Tenenbaum, Kamata, & Hayashi, 2007, for detailed summary of this issue).

Several authors in this book have noted that behavioral analysis, which takes place during a designated time frame, must be evident through a triangulation of measures, observations, and reflections. This process is illustrated in Fig. 15.1. A practitioner starting work with an athlete or a team must first identify and diagnose the psychological and social components of interest (see Chapters 1, 2, 4, 5, 11, 12, and 14 in this book). Once these components are defined, the practitioner selects the measurement methods and tools to establish a baseline measure. More than one relevant variable is usually selected. Regardless of applying any intervention, during the practitioner's involvement with the performer/team, evidenced-based practice must be accompanied by the use of valid and reliable measures that are appropriate to the given situation. Such measures include observations (in practices and

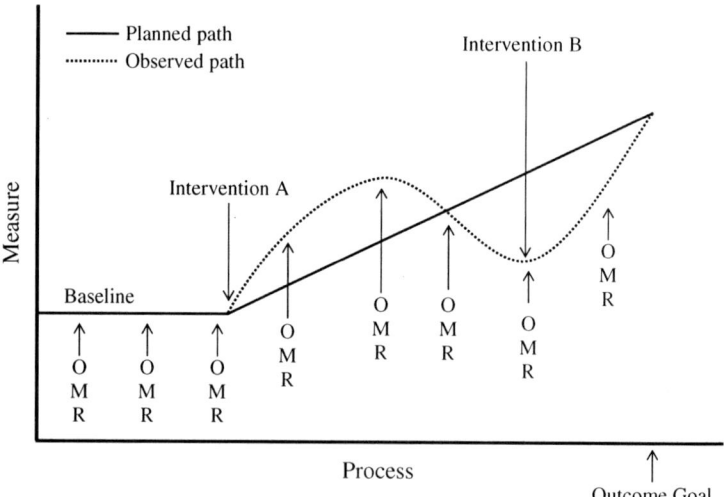

**Fig. 15.1** Observation (O), measure (M), and reflections (R) during a given time frame. Adjustment of intervention depends on the evidence gathered through O, M, and R

competitions), introspective questionnaires during competition when possible (or retrospectively while watching footage using video), and reflections, which are triggered and probed by the practitioner. Collecting relevant data through an ongoing triangulated process enables one to make needed changes and adjustments in order to achieve goals.

One should assume that the structural components of human performance, such as emotional processes (i.e., feelings, mood), cognitive processes and structures (e.g., knowledge architecture, long-term working memory), motor processes (coordination, endurance), and the neurophysiological basis of these structural components (i.e., activation of cortical areas), have been studied independently. Tenenbaum and Land (2009) postulated that

> every action made by humans is a consequence of response selection, whether intentional or unintentional. By definition, response selection indicates adaptive behavior based upon the capacity to solve problems. Cognitive processes and mental operations underlie this "behavioral effectiveness." The effectiveness of these processes consists of the richness and variety of perceptions processed at a given time; that is, the system's capacity to encode (store and represent) and access (retrieve) information relevant to the task being performed ...Under pressure, changes in each functional component may occur. These changes can affect the perceptual components, continuing with the cognitive components, and ending with the motor system ...To capture changes in the perceptual-cognitive–motor linkage under varied conditions of pressure and evoked emotions, we must use research paradigms that integrate the cognitive structure components and processes (cognitive appraisal), emotional system, and the self-regulation structure (i.e., emotional control, motivation control, attentional control, etc.) ... allowing for detection of a collapse in the perceptual-cognitive linkage under altered emotional states, and their subsequent effects on the motor system (pp. 251, 252).

Thus, an evidenced-based practice is one that captures all relevant components simultaneously – not in isolation. Interventions aimed at controlling emotions or solving problems, for example, must incorporate not only "emotional measures" but also measures of visual-perceptual behaviors, information processing, attention and anticipation, as well as measures of the motor system. These must also be observed during competition when pressure is evident and later reflected upon by the performer. A conceptual framework of each task is necessary for defining its components and observing them under varying conditions. One should keep in mind that all types of information, including emotions' primed cognition and actions, are stored in long-term memory in the form of a mental representations hierarchy (Ericsson & Kintsch, 1995). Choking under pressure, or alternatively performing optimally, depends on the extent to which appropriate neural schemas are retrieved, along with effective activation of the motor system. Evidenced-based practice must develop the tools to capture the components that are enhanced when an intervention takes place, including sensational-perceptual, cognitive, motor, or any other combination. These ideas are captured in Fig. 15.2, and further elaborated in Tenenbaum et al. (2009) and Tenenbaum and Land (2009). In a recent publication, Schack (in press) described how mental representations can be measured and how changes in these structures can indicate the efficacy of an intervention. Once this concept is applied to the behavioral analysis practice, effects of cognitive interventions such

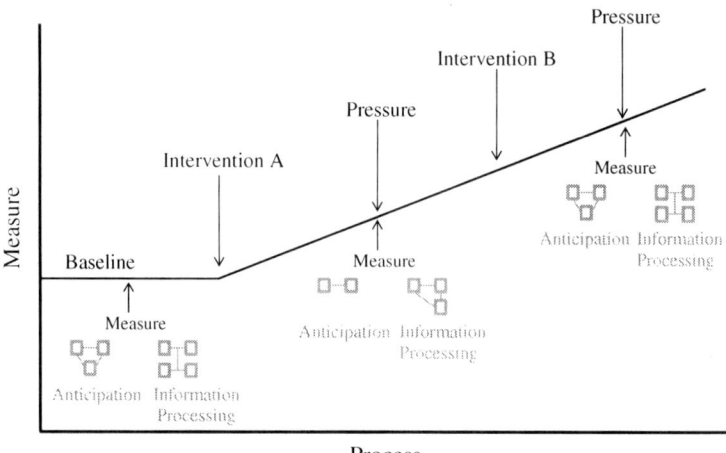

**Fig. 15.2** Baseline measures of mental-representations (i.e., mental schemas/maps) at baseline (no pressure) following intervention A (pressure causing schema impairment) and intervention B (pressure unaffecting the original schema structure)

as self-talk and imagery can be more reliably elicited in integrating *in vivo* and *enhanced-memory* techniques in practice (see Donohue, Dickens, & Del Vecchio in Chapter 5).

## An Innovative Idiographic Approach

One of the innovative ideas developed in the sport psychology domain was captured first by Hanin's (2000) conceptualization of defining the Individual Zone of Optimal Functioning. This idea was introduced several decades earlier, but was enhanced 11 years ago when not only "anxiety" but also the entire spectrum of emotions was believed to be associated with performance quality. The idea was that each individual feels and thinks in a certain manner while "in the zone" and in another manner while being out of the zone. Thus, the practitioner/performer can first define the affect-related performance under which the performer is most likely to be in or out of the zone. Once the zones are defined, an intervention strategy for securing more occurrences of the former than the later can take place. A challenge, however, is in measuring the affective variables and the performance variables, and then contrasting them each against the other to define the zone. Hanin's conceptualization is based on retrospectively recalling emotions associated with outstanding (i.e., optimal) and poor performances. The main shortcoming of this methodology is that in retrospect, emotions are very much influenced by performance outcomes and that similar emotions can be felt in all zones of functioning, and thus cannot be considered deterministically. To better define the zones of functioning, Kamata, Tenenbaum, and Hanin (2002) developed the probabilistic method for defining the

15 Conclusions and Recommendations: Toward a Comprehensive Framework... 255

Individual Affect-Related Performance (IAPZ) for each performer. It consists of measuring in real time (or while watching the performance on video, which is a more biased methodology, but in most cases unavoidable) the affective valence and intensity (using an affect grid), along with any subjective or objective measure of performance simultaneously. When repeating this process many times in one competition, and across many competitions, affect and performance measures are contrasted to each other via ordinal logistic regression. The resulting regression coefficients are then used as an input in a graphic algorithm, which defines all affect-related performance zones for each single athlete. Each functional zone is probabilistic in nature; i.e., it provides the range of the affective values associated with poor performance and its probability to occur if the performer feels within this range. Similarly, it provides the value range for moderate and optimal performance zones – all probabilistic in nature. Once the IAPZs are defined, the practitioner can draw the functional zone on a figure and then the state of the performer at each point of observation time. Such an illustration is presented in Fig. 15.3.

As one can notice, after defining the probabilistic zones' values, these values are transposed onto the $y$-axis (see Fig. 15.3). The single-affect observations are then inserted into the figure at the time they were taken, thus creating a profile where shifts among the zones are illustrated. One should keep in mind that affective state can be replaced or accompanied simultaneously by other measures of emotions, or physiological measures, such as heart rate (HR), heart rate variability (HRR), breathing pattern (frequency and depth), galvanic skin response (GSR), EEG measures, and others. As illustrated in Fig. 15.3, the ideal state would be when the performer shows consistent behavior and stays in the optimal zone. However, the illustrated performer showed intense arousal at the outset of the competition,

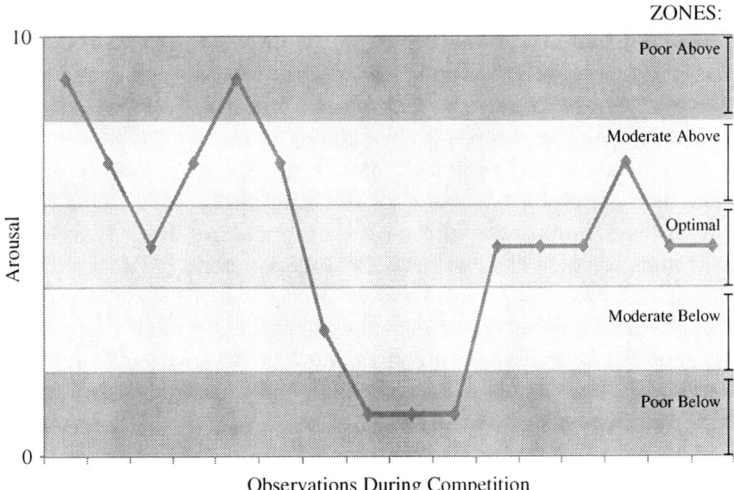

**Fig. 15.3** An observational profile of a single performer in competition: Fluctuations among individual affect-related performance zones (IAPZs)

which placed him/her above the optimal zone of functioning; he/she returned to the optimal zone and then continued to fluctuate among the high and moderate zones above and below the optimal zone until achieving a relatively stable state within the optimal zone. As the practitioner and the performer watch the competition on a video, the practitioner may stop the film at each of the observation points and ask the performer to reflect upon his feelings and thoughts in detail at this point. When many reflections are gathered, some generalizations about the affective states and performance can be made and linked into the environmental and social conditions. In this way, when one designs an intervention, such a method can provide platforms for detecting difficulties or successes in the implementation of the intervention and enables modifications and changes in the intervention to be made. The practitioner who wishes to systematically collect evidence of the intervention implemented, whether it is through goal setting and performance feedback (see Ward in Chapter 6), cognitive–behavioral strategies (see Brown in Chapter 7), detecting behavioral markers of momentum shift (see Roane in Chapter 9), or examination of fluency, efficiency, and automaticity of performance under pressure and evoked emotions (see Martens & Collier in Chapter 10), is encouraged to integrate the IAPZ method into the intervention paradigm so that a clear picture of what intervention outcomes and process will emerge.

## Using the Idiosyncratic Probabilistic Approach

Several practitioners and scholars have used the IAPZ idiosyncratic concept in both research projects and practice using introspective and physiological measures of arousal and defining the IAPZs of the performer. We briefly describe their work below, according to sport type.

*Golf.* Van der Lei (2010) implemented a multimodal assessment approach in which the probabilistic relationship between affective states and both performance process and outcome measures was determined. Three male golfers of a varsity team were observed during three rounds of competition. Introspective (i.e., verbal reports) and objective (heart rate and respiration rate) measures of arousal were incorporated to examine the relationships between arousal states and process components (i.e., routine consistency, timing) and outcome scores related to golf performance in competition. Results revealed distinguishable and idiosyncratic IAPZs associated with physiological and introspective measures for each golfer. The associations between the IAPZs and decision-making or swing/stroke execution were strong and unique for each golfer. While observing the golfers, Van Der Lei uncovered two pre-routine time phases (e.g., *information processing* and *confirmation*) and two post-routine time phase (*evaluation* and *reorientation*). Comparison of the temporal patterns associated with the four functional time phases indicated more consistent time use by the golfers during the confirmation and evaluation phases immediately preceding and following the task execution (i.e., swing or stroke), respectively, compared to the information-processing phase and the reorientation phase preceding and ensuing the task execution (i.e., swing or stroke), respectively. Consequently, an hourglass performance (HP) model for golf was developed to illustrate the relationship between a golfer's information-processing pattern and the functional performance phases in golf.

Cohen, Tenenbaum, and English (2006) applied the probabilistic approach in a study involving female collegiate golfers. They were interested in defining the relationship between two dimensions of affect (i.e., arousal level and pleasantness) and functionality (i.e., how helpful the affective state was to performance) in relation to objective and perceived performance levels. In addition, they examined how perceived affect and golf performance change following a psychological skills training (PST) intervention. Cohen et al. (2006) utilized a multiple case study format to identify and refine individual IAPZs for the participants. The profiles and assessment of psychological strategies employed during practice and competition were used to develop a brief PST intervention. The PST intervention targeted the psychological and emotional strategies of self-talk, emotional control, imagery, relaxation, activation, resistance to disruption, negative thinking, attention control, and automaticity. Results indicated that the IAPZ concept was supported via probabilistic estimations in that varying levels of affect were associated with different levels of performance within and between the participants (i.e., each participant maintained unique and idiosyncratic IAPZs). Additionally, the PST intervention resulted in the participants' attainment of optimal affective states via psychological and emotional self-regulation strategies, which ultimately led to improved performance.

*Race-car simulation.* Edmonds, Mann, Tenenbaum, and Janelle (2006) conducted an exploratory investigation of the IAPZ model by integrating perceived affective states (i.e., arousal, pleasantness) and physiological measures of arousal (i.e., heart rate and skin resistance) online in a competitive driving simulator. Participants in the study were given the same race settings on the race simulator and were required to drive a total of five race trials (i.e., one trial equaled four laps), with the main goal to reach the finish line as fast as possible. Participants completed all four laps of each trial in succession; however, between trials they were able to take a 3-min break. Indicators of heart rate and skin conductance were taken simultaneously with the perceived measures of arousal pleasantness at three different stages of a lap. Results indicated that athletes maintained idiosyncratic performance zones. The distinct IAPZ profiles linking arousal and performance that were revealed in the driving simulation are also indicative of relative changes in driver performance, which were indexed by changes in physiological parameters. Furthermore, a driver's performance could be determined by the driver's level of arousal or activation.

Edmonds, Tenenbaum, Mann, Johnson, and Kamata (2008) used the IAPZ probabilistic method to verify the utility and effectiveness of a biofeedback intervention by manipulating affective performance states in a race-car simulator. Nine males completed five separate time trials of a simulated racing task and were then randomly assigned to one of three arousal regulation treatment conditions: (1) optimal, (2) poor, and (3) attention control. Following the biofeedback intervention, participants underwent another series of race trials to determine the effectiveness of the arousal regulation intervention. The results indicated relative similarities in the strength and direction of the perceived and physiological states between the participants; however, the subtle details of the participants' unique performance zones and the probability of achieving each zone were revealed to be unique among the participants. The results also indicated that the biofeedback manipulation resulted in the expected changes for each participant, though some large individual differences among them were noted.

*Tennis.* Golden, Tenenbaum, and Kamata (2004) conducted a study utilizing the probabilistic approach with collegiate female tennis players. They established IAPZs for each player across an entire season of tennis. Additionally, throughout the season after each match, they administered positive–negative affect scales (PNA; Hanin, 2000) and flow state scales (FSS; Jackson & Marsh, 1996). Results revealed that the IAPZs for each athlete were unique and distinct. In addition, they found that when the athletes were performing at optimal or near-optimal levels, they were experiencing elevated levels of flow. The results from the PNA revealed that during optimal performances, pleasant emotions perceived to be helpful were most prevalent. However, during moderate and poor performances, unpleasant emotions perceived to be harmful became elevated.

Johnson, Edmonds, Tenenbaum, and Kamata (2007) extended the examination of the IZOF model by utilizing the IAPZ model to determine IAPZs in male collegiate tennis players. They observed the athletes across an entire season and found that the linkage between affect and performance was of a dynamic nature, where affect level during competition has an effect on performance, though this effect is unique for each player. The athletes in the study demonstrated distinguishable and unique IAPZs for the two affect dimensions (e.g., arousal and pleasantness) and functionality (e.g., how do affect and pleasantness are functional for the performance). This research is in line with Hanin's (2000) IZOF model, which is built upon the pillar that the affect–performance linkage is unique to each individual.

*Archery.* Johnson, Edmonds, Moraes, Filho, and Tenenbaum (2007) used the probabilistic IAPZ method to explore the dynamic nature of within-competition perceived affect-performance and heart-rate performance linkage in one world-class archer. Multiple competitions at five different shooting distances (18, 30, 50, 60, and 70 m) were observed throughout the entire competitive international season. The findings illustrated the archer's unique IAPZs at each shooting distance. Furthermore, affective state fluctuations were noticed among the IAPZs during competition, which necessitated the utilization of different self-regulatory methods when these were noticed by the archer.

Filho, Moraes, and Tenenbaum (2008) applied the IAPZ method for studying the link between affective states and athletic performance for the purpose of determining graphic profiles associated with optimal and nonoptimal performance in three Brazilian male archers. Data were collected throughout a whole competitive season during competitions at different shooting distances. The archers reported their perceptions of arousal and pleasure and had their heart rate responses recorded. Results indicated that (a) the archers possess unique IAPZs for the different archery shooting distances, (b) they fluctuated among their optimal and nonoptimal IAPZs throughout the season, and (c) a consecutive optimal performance was not prevalent following an initial optimal performance.

*Tutorial on IAPZ.* Practitioners and researchers interested in the use of the IAPZ method are encouraged to read the development of the theoretical and mathematical components of it in Kamata et al. (2002). However, a clear and easy-to-read and -capture tutorial of the IAPZ method can be found in the article of Johnson, Edmonds, Tenenbaum, and Kamata (2009). The methodology described in this tutorial consists of eight steps: (a) collecting data, (b) categorizing affect and performance level, (c) converting the data, (d) performing logistical ordinal regressions, (e) creating IAPZ curves, (f) creating IAPZ profile charts, (g) plotting within competition states onto IAPZ profile charts, and (h) utilizing IAPZs to select, implement, and evaluate performance enhancement strategies.

## Linking the IAPZ to the Individual Psychological Crisis Theory

In a recent publication Tenenbaum, Edmonds, and Eccles (2008) linked the IAPZ to the Individual Psychological Crisis Theory (IPCT; Bar-Eli & Tenenbaum, 1989), which is congruent with the concepts of behavioral analysis and evidenced-based practice. The IPCT views the athlete as a dynamic and open system that responds to environmental stimuli with certain probability levels. The athlete continuously processes information and makes decisions (DM) aimed at maximal adaptation to the environmental conditions via the reduction of event uncertainty. Physiological arousal is viewed as the energizing component of motivation, with the cognitive component providing its direction. Their relationship is viewed within a bilateral transaction process (Nitsch, 1982). Physiological arousal may be unaffected by cognitive directional mechanisms or, alternatively, controlled or regulated by them. Continuous exposure to similar situations and conditions shifts the operational mode of the system from intentional to an automated mode. According to Nitsch, automaticity via the adaptation process reduces the vulnerability of the system to "choking" under pressure and/or uncertainty. Therefore, performance expertise may be determined through the extent to which an athlete has assimilated and accommodated the arousal-coping strategies, which are linked through exposure to practice and competition. In this respect, the acquisition of expertise in an anxiety-provoking setting requires deliberate practice under conditions of high arousal and uncertainty. The extent to which vulnerability to crisis depends on experience and expertise level is related to the quality and quantity of cognitive mechanisms available to cope with the emotional state of the athlete, the level of attained simplification and routine of relevant responses, and the point of balance between damaging and contributing effects resulting from the emotional state of the athlete.

The IPCT was the first theoretical concept to describe the emotion–performance relationship in a probabilistic nature and a continuous time frame. In other words, when a performer is in a given stressful situation, experiences high pressure and anxiety, cannot pay attention to the task, and lacks self-regulatory mechanisms to reduce pressure, it is highly probable that he/she will choke or face a significant performance decline. Though the IPTC referred merely to arousal/activation levels of the athlete at a certain time point during competition, other emotions have similar relevance in the emotion–performance linkage. Relying on the classical inverted "U" function, the athlete was considered to be in a phase of hypoactivation, optimum activation, or hyperactivation at any moment in time. The probability of a psychological crisis occurring increases as the individual shifts away from the optimal state toward the hypo- or hyperactivation states. However, these can be determined by the IAPZ concept, as a descriptive method, the changes in cognitive schema (Schack, in press), and the classical behavior analysis methods advocated in this book.

## Additional Thoughts

We believe that the IAPZ method and the IPCT conceptual framework, along with the concept of triangulation of measures, provide a sound framework for practitioners who work with performers. An important issue, which was not addressed in this chapter, is the quality and soundness of the interventions practitioners use to enhance the mental, cognitive, and emotional states of the performer. Interventions must share theoretical, scientific, and empirical soundness as one expects from measures used to quantify feelings, states, thoughts, and disposition. The scientist is eager to explore the underlying mechanism of a phenomenon under investigation. Medical interventions, for example, cannot be implemented without being able to explain *how* and *what* changes have occurred in the biological and/or mental states of the patient. Interventions with performers are aimed at changing a mental, behavioral, emotional, or motor status quo, or alternatively maintaining a desired state to secure high-level performance, a state that will allow mental schemas to remain intact and retrievable. Consistent monitoring of outcome and process behaviors inherent in behavioral analysis is an important measure toward establishing an evidenced-based intervention.

One of the most paramount approaches to the design of evidenced-based intervention is presented in Chapter 14 by Smith and Smoll. In the outset of their chapter, Smith and Smoll write, "In this chapter, we describe the evolution of a program of research on coaching behaviors and interventions that has spanned more than three decades and has resulted in an empirically-supported coach training program. We describe the manner in which a theoretical model derived from the areas of learning, social and personality psychology, and developmental psychology has helped guide a program of basic and applied research. Research results derived from the basic and applied research have guided the intervention program's development, and research results from basic research and program evaluations address important theoretical issues." The approach Smith and Smoll have taken is based on an integrated theoretical framework, which they used for designing measures and interventions. However, they believed that without first designing reliable and valid measurement tools, they would have been unable to validate or refine their theoretical framework. Each tool that was developed underwent a rigorous process of experimentation using large samples of young athletes and coaches. Only at this stage they concluded, "Data from our basic research indicated clear relations between coaching behaviors and the reactions of youngsters to their athletic experience. Along with findings from research inspired by achievement goal theory, these relations provided a foundation for developing a set of coaching guidelines that formed the basis for an intervention that was initially called Coach Effectiveness Training. With the later emergence of achievement goal theory and the wealth of research it inspired, we incorporated its principles into an evolved program called the Mastery Approach to Coaching (MAC) that explicitly focuses on the development of a mastery motivational climate. This emphasis is highly consistent with principles (particularly our conception of success as doing one's best and striving to maximize one's potential) that have been emphasized in CET from the beginning." When this stage was accomplished, an extensive outcome research was planned and performed to refine all aspect of the interventions design for coach education. Since then, 500 CET and MAC workshops have been provided to more than 25,000 coaches.

There is no doubt that three decades of experimentation, practice, and development of a sound intervention is a life-long job of the scientist-practitioner who wishes to be accountable and helpful to performers. It is not always the desire of the practitioner who must provide immediate and reliable intervention to a performer or a team. However, the practitioner should have in mind that both the interventions and the measurement tools he/she uses must be related to a sound theoretical framework that was proven to be accountable and reliable. He or she must also follow a scientific reasoning when implementing interventions and measuring overt and covert behaviors. We attempted to introduce such a framework in this concluding chapter.

## References

Bandura, A. (2006). Guide for creating self-efficacy scales. In F. Pajares & T. Urdan (Eds.), *Self-efficacy beliefs of adolescents* (pp. 307–337). Greenwich, CT: Information Age Publishing.

Bar-Eli, M., & Tenenbaum, G. (1989). A theory of individual psychological crisis in competitive sport. *Applied Psychology, 38,* 107–120.

Borg, G. (1998). *Borg's perceived exertion and pain scales*. Champaign, IL: Human Kinetics.

Cohen, A. B., Tenenbaum, G., & English, R. W. (2006). Emotions and golf performance: An IZOF-based applied sport psychology case study. *Behavior Modification, 30,* 259–280.

Edmonds, W. A., Mann, D. T. Y., Tenenbaum, G., & Janelle, C. M. (2006). Analysis of affect-related performance zones: An idiographic approach using physiological and introspective data. *The Sport Psychologist, 20,* 40–57.

Edmonds, W. A., Tenenbaum, G., Mann, D. T. Y., Johnson, M., & Kamata, A. (2008). The effect of biofeedback training on affective regulation and simulated car-racing performance: An experimental study. *Journal of Sport Sciences, 26,* 761–773.

Eldar, E. (2005). Single subject research: Roots, rational and methodology. In G. Tenenbaum & M. P. Driscoll (Eds.), *Methods of research in sport sciences: Quantitative and qualitative approaches* (pp. 543–573). Oxford: Meyer & Meyer Sport.

Ericsson, K. A., & Kintsch, W. (1995). Long-term working memory. *Psychological Review, 102,* 211–245.

Filho, E. S. M., Moraes, L. C., & Tenenbaum, G. (2008). Affective and physiological states during archery competition: Adapting and enhancing the method of performance zones. *Journal of Applied Sport Psychology, 20*, 441–456.

Golden, A., Tenenbaum, G., & Kamata, A. (2004). Performance zones: Affect-related performance zones: An idiographic method linking affect to performance. *International Journal of Sport and Exercise Psychology, 2*, 24–42.

Hanin, Y. L. (2000). *Emotions in sport*. Champaign, IL: Human Kinetics.

Jackson, S. A., & Marsh, H. W. (1996). Development and validation of a scale to measure optimal experience: The flow state scale. *Journal of Sport and Exercise Psychology, 18*, 17–35.

Johnson, M. B., Edmonds, W. A., Moraes, L. C., Medeiros-Filho, E. S., & Tenenbaum, G. (2007). Linking affect and performance of an international level archer incorporating an idiosyncratic probabilistic method. *Psychology of Sport and Exercise, 8*, 317–335.

Johnson, M., Edmonds, W. A., Tenenbaum, G., & Kamata, A. (2007). The relationship between affect and performance in competitive intercollegiate tennis: A dynamic conceptualization and applications. *Journal of Clinical Sport Psychology, 1*, 130–146.

Johnson, M. B., Edmonds, W. A., Tenenbaum, G., & Kamata, A. (2009). Determining individual affect-related performance zones (IAPZs): A tutorial. *Journal of Clinical Sport Psychology, 3*, 34–57.

Kamata, A., Tenenbaum, G., & Hanin, Y. (2002). Individual zone of optimal functioning (IZOF): A probabilistic conceptualisation. *Journal of Sport and Exercise Psychology, 24*, 189–208.

Martin, G. L., & Pear, J. J. (2011). *Behavior modification: What it is and how to do it* (9th ed.). Upper Saddle River, NJ: Pearson-Prentice Hall.

Nitsch, J. R. (1982). Handlungspschologische snsaetze im sport. In A. Thomas (Ed.), *Sportpsychologie: Ein handbuch in schluesselbergiffen* (pp. 26–41). Munchen: Urban & Schwazenberg.

Schack, T. (in press). Mental representation of motor action. In G. Tenenbaum, R. C. Eklund, & A. Kamata (Eds.), *Handbook of measurement in sport and exercise psychology*. Champaign, IL: Human Kinetics.

Skinner, B. F. (1969). *Contingencies of reinforcement: A theoretical analysis*. New York: Appelton-Cantury-Crofts.

Tenenbaum, G., Edmonds, W. A., & Eccles, D. (2008). Emotions, coping strategies, and performance: A conceptual framework for defining affect-related performance zones. *Journal of Military Psychology, 20*, 11–37.

Tenenbaum, G., Hatfield, B., Eklund, R. C., Land, W., Camielo, L., Razon, S., et al. (2009). Conceptual framework for studying emotions-cognitions-performance linkage under conditions which vary in perceived pressure. In M. Raab, J. G. Johnson, & H. Heekeren (Eds.), *Progress in brain research: Mind and motion-the bidirectional link between thought and action* (pp. 159–178). Amsterdam, Nederland: Elsevier Publication.

Tenenbaum, G., Kamata, A., & Hayashi, K. (2007). Measurement in sport and exercise psychology: A new outlook on selected issues of reliability and validity. In G. Tenenbaum & R. C. Eklund (Eds.), *Handbook of sport psychology* (3rd ed., pp. 757–773). Hoboken, NJ: Wiley.

Tenenbaum, G., & Land, W. M. (2009). Mental representations as an underlying mechanism for human performance. In M. Raab, J. G. Johnson, & H. Heekeren (Eds.), *Progress in brain research: Mind and motion-the bidirectional link between thought and action* (pp. 251–266). Amsterdam, Nederland: Elsevier Publication.

Van der Lei, H. (2010). Applied psychophysiology research in the study of affect-performance relationship in sport. Unpublished doctoral Dissertation. Florida State University, USA.

# Index

Note: Letters 'f' and 't' following the locators refers to figures and tables cited in the text.

**A**
AAN, *see* American Academy of Neurology (AAN)
AASP, *see* Association for Applied Sport Psychology (AASP)
ABA, *see* Applied behavior analysis (ABA)
A-B-A-B design, 65–68
    A-B-A-B-B+C-A-B+C design, 66f
    A-B+C-A-B+C-B-A-B design, 66f
    hypothetical data, 65f
    one-day reversal effect, 67f
    research examples, 67–68
ABC model, 89
Acceleration-deceleration force, 180, 184
Achievement Goal Scale for Youth Sports (AGSYS), 241, 243
Acrophase, 39
Across-sport behavioral checklist
    athletic coping skills inventory-28, 15
    post-competition evaluation form, 15
    psychological skills inventory for sport, 15
ACSM, *see* The American College of Sports Medicine (ACSM)
Actigraphs
    advantages
        proportionality, 37
        time-locked repeated measurements, 37
    circadian applications, 38–39
    diurnal activity, 39–40
    sleep, importance, 37–38
    sleep, improvement, 39
    vendors and devices, 28t–29t
Actigraphy
    application to sports, 34–40
        actigraphs, 37–40
        pedometers, 34–37
    human activity, measurement, 25–34
        direct methods, 26–30
        indirect methods, 25–26
        methodological issues, 30–34
ActiTrainer Solution Package, 39
A/D, *see* Analog-to-digital (A/D) converters
Aggressive behavior
    conceptual and operational criteria of, 203
    self report, athlete, 204–205
    *See also* Direct observation method; Methodologies, sport-specific aggression; Prevention-based intervention
Alternating treatments design (ATD), 75–77, 76f
    behavior-altering effect, 75
    research examples, 76
American Academy of Neurology (AAN), 179
The American Academy of Sleep Medicine, 37
The American College of Sports Medicine (ACSM), 35
Amyotrophic lateral sclerosis, 191
Analog-to-digital (A/D) converters, 30
Analysis of variance (ANOVA), 31, 62
ANAM, *see* Automated Neuropsychological Assessment Metrics (ANAM)
ANOVA, *see* Analysis of variance (ANOVA)
APoE-e4 allele, 189
Application, major areas, 8–16
    athletes, decreasing problem behaviors, 10–11
    athletic performance, managing emotions, 11–12
    confidence and concentration, maximizing, 14–15
    decreasing persistent errors, 10
    motivating practice and fitness training, 8–9

Application, major areas (*cont.*)
   new sport skills, 9–10
   self-talk/imagery training, 12–14
   user-friendly behavioral assessment tools, development, 15–16
   user-friendly sport psychology manuals, development, 16
Applied behavior analysis (ABA), 7–8, 106
Archery, 258
Archival methodology, 201–202
Arena Football League, 50
Arousal management, 81–82
   anxiety and self-confidence, relation, 82
   influencing factors, 81
   optimum, 82
Association for Applied Sport Psychology (AASP), 8, 77, 117
ATD, *see* Alternating treatments design (ATD)
Athlete
   cognitive–behavioral attitudes, 239–240
   coping skills inventory-28, 15
   self report, 204–205
   decreasing problem behaviors, 10–11
   interaction, coach, 228
   perceived behavioral ratings, 239
   performance managing emotions, 11–12
   self-esteem, 234–235
   *See also* ABC model; Prevention-based intervention; Proficiency techniques
Athlete-perceived behavioral ratings, 239
Athletic Achievement Motivation Scale, 86
Athleticism, 115
Attitudes
   help follow-through, 83
   help-seeking, 83
Attrition, 242–243
Autocorrelation, 31
Automated Neuropsychological Assessment Metrics (ANAM), 188
Automatic repertoires
   in changing situations, 159
   neuromuscular adaptations, 168
   stretching or flexibility training, 171–172
   *See also* Deliberate practice; Muscular adaptations

# B

Bag of tricks mentality, 119
*The Baseball Economist: The Real Game Exposed*, 45
*Baseball Is Played All Wrong*, 44
Baseline assessment model, 185
Basic research on coaching behaviors
   behavioral signatures, 230–231
   coaching behaviors, measurement
     behavioral assessment techniques, 229
   coaching behaviors and children's evaluative reactions, 231
   situational and personality moderators of behavior–attitude relations
     game situation, 232–233
     motivational climate, 233–234
   theoretical underpinnings
     athlete self-esteem, 234–235
     coach–athlete interactions, 228
     cognitive revolution, 228
Basic science, 227
BDNF, *see* Brain-derived neurotrophic growth factor (BDNF)
Behavioral coaching intervention
   imitation, 67
   modeling, 67
   performance feedback, 67
   positive and negative reinforcement, 67
   systematic verbal instructions, 67
Behavioral goal, 121, 135, 239
Behavioral momentum
   metaphor extension to other sports, 151–154
     coaching tactics, 153
     reinforcement rates, 152
   momentum and behavior analysis, 146–147
     evaluation, 146
     low-probability *vs.* high-probability tasks, 147
     metaphorical application, 146
   previous research, 147–151
     commencing events, 148
     conceptualization, 148
     data analysis procedure, 150
     data collection, 148–149
   property, application, 143
   psychological aspects, 144–146
     complex models, 145
     conceptualization and quantification, 145
     multidimensional definitions, 144–145
   technical application, 144
Behavioral momentum principle, 53
Behavioral observation
   intent to harm, 204–205
   role, in prevention based intervention, 206–208
   *See also* Direct observation method
Behavior-altering effect, 75

Behavior-reduction measure, 62
Between-group statistical analyses, 62
BMI, *see* Body mass index (BMI)
Body mass index (BMI), 35–36
Brain-derived neurotrophic growth factor (BDNF), 128
Bredemeier Athletic Aggression Inventory (BAAGI), 200
BuzzBee™ actigraph, 33

C

Calling a time-out strategy, 149, 151–153
*The Canadian Society for Psychomotor Learning and Sport Psychology*, 3
CDC, *see* The Center for Disease Control (CDC)
The Center for Disease Control (CDC), 129, 181, 192–193
Cerebral concussion
  epidemiology, 181–185
    acute effect of history, 183–184
    animals *vs.* humans, 184
    gender, 182–183
    head injury, emergency room admissions, 182t
    physical forces, 184–185
    soccer players *vs.* football players, 182
CET and MAC workshops in U. S and Canada, 243
CET/MAC intervention, 238–239, 242–243
CG, *see* Control group (CG)
Changing criterion design, 73–75
  hypothetical data, 74f
  research examples, 74–75
  rewarding, 75
Chronic traumatic encephalopathy (CTE), 191
Church-based health-promotion intervention, 131
CINAHL, 36
Clinical repeatability, 33–34
Coach effectiveness training, 236, 261
Coaches
  good behavior contracts, 206–207
Coaching Behavior Assessment System (CBAS), 229–231, 238–239
Cochrane Library, 36
Coefficient of variation (CV), 32
Cognitive assessment
  common factors affecting, 79–83
    *See also individual entries*
  empirically guided method, description, 83–91
    ABC models for use in athletes, 89t

behavioral observation, 87–88
cognition, frequency recording, 89
collateral informants, 83–84
functional assessment and analysis, 89–90
functional hypotheses, testing, 90–91
observational effects, 88
psychometrically validated scales, 84–87
SARI sample items, 86t
self-monitoring, 88–89
setting, 83
SIC sample items, 85t
familial relationships, 82
primary focus, 82
Cognitive–behavioral coach training
  basic research on coaching behaviors
    coaching behaviors, measurement, 229–231
    coaching behaviors and children's evaluative reactions, 231
    situational and personality moderators of behavior–attitude relations, 232–235
    theoretical underpinnings, 228–229
  outcome research
    achievement goal orientation, 240–241
    athlete attitudes, 239–240
    coaching behaviors, 238–239
    dropout rate, 242–243
    performance anxiety, 241–242
    self-esteem, 240
  translating basic research findings into coach intervention
    Coach Effectiveness Training, 236
    MAC principles and goals, 236–238
    "positive approach" to coaching, 236–237
Cognitive–behavioral strategies
  alliance building, 115–117
    clients and their language, relation, 116
    and sport psychology, brief history, 116–117
  behavioral interventions, 120
  development, 117
  evidenced-based self-talk, 122–123
  goal setting, 120–122
  imagery, 123–124
  psychological advice, 114–115
    session with college football player, 114
    use by athletes, 115t
  theory and athlete, protection, 117–120
    myth 1: collection of tricks, 118

Cognitive–behavioral strategies (cont.)
  myth 2: immediate effects, 118
  myth 3: physical training, comparison, 118–119
  myth 4: psychopathological conditions, 119
  myth 5: competent professional, 119–120
Cognitive–behavior therapy, 7
Cognitive processes
  experimentation, 118
  practice, 118
  restructuring, 118
  self-monitoring, 118
Cognitive processes, assessment, 251
Cognitive tracking assignment, 88
CogSport, 188
Collision frequency, 181
Community-based program, 135
Competitive State Anxiety Inventory-2, 87
CompuSports©, 56
Computed tomography (CT), 180
Computerized neurocognitive screening measure, 186
Computer simulation model, 184
Concentration, 12, 14–15, 17, 87, 171–172, 188, 215–216, 221, 223, 242
Concussion Resolution Index (CRI), 188
Conditioned seeing, 13
Confidence, 14–17, 34, 36–37, 81, 84, 87, 124, 250
Congruence method, 88
Consumer-driven evidence-based care, 91
Contact sports, 143
Contingent musical reinforcement, 109
Control group (CG), 38, 128, 136, 185, 240–241
Control theory (CT)
  hierarchical organization, 132
  key intervention components
    feedback, 132
    goal review, 132
    goal setting, 132
    self-monitoring, 132
  loop functions, 132
  meta-regression, 133
Cook-book methodology, 119
Coping Inventory for Sport, 87
Core body temperature, 26
Covert behaviors, 4, 7, 250, 261
CPSC, see The United States Consumer Product Safety Commission (CPSC)
CRI, see Concussion Resolution Index (CRI)
Criterion, 73
Cronbach's alpha, 32
Cross-fit programs, 171
40 CSA Model 7164 actigraph, 33
CT, see Computed tomography (CT); Control theory (CT)
CTE, see Chronic traumatic encephalopathy (CTE)
CV, see Coefficient of variation (CV)

**D**

Deceptive advertising practices, 211
Delayed onset muscle soreness (DOMS), 171
Deliberate practice
  goals, 161–165
  physiological concepts, 168
  as proficiency technique, 167–168
  RESAA, benefits of, 163–164
  strategies, 160
  See also Proficiency techniques
Department of Health and Human Services, 129
Descriptive and verbal feedback (DF + VF), 72
Descriptive (nonverbal) feedback (DF), 72
Desire for Sport Psychology Scale (DSPS), 84
*The Developmental and Control of Behavior in Sport and Physical Education*, 3
Dietary and nutritional supplements, 213–214
Dietary Supplement and Nonprescription Drug Consumer Protection Act, 212
Dietary Supplement Health and Education Act of 1994 (DSHEA), 212–213
Dietary supplements, effects, 212
Difficult-to-complete instruction, 147
Digital step counters, 26–28
Direct observation method
  acquisition of, aggressive behavior, 205–206
  advantages of, 203–204, 206
  as data collection tool, 205
  multiple coders, 203
  rule violation, athletes, 208
  socialization process in, 205–206
  validity measurement, 202–204
  videotape, using of, 203
Disengagement-oriented coping, 87
Dispositional Flow Scale, 87
Distraction-oriented coping, 87
Dose–response effect, 128
Doubly labeled water, 26
DSPS, see Desire for Sport Psychology Scale (DSPS)

# Index

## E

Early development, 3–4
Easy-Scout XP Plus©, 56
Easy-Scout XP Professional©, 56
Ecological validity, 102, 105, 200–201, 204
Electrophysiological technique, 180
EMBASE, 36
Enhanced-memory techniques, 254
Environmental–behavioral relations, 46
ERIC, 36
Error variance, 251
Estrogen, 183, 223
ETG, *see* Evening training group (ETG)
Evening training group (ETG), 38
Evidenced-based practice with performers
   additional thoughts, 260–261
   Innovative Idiographic Approach, 254–256
   linking IAPZ to Individual Psychological Crisis Theory, 259–260
   measurement issues, 249–254
   using the Idiosyncratic Probabilistic Approach, 256–259
Evidenced-based self-talk
   cognitive errors, 123
   intervention and discussion, 122–123
   sample self-talk log, 123t
   vignette, 122
   *See also* Cognitive–behavioral strategies
Exercise induced muscular damage (EIMD), 222
Exogenous *vs.* endogenous estrogen, 183
External validity, 63

## F

Fact-to-face intervention, 136
Fear of failure (FF), 87, 236
*The Feeling Good Handbook*, 123
FF, *see* Fear of failure (FF)
Flow state scale (FSS), 87, 258
fMRI, *see* Functional MRI (fMRI)
Force–mass relationship, 183
Form training intervention, 70
Four-step strategy, 12
Freeze strategy, 106
FSS, *see* Flow state scale (FSS)
Functional MRI (fMRI), 180
Function-based behavior, 101

## G

Gadd Severity Index, 184
Gender-discrepant incidence, 183
Goal-directed activity, 127
Goal setting
   behavior, consequences, 102–103
   combined with performance feedback, 103
   commitment, gaining, 104
   definition, 99–105
      evidenced-based principles, 101–103
      interventions principles without direct assessment, 103–105
      presentation statements, 100
   definition from psychologist, 120
   intervention and discussion, 121–122
      brief interchange, example, 121
      two-question test, 121
   literature examination, 100–101
   public goals *vs.* private goals, 103–104
   as a rule, 100
   single-subject design studies, 102
   types
      behavioral, 121
      outcome, 121
      performance, 121
   vignette, 120
   *See also* Cognitive–behavioral strategies
Gold standard criterion, 38
GraphPad Prism®, 57
GT3X model, 39–40

## H

Hands-on method, 83
Hanin's conceptualization, 254
Head Injury Criterion (HIC), 184–185
Heart rate, 26
Heel-toe transition, 26
HIC, *see* Head Injury Criterion (HIC)
Hourglass performance (HP) model, 257
Human performance, structural components, 253
Human physique changes, 118

## I

IAPZ, *see* Individual Affect-Related Performance (IAPZ)
IAPZ fluctuations, 255f
IBM SPSS Statistics Base®, 57
Idiosyncratic Probabilistic Approach, 256–259
Imagery, 81
   controllability, 124
   facilitating factors, 81
   intervention and discussion, 124
   kinesthetic movement, 81
   positive experiences, 81
   vignette, 124
   vividness, 123

Immediate Measurement of Performance and Cognitive Testing (ImPACT), 188
ImPACT, see Immediate Measurement of Performance and Cognitive Testing (ImPACT)
Individual Affect-Related Performance (IAPZ), 255–260
Individual-player basis, 152
Individual Psychological Crisis Theory (IPCT), 259–260
Individual Zone of Optimal Functioning, 254
In-game performance, 72
Injuiries, classification
   grade I (mild), 179
   grade II (moderate), 179
   grade III (severe), 179
Innovative delivery mechanism, 136
   behavior change principles, 136
Innovative Idiographic Approach, 254–256
Instrument reliability, 31–33
Instrument validity, 34
Interdisciplinary cybernetic control theory, 132
Internal validity, 63
The *International Society of Sport Psychology*, 3
Intervention techniques, 73
Inverted-U relationship, 12
IPCT, see Individual Psychological Crisis Theory (IPCT)
iPod Touch™, 137
Irritable bowel syndrome, 119
IZOF model, 258

**J**
*Journal of Applied Behavior Analysis*, 3, 77
*Journal of Clinical Sport Psychology*, 77
*Journal of Quantitative Analysis in Sports*, 45
*Journal of Sport Behavior*, 77
Judgments About Moral Behavior in Youth Sport Questionnaire (JAMBYSQ), 200
JW200 pedometer engine, 33

**K**
KS10 pedometer engine, 33

**L**
Large N method, 61
LOC, see Loss of consciousness (LOC)
*Los Angeles Times*, 191
Loss of consciousness (LOC), 179, 189–190
Low-effort inexpensive intervention, 134–135
Lower-order goal, 132

**M**
MAC, see Mastery Approach to Coaching (MAC)
Magnetic resonance imaging (MRI), 180
Major League Baseball (MLB), 43, 55
Manhattan Project, 44
Manpo-meter, 26
MAPS, see Mastery Approach to Parenting in Sports (MAPS)
Marked-ball intervention, 76
Massive cellular excitation, 180
Mastery Approach to Coaching (MAC), 236, 261
   intervention, 238, 240–243
   principles, 236–237
Mastery Approach to Parenting in Sports (MAPS), 244
Mastery climate promotion in CET and MAC programs, 241
MBD, see Multiple baseline design (MBD)
Measor, 39
Measurement methods
   duration, 62
   event recording, 62
   interval recording, 62
Measures of effort, 187
*Medicine and Science in Sports and Exercise*, 36
MEDLINE, 36
Mental imagery, strategies, 13–14
Mental practice, 13
Mental rehearsal, 13–14
Mental training, 16, 119
Methodologies, sport-specific aggression
   archival, 201–202
   behavioral observation, 204–205
   direct observation, 202–206
   self-report, 200–201
Microsoft Office Excel®, 56
12-Min demonstration video, 244
MIT Sloan Sports Analytics Conference, 44
MLB, see Major League Baseball (MLB)
Model attentional redirection, 130
*Moneyball: The Art of Winning an Unfair Game*, 43
Mood congruence, 232
Morning training group (MTG), 38
MotionLogger™ actigraph, 33
Motivational Climate Scale for Youth Sports (MCSYS), 240
MRI, see Magnetic resonance imaging (MRI)
MTG, see Morning training group (MTG)

Multiple baseline design (MBD), 68–73
  across behaviors, 68
  hypothetical data, 69f–71f
  research examples, 69–73
  three coaching interventions across individuals, evaluation, 72f
Multiple-schedule paradigm, 146
Multiple treatment interference, 76–77
Muscular adaptations
  central nervous system (CPGs), role in, 168
  exercise-limiting factors, 170
  fatigue mechanisms and, 169
  fiber recruitment and, 169
  gender difference in, 171
  SAID principle (Specific Adaptation to Increased Demand) and, 169–170
  skeletal plasticity in, 169–170
  stretching excercises, benefits of, 171–172
  training regimen, 170–171

**N**
NAN, see National Academy of Neuropsychology (NAN)
NATA, see National Athletic Trainers Association (NATA)
National Academy of Neuropsychology (NAN), 192
National Athletic Trainers Association (NATA), 192
National Basketball Association (NBA), 44, 55
National Collegiate Athletic Association (NCAA), 49–50, 70, 84, 162, 181, 192
National Council of Youth Sports (NCYS), 181
National Football League (NFL), 50–52, 55, 186, 192
National Health and Nutritional Examination Survey (NHANES), 129
National Hockey League (NHL), 186, 192
National Women's Football Association (NWFA), 50–51
NBA, see National Basketball Association (NBA)
NCAA, see National Collegiate Athletic Association (NCAA)
NCYS, see National Council of Youth Sports (NCYS)
Neurocognitive performance, 185–186
Newton's second law of motion, 143
NFL, see National Football League (NFL)
NHANES, see National Health and Nutritional Examination Survey (NHANES)
NHL, see National Hockey League (NHL)
NHL Players Association, 192
Non-concussed control group, 185
Non-contact sports, 143
*The North American Society for the Psychology of Sport and Physical Activity*, 3
NWFA, see National Women's Football Association (NWFA)

**O**
Obsessive compulsive disorder, 119
One-day reversal effect, 67
One-on-one interaction, 186
Operant conditioning, 3, 5–6, 11, 13, 17, 135, 249
Optimal play calling, 153
Outcome expectancies
  physical areas, 130
  self-evaluative areas, 130
  social areas, 130
Outcome goal, 121
Overmatching, 48–49
Overt behaviors, 4, 7, 200, 250

**P**
Parents, good behavior contracts, 206–207
Pavlovian conditioning, 5–6
Pavlovian extinction process, 5
Peak performance, 14–15
Pedometers, 26–28
  general fitness using, 34–37
*Percentage Baseball*, 43, 57
Performance-enhancing effect, 212
Performance Failure Appraisal Inventory, 87
Performance feedback
  behavioral coaching, 105–106
    instructions, 106
    verbal feedback, 106
  performance, public posting, 106–107
    components, 106
  self-monitoring, 107–108
    effect on participant's behavior, 107
  technology, 108–109
Performance goal, 74, 102, 104, 121–122
Performance measures, 62, 65, 67–69, 71–74, 251, 255
Personal consultant model, 115, 117
PET, see Positron emission tomography (PET)
Physical exercise, establishment and maintenance
  baseline levels and recommendations, 129
  benefits, 127–128
    central nervous system functioning, 128
    impact, 127–128

Physical exercise (cont.)
  interventions, 128
    psychological ability, 128
    subjective psychological, 128
  health promotion, theoretical models, 129–134
    Michie and colleagues' taxonomy of intervention components, 133t
    proxy indicator, 127
    typical intervention delivery mechanisms, 134–136
      additive effect, 134
      baseline patient characteristics, 134
Piezoceramic accelerometer, 30
Poisson distribution, 31
Polysomnography (PSG), 37–38
Positron emission tomography (PET), 180
Post-concussion effect, 183
Post-concussion testing, 187
Post-head injury performance, 185
Post hoc determination, 189
Post-routine time phase, 256
Posttraumatic amnesia (PTA), 179
Potential cognitive domains, 84
Potential long-term morbidity, 184
Pre-routine time phase, 256
Preseason baseline testing, 192
Prevention-based intervention
  athletes, 208
  by coaches, 206–207
  by game officials, 207–208
  by parents, 206–207
Problems in Sport Competition Scale (PSCS), 84
Problems in Sport Training Scale (PSTS), 84
Proficiency techniques
  attentional focus, 166–167
  component behavior as, 161–162, 166–167
  deliberate practice, reinforcement of, 167–168
  elite status, 165, 168
  expert models, 165
  instructional hierarchy as, 161
  metophors usage, 165–166
  rhythmic priming, 167
  stimulus control as, 161–162, 164, 173
  See also Muscular adaptations
Progesterone, 183
Prominent characteristics, 4–8
  behavior, common synonyms, 4
  external stimuli vs. internal stimuli, 4
  Pavlovian conditioning of fear, 6f
  stimulus discrimination training, 7f

Proprietary blend, 211–212
PSCS, see Problems in Sport Competition Scale (PSCS)
PSG, see Polysomnography (PSG)
PSTS, see Problems in Sport Training Scale (PSTS)
PsycINFO, 36
PTA, see Posttraumatic amnesia (PTA)
PubMed, 37, 182

## Q

QOL, see Quality of life (QOL)
Quality of life (QOL), 128
Quantitative analyses
  of behavior, 46–47
  data, analysis, 56–57
  data, sources, 55–56
  data considerations, 54–55
  matching law, 47–53
    data on generalized equation, bar graph, 52f
    plotted on coordinate plane, 48f
    Reed et al.'s analysis of teams' bias, 51f
    three analyses using generalized, 48f
    two- and three-point shots, 49
    two generalized equation analyses, 50f–51f
    Vollmer and Bourret's concatenated analyses, 50f
  other models, 53
  situational data, 55
  translating to sports applications, 53–54

## R

Race-car simulation, 257–258
Randomized controlled trial (RCT), 36, 128, 134
Rational emotive behavior therapy, 117
RCT, see Randomized controlled trial (RCT)
Reactive behaviors, 230
RE-AIM dimension, 138
Research-based behavioral intervention, 115
Research Quarterly for Exercise and Sport, 36
Respondent conditioning, see Conditioned seeing
Response-acquisition program, 147
Return-to-play protocol, 189–190
Reversal design, see A-B-A-B design
Reversal-to-baseline phase, 67–68, 73, 75
Robust efficacy, 123
Rotational acceleration, 180, 185
RT3, 39

# Index

## S

*The Sabermetric Manifesto*, 43, 46
SARI, *see* Student–Athlete Relationship Instrument (SARI)
School-based intervention, 135–136
  physical activity promotion, 135
  SCT and CT, principles, 135
  self-management strategies
    goal setting, 135
    self-monitoring, 135
    self-reinforcement, 135
    stimulus control, 135
  SPARK program, 135
SCN, *see* Suprachiasmatic nucleus (SCN)
ScoreKeeper©, 56
SCT, *see* Social Cognitive Theory (SCT)
SD, *see* Standard deviation (SD)
Second impact syndrome, 184
Self-defeating thought, 90
Self-efficacy, 80, 87, 90, 130–132, 134–135, 137, 145, 252
Self-Efficacy in Sport Scale, 87
Self-esteem in children, 240
Self-monitoring
  individual program components, importance, 133
  pedometer, 134
Self-regulation, 131, 137, 253, 257
Self-report methodology, 200–201
  instruments used in, 200
  validity and reliability of, 200–201
Self-talk, 79–81
  attributional statements, 80
  comparisons with others, 80
  nonverbal speech, assessment, 80
  self-statements, timing, 80–81
  specific content, assessment, 80
SEM, *see* Structural equation modeling (SEM)
Semi-structured behavioral interview format, 84
Shaping procedure, 108
SIC, *see* Sport Interference Checklist (SIC)
SigmaPlot®, 57
Single-case evaluation designs
  behavior trends during baseline measurement, 64f
  decreasing trend *vs.* increasing trend, 63
  description, 65–77
    *See also individual entries*
  principles and operations, 62–64
    baseline evaluation, 63
    internal and external validity, 63–64
    intervention, 63
    measurement, 62–63
    visual inspection, 62
Single-case research designs, *see* Single-case evaluation designs
Single-subject design, 3–4, 7–9, 100, 102, 213
Single Subject Research (SSR), 7, 17, 213, 249
SIQ, *see* Sport Imagery Questionnaire (SIQ)
SIQ-C, *see* Sport Imagery Questionnaire for Children (SIQ-C)
Site of attachment, 30–31
Skepticism, 83
Skinnerian analysis, 4
SMTQ, *see* Sports Mental Toughness Questionnaire (SMTQ)
Soccer-specific concussion, 182
Social Cognitive Theory (SCT), 129–130, 228, 230
  core factors, 130–131
Social learning theory, 132
Social validation, 8
SPARK program, *see* Sports, Play, and Active Recreation for Kids (SPARK) program
Spearman–Brown prophecy formula, 34
Spontaneous (emitted) behaviors, 230
Sport Anxiety Scale-2 (SAS-2), 242
Sport Behavior Inventory (SBI), 200
SportDiscus, 36
Sport Imagery Questionnaire for Children (SIQ-C), 124
Sport Imagery Questionnaire (SIQ), 124
Sport Interference Checklist (SIC), 84–85
Sport neuropsychology
  areas of research and practice, 178
  common neuropsychological tests, 187t
  concussion pathophysiology, 178–181
  educational approaches, 192–193
    public policy changes, 192
    self-evident problems, 193
  management programs, 186–188
    baseline testing, 186
    concussion management, computerized instruments, 188
    trauma testing, 186–188
  related concussion, 178–180
    definition, 178
    severity grading guidelines, 179t
    resolution of symptoms: normal recovery curve and complications, 188–191
    length of recovery, 188–189
    repetitive head trauma, effects, 190–191
    return to play protocol, 189–190

Sport neuropsychology (cont.)
    Zurich conference consensus recommendations, 190t
    SLAM: gold standard for studying sport concussion, 185–186
    sport psychology vs. sport science disciplines, comparison, 178t
Sport nutritional supplements, behavioral effects of, 220–222
    general considerations, 213–214
    recovery drinks, 217–218
    research support, 214–223
        caffeine, 220–222
        carbohydrate-protein drink, 217
        creatine, 219–222
        nonsupported supplements, 222
        sports drinks, 214
        testosterone levels raised, 223
        testosterone prohormone supplements, 222–223
        whey protein, 218–219
Sport psyching, 16
Sport-related aggression., see Aggressive behavior
Sports, Play, and Active Recreation for Kids (SPARK) program, 135
Sports drinks
    carbohydrate–sodium drink ingestion, 215
    dehydration, 214
    increased blood flow to skin, 214
*Sports Medicine*, 36
Sports Mental Toughness Questionnaire (SMTQ), 87
SSR, see Single Subject Research (SSR)
Standard deviation (SD), 31–33, 36
Structural equation modeling (SEM), 131
Student–Athlete Relationship Instrument (SARI), 16, 84, 86t
Suprachiasmatic nucleus (SCN), 39
Symptoms Check-List-90-Revised, 87

T
TAG, see Teaching with acoustical guidance (TAG)
Task-oriented coping, 87
Teaching with acoustical guidance (TAG), 72
Test–retest temporal stability, 32
Theory of Planned Behavior, 129
Theory of Reasoned Action, 129
Third-variable confounds, 55
Thompson Scientific, 36
Topographical-based behavior, 101
Transient neurocognitive impact, 185
Traumatic biomechanical force, 178
True variance, 251
t-tests, 31, 62
TurboStats©, 56
TurboStats Software Company©, 56
Turnover rate index, 51
Tutorial on IAPZ, 259

U
Unique discriminative stimulus, 146
The United States Consumer Product Safety Commission (CPSC), 181
United States Olympic Committee (USOC), 117
USOC, see United States Olympic Committee (USOC)

V
Video
    feedback effect, 73
    modeling effect, 73
Visualization, see Imagery

W
Web of Science, 36
9-Week program, 136
Weight-related criticism, 130
Win-at-all-cost culture, 119
Winning Profile Athlete Inventory, 87
Within-game performance, 153
Within-sport behavioral checklist, 15
Worn-out cognitive distortion, 116

Y
24 Yamax MLS-2000 digital pedometer, 33
Yard-stick, 250

Z
Zeo (sleep-monitoring system), 39

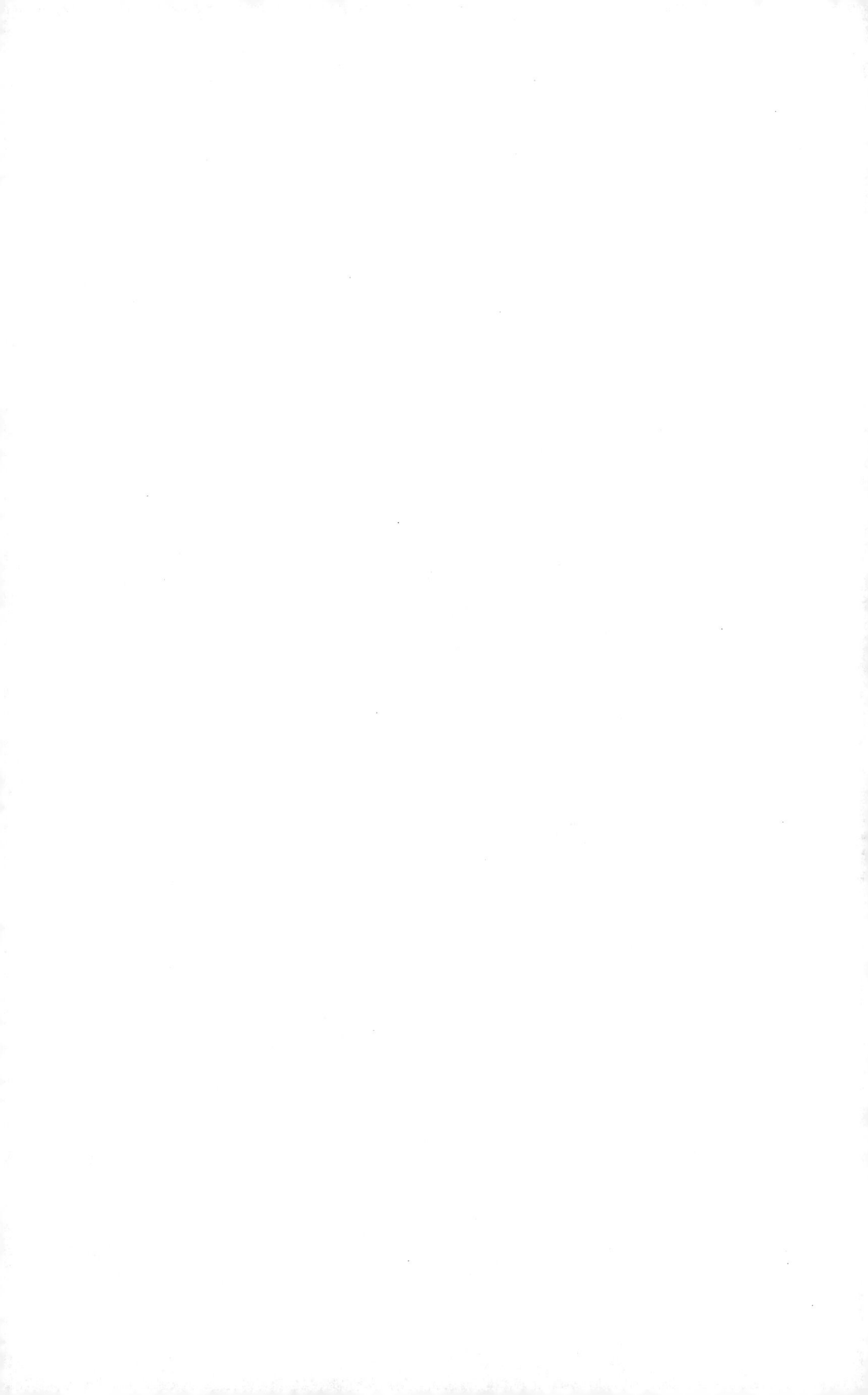